D0207805

Classical Genetic Research and its Legacy

With the rise of genomics, the life sciences have entered a new era. Maps of genomes have become the icons for a comprehensive knowledge of the organism on a previously unattained level of complexity. This book provides an in-depth history of mapping procedures as they were developed in classical genetics.

The book shows that the technology of genetic mapping is by no means a recent acquisition of molecular genetics or even genetic engineering. It demonstrates that the development of mapping technologies has accompanied the rise of modern genetics from its very beginnings. In Part I, Mendelian genetics is set in perspective from the viewpoint of the detection and description of linkage phenomena. Part II addresses the role of mapping for the experimental working practice of classical geneticists, their social interactions, and for their laboratory "life worlds."

With its detailed analyses of scientific practices and its illustration of the diversity of mapping, this book is a significant contribution to the history of genetics.

A companion volume from the same editors—*From Molecular Genetics to Genomics: The Mapping Cultures of Twentieth-century Genetics*—covers the history of molecular genetics and genomics.

Hans-Jörg Rheinberger is Director at the Max Planck Institute for the History of Science in Berlin. He has published numerous papers and books on molecular biology and the history of science, including a co-edited collection, *The Concept of the Gene in Development and Evolution* (2000).

Jean-Paul Gaudillière is a senior researcher at the National Institute of Health (INSERM), Paris. His work has addressed many aspects of the history of molecular biology and of the biomedical sciences during the twentieth century. His actual research focuses on the history of biological drugs. He is the co-editor of *Heredity and Infection: A History of Disease Transmission* (2002).

Routledge studies in the history of science, technology and medicine

Edited by John Krige

Georgia Institute of Technology, Atlanta, USA

Routledge Studies in the History of Science, Technology and Medicine aims to stimulate research in the field, concentrating on the twentieth century. It seeks to contribute to our understanding of science, technology, and medicine as they are embedded in society, exploring the links between the subjects on the one hand and the cultural, economic, political, and institutional contexts of their genesis and development on the other. Within this framework, and while not favouring any particular methodological approach, the series welcomes studies which examine relations between science, technology, medicine and society in new ways, e.g. the social construction of technologies, large technical systems etc.

1 **Technological Change**
Methods and themes in the history of technology
Edited by Robert Fox

2 **Technology Transfer out of Germany after 1945**
Edited by Matthias Judt and Burghard Ciesla

3 **Entomology, Ecology and Agriculture**
The making of scientific careers in North America, 1885–1985
Paolo Palladino

4 **The Historiography of Contemporary Science and Techonology**
Edited by Thomas Söderquist

5 **Science and Spectacle**
The work of Jodrell bank in post-war British culture
Jon Agar

6 **Molecularizing Biology and Medicine**
New practices and alliances, 1910s–1970s
Edited by Soraya de Chadarevian and Harmke Kamminga

7 Cold War, Hot Science
Applied research in Britain's defence laboratories 1945–1990
Edited by Robert Bud and Philip Gammett

8 Planning Armageddon
Britain, the United State and the command of Western nuclear forces 1945–1964
Stephen Twigge and Len Scott

9 Cultures of Control
Edited by Miriam R. Levin

10 Science, Cold War and the American State
Lloyd V. Berkner and the balance of professional ideals
Alan A. Needell

11 Reconsidering Sputnik
Forty years since the Soviet satellite
Edited by Roger D. Launius

12 Crossing Boundaries, Building Bridges
Comparing the history of women engineers, 1870s–1990s
Edited by Annie Canel, Ruth Oldenziel and Karin Zachmann

13 Changing Images in Mathematics
From the French revolution to the new millennium
Edited by Umberto Bottazzini and Amy Dahan Dalmedico

14 Heredity and Infection
The history of disease transmission
Edited by Jean-Paul Gaudillière and Llana Löwy

15 The Analogue Alternative
The electric analogue computer in Britian and the USA, 1930–1975
James S. Small

16 Instruments, Travel and Science
Itineraries of precision from the seventeenth to the twentieth century
Edited by Marie-Noëlle Bourguet, Christian Licoppe and H. Otto Sibum

17 The Fight Against Cancer
France, 1890–1940
Patrice Pinell

18 Collaboration in the Pharmaceutical Industry
Changing relationships in Britain and France, 1935–1965
Viviane Quirke

19 Classical Genetic Research and its Legacy
The mapping cultures of twentieth-century genetics
Edited by Hans-Jörg Rheinberger and Jean-Paul Gaudillière

20 From Molecular Genetics to Genomics
The mapping cultures of twentieth-century genetics
Edited by Jean-Paul Gaudillière and Hans-Jörg Rheinberger

21 Interferon
The science and selling of a miracle drug
Toine Pieters

22 Measurement and Statistics in Science and Technology
1930 to the present
Benoît Godin

Also published by Routledge in hardback and paperback

Science and Ideology
A comparative history
Mark Walker

Classical Genetic Research and its Legacy

The mapping cultures of twentieth-century genetics

Edited by
Hans-Jörg Rheinberger and Jean-Paul Gaudillière

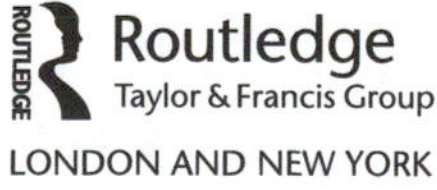

LONDON AND NEW YORK

First published 2004
by Routledge
2 Park Square, Milton Park, Abingdon, Oxon OX14 4RN

Simultaneously published in the USA and Canada
by Routledge
270 Madison Ave, New York, NY 10016

Routledge is an imprint of the Taylor & Francis Group

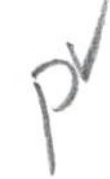

Typeset in Baskerville MT by
Newgen Imaging Systems (P) Ltd, Chennai, India
Printed and bound in Great Britain by
MPG Books Ltd, Bodmin

British Library Cataloguing in Publication Data
A catalogue record for this book is available
from the British Library

Library of Congress Cataloging in Publication Data
A catalog record for this book has been requested

ISBN 0–415–32849–7

This book is dedicated to the memory of Lily E. Kay

Contents

Figures

Notes on contributors

Christophe Bonneuil is Historian of Science at the Centre Koyré (CNRS, Paris). He has published in the following areas: Science, Nature, and Colonialism; the social history of plant breeding and genetics; and the public controversy on GM crops.

Raphael Falk is Professor of Genetics (retired) at the Hebrew University of Jerusalem. He has been studying the concept of the gene and the development of genetic thought. He co-edited with P. Beurton and H.-J. Rheinberger, *The Concept of the Gene in Development and Evolution: Historical and Epistemological Perspectives* (2000).

Lisa Gannett is Assistant Professor in the Department of Philosophy at St Mary's University, Halifax. Her research interests in the history and philosophy of genetics are focused particularly on value questions. She is beginning a book project on population concepts in genetics.

Jean-Paul Gaudillière is a Senior Researcher at INSERM, Paris. His work has addressed many aspects of the history of molecular biology and of the biomedical sciences during the twentieth century. His contemporary research focuses on the history of biological drugs. He is the co-editor of *Heredity and Infection: A History of Disease Transmission* (2002) and the author of *Inventer la biomédecine. La France, l'Amérique et la production des savoirs du vivaut (1945–1965)* (2002).

James R. Griesemer is Professor of Philosophy and a member of the Center for Population Biology at the University of California, Davis. In addition to empirical research in population biology, he is interested in philosophical and historical problems of natural history, genetics, development, and evolution. He is a co-editor of *The Principles of Life* (2003). He is currently writing a book, *Reproduction and the Evolutionary Process.*

Jonathan Harwood is Reader in the Centre for History of Science, Technology & Medicine, University of Manchester (UK). He is the author of *Styles of Scientific Thought: The German Genetics Community, 1900–1933* (UP 1993) and is currently completing a book on the agricultural sciences in early twentieth-century Germany.

Lee B. Kass is Visiting Professor at Cornell University, where she is writing an intellectual biography of Nobel Laureate Barbara McClintock. She recently retired from college teaching (1979–2000). As a Fulbright Scholar (1995–96), she established the National Herbarium for the Bahamas. She has published histories of nineteenth- and twentieth-century American botanists and conducts research on plant diversity and pollination biology. Her field guide to plants of San Salvador Island, Bahamas (1991) is currently in revision.

Jens Lachmund is a Lecturer at Maastricht University, the Netherlands. Among his publications are *Der abgehorchte Körper. Zur historischen Soziologie der medizinischen Untersuchung* (1997). His current research is on the history of representations of space in urban ecology. Together with S. Dierig and A. Mendelsohn he edited a collection of essays on the theme *Science and the City* (OSIRIS 2003).

Hans-Jörg Rheinberger is Director of the Max Planck Institute for the History of Science in Berlin. He has published numerous articles on molecular biology and the history of science. He has written, among other books, *Toward a History of Epistemic Things: Synthesizing Proteins in the Test Tube* (1997); edited (together with P. Beurton and R. Falk) *The Concept of the Gene in Development and Evolution* (2000); *Experimentalsysteme und epistemische Dinge* (2001); edited (together with F.L. Holmes and J. Renn) *Reworking the Bench: Research Notebooks in the History of Science* (2003).

David Turnbull is a Research Fellow in the Arts Faculty, Deakin University; History and Philosophy of Science, University of Melbourne; the Centre for Australian Indigenous Studies, Monash University; and Sociology, Lancaster University. His most recent publications include *Masons, Tricksters, and Cartographers: Comparative Studies in the Sociology of Scientific Knowledge* (2000); 'Performance and Narrative, Bodies and Movement in the Construction of Places and Objects, Spaces and Knowledges: The Case of The Maltese Megaliths', Special Issue on Sociality and Materiality of *Theory, Culture and Society*; 'Travelling Knowledge: Narratives, Assemblage and Encounters', in M.-N. Bourget, C. Licoppe, and H.O. Sibum, *Instruments, Travel and Science: Itineraries of Precision from the Seventeenth to the Twentieth Century* (2002). He is currently working on narratives of prehistory and on indigenous knowledge assemblage and databases.

Acknowledgments

We wish to thank all the contributors to this volume for sharing their expertise and having been so cooperative and patient in the process of finalizing the manuscript. We would also like to express our gratitude to Gabriele Brüß and Antje Radeck for helping with the difficult task of making everything ready for press. We thank John Krige as the Series Editor for his interest, and two anonymous referees for their valuable comments. Finally, we would like to acknowledge Jo Whiting, Terry Clague, and Amritpal Bangard from Routledge and Vincent Antony from the Production Office for guiding us so smoothly through the production stages.

The editors
Hans-Jörg Rheinberger
Jean-Paul Gaudillière

Introduction

Hans-Jörg Rheinberger and Jean-Paul Gaudillière

This book is about the mapping cultures of twentieth-century genetics. *Classical Genetic Research and its Legacy* is the first volume of a collection of papers resulting from a conference that was held at the Max Planck Institute for the History of Science in Berlin in March 2001. It covers the mapping procedures developed in the period of classical genetics, that is, roughly, in the first part of the twentieth century. An accompanying second volume—*From Molecular Genetics to Genomics*—covers the latter part of the twentieth century. We felt that a detailed history of genetic mapping was timely, if not overdue, in view of the recent developments in genomics epitomized by the announcement of a first draft of the structure of the human genome in the summer of 2000, which was eventually made public in February 2001, a month before the workshop from whose deliberations this book took shape.

It is possibly not too far-fetched to postulate that the spaces of our genetic knowledge about living beings have been organized around two major fields of metaphor, metonymy, and model with their concomitant practices. One of these fields gravitates around the theme of mapping, the other around that of information and communication. Whereas the concept of information has been given wide attention by historians and philosophers of science, particularly as far as the history of molecular biology is concerned, mapping has not. This book is about mapping. Both themes have not only transformed biology, they have also created powerful public images and icons associated with contemporary genomics, its potential uses and abuses: that is, the genetic map and the genetic program. Whereas the notion of information has become firmly embedded within the space once defined and confined by quite different conceptions of biological specificity and function, the idea of the map resides and exerts its power predominantly at the level of structure, organization, and correlation. And whereas mapping is clearly associated with the activity of organizing and of performing a certain kind and form of research, with its instruments and practices circulating in specific communities—that is, with a distinctly epistemological and performative meaning—the concept of information carries the burden of the new molecular genetic ontology. It should be an interesting exercise to ask why these two metaphorical realms could obviously coexist in such a productive manner and why they could develop such an enormous impact on the representation and the manipulation of life over the past century, although they do not have any obvious theoretical linkage to each other.

The year 1953 was remarkable in the history of the life sciences. It was the year that Francis Crick and James Watson first presented their model of the double helical structure of DNA, to whose fiftieth anniversary this book is a contribution. With it, the way was open to define the classical gene on the molecular level. It was a turning point for the molecular genetic meaning of information, and for genetic mapping as well. But it was also a remarkable year for mapping in the philosophy of science, albeit perhaps less spectacularly, and certainly less well known than the advent of the double helix. In 1953, a British philosopher in the tradition of Ludwig Wittgenstein, Stephen Toulmin, published a little book with a very ambitious title: *The Philosophy of Science: An Introduction.* In it, Toulmin tells us that in physics as elsewhere in science, we draw consequences by drawing lines (Toulmin 1953: 25). In a chapter entitled "Theories and Maps," Toulmin extended this general epistemological claim. He argued that the comparison of scientific laws with generalizations, and the logical structure in which generalizations are framed, had for a long time misled philosophers of science in their search for models of scientific activity. Instead, he postulated, physical theories should be compared with maps. He contended that diagrams and equations could be seen as a means for setting up "maps of phenomena" (Toulmin 1953: 108), and that the mapping metaphor could be used to shed fresh light on dark and dusty corners and impasses in the philosophy of science.

Maps, for those who know to read them are, first of all, a means of orientation. But they also condense and depict phenomena in relation to each other. Thus, they create meaning through condensation and relating—that is, through the power of synopsis—as much as through representation and reference—that is, through the ongoing traffic between the map and the mapped territory. It has become a common observation in the history of science that models and tools have a life of their own and may profoundly transform the phenomena they are supposed to represent. As Georges Canguilhem once wrote about "life" in the laboratory: "We must not forget that the laboratory itself constitutes a new environment in which life certainly establishes norms whose extrapolation does not work without risk when removed from the conditions to which these norms relate. For the animal and for man the laboratory environment is one possible environment among others (...) for the living being apparatuses and products are the objects among which it moves as in an unusual world. It is impossible that the ways of life in the laboratory should fail to retain any specificity in their relationship to the place and moment of the experiment" (Canguilhem 1966, quoted from 1991: 148).

The transformational role of models and tools is especially true for maps in general and genetic maps in particular. This form of biological research could only take off when geneticists worked out a strong linkage between the vision of hereditary factors as being linearly arranged on chromosomal threads, and the breeding procedures for producing standardized strains of organisms with stable distances between genetic factors. Since their arrival genetic maps have delivered powerful images of relations between things within and outside the confines of the laboratory. A century of research testifies to this performative power of chromosomal genetics. Throughout the chapters in these volumes, we will see how differently genetic items can be related, not only to each other, but also to matters technical, economical, or political. Yet this diversity was kept under control. The heterogeneity of purposes, organisms, and epistemic entities was homogenized to varying degrees, thus giving birth to the integrated mapping cultures of genetics described and analyzed in this book. The basic mapping conception of linearly arranged genetic elements proved more robust than any of its early advocates might have thought. But it also proved deceptive, channeling huge research energies into a one-dimensional genetic vision, which supposedly accounted for the entire organism.

It has generally been taken for granted by historians of the life sciences that the first genetic mapping culture, originating in early Drosophila genetics research, had a very strong impact on twentieth-century biology. Hence, the more or less tacit assumption that it was passed on from the fly group—so forcefully described by Robert Kohler (1994) in *The Lords of the Fly*—to other research communities. Because groups of mappers such as the phage group or the bacterial geneticists of the 1950s—analyzed in the next volume—played a critical role in the history of molecular biology, the idea of an epistemic, technological, and social continuity was attractive. All the more so as the very recent human genome research consortia—or their forerunners of the 1970s, consisting of immunogeneticists and medical geneticists—seemed to use the same methods of searching. The assumption of continuity has been a valuable basis for posing questions and designing projects. However, it has resisted deeper historical investigation, which suggests that much of retrospective streamlining has gone into it. Accordingly, the contributors to this volume take pains to assess in detail *the different mapping traditions* as they developed in their respective areas, with their separate origins, their points of connection, and the spaces of knowledge they helped to shape, to connect, and to differentiate.

By the eve of the First World War, genetic mapping seemed to be set on a good footing in Thomas Hunt Morgan's laboratory at Columbia University in New York. The theoretical backbone of mapping work were the notion of *linkage* between genes, the idea of *crossing over* between homologous chromosomes leading to rare rearrangements of linked traits, and the concept of the *frequency of recombination* which was employed to measure the relative distances between genes. The emergence of these notions will be assessed in detail in Part I of this book—Mendelian Genetics and Linkage Mapping—which also explores the historical preconditions under which they could gain meaning and momentum.

Part II examines Mapping Work, Mapping Collectives, and Mapping Cultures. Four broad themes characterize the mapping culture of classical genetics. First, *experimental practice.* Drosophila mapping was based on selecting and breeding mutant strains of the fruit fly and counting and sorting out the huge progeny of innumerable crosses. Historians of biology have stressed that this form of cooperative research, which centered on a particular technology, and which acted on a particular organism, was a rare development in the context of early twentieth-century biology. As Robert Kohler has convincingly shown, the Drosophila mapping culture rested on innovative practices, which were simultaneously literary, social, technological, and epistemological. The integrated maps of the four Drosophila chromosomes showing dozens of genes aligned on linear segments were only the visible tip of an iceberg resting on a deep-floating infrastructure of specific arrangements of tools, cooperating people, strains of flies, and inscriptions.

Second, mapping involved establishing and producing a new form of *biological material.* During the early days of the work of the fly group, results were usually not stable, a fact that continually raised concerns about the postulated relationship between chromosomal distances and the recombination rates used to evaluate these distances. The choice and appropriate inbreeding of peculiar mutants, the standardization of breeding conditions, and even the construction of specific, well-designed mapping strains were all critical in establishing the practical feasibility and scientific legitimacy of mapping.

Mapping was also a matter of *representation.* This statement is rather tautological in principle, but less so in practice. Work in the Morgan laboratory was both facilitated by and organized around a series of devices depicting material entities and the results of their manipulation as one-dimensional images of chromosomes. Different media were used at different stages of representation, whose final expression was a chart. Representational devices like catalogues of reference strains or so-called construction maps showing the progressive ordering of mutants were critical in making sense of the diversity and flexibility of laboratory work. They depended on the physical infrastructure, and served to organize this infrastructure into coherent registers to be employed as reference maps. They in turn guided decisions on further breeding experiments, that is, additional displacements within the mutational landscape. To use the words of cognitive anthropologist Edwin Hutchins: the setting evolved "over time as partial solutions to frequently encountered problems [were] crystallized and saved in the material and conceptual tools of the trade and in the social organization of the work" (Hutchins 1995: 374).

Finally, characterizing mapping also involves social factors. Mapping is a peculiar research enterprise in the sense that it not only allowed, but also depended on in-depth integration of the work of all participants in a network of mappers. The amalgamation of Drosophila researchers into one mapping network was facilitated by the fact that many participants were trained in Morgan's laboratory. Diversification of settings, and hence practices nevertheless emerged. The subsequent and ongoing reintegration of divergent systems was associated with the regular exchange of mutants, the continuous flow of information culminating in the highly regarded *Drosophila Information Service*, regular visits by members of the network to other people's laboratories, and collective experimentation. Mapping became a material network of cognition similar to the one for navigation described by Hutchins, with its crystallization of practices in physical artifacts wired into collaborative performances.

The Drosophila exemplar has been widely researched. We thought it useful to recapitulate major features of this research here because the book does not include a chapter specifically dealing with Morgan's research. Part I of this volume focuses on the origin of genetic mapping culture of the twentieth century, viewed in its broader context. Both Hans-Jörg Rheinberger and Jonathan Harwood place it within the perspective of early attempts to analyze co-transmission patterns, and more particularly within the context of plant breeding research. As we have learned from many studies, Morgan's theory of linkage and crossing-over was one of several possible schemes. Its acceptance certainly correlated with the stabilization and further development of the Drosophila form of experimentation within the Columbia laboratory. Raphael Falk's chapter (Chapter 3) demonstrates that it was also facilitated by the circulation of new representations, which in turn gave multiple meanings to the notion of genetic linkage. Moreover, mapping was not—even in Morgan's setting—confined to the analysis of chromosomal locations. In Chapter 4, Lisa Gannett and James Griesemer show how work in the laboratory and work in the field were combined to draw geographical and evolutionary maps of the flies.

Part II of this volume—Mapping Work, Mapping Collectives, Mapping Cultures—gathers studies which argue that the mapping practices of classical genetics should not be confined to the fly work. Lee Kass and Christophe Bonneuil (Chapter 5) analyze how mapping in maize genetics took on a novel shape rooted in the articulation of linkage studies and cytology, although strongly influenced by the Drosophila exemplar. The early form of mapping human genes, dicussed by Lisa Gannett and James Griesemer (Chapter 6), was also unique as it crystallized at the boundary between serology and physical anthropology. Finally, the case of mouse genetics investigated by Jean-Paul Gaudillière (Chapter 7) reveals another area in which mapping technologies existed, but which were used as research tools in modeling human diseases. The use of mapping as a discrete project within mice genetics only emerged after the Second World War when the scale of biomedical research changed.

These diverse contexts could be extended. They stand as an indication of a historical proliferation of related work that will never be fully understood if only seen from the perspective of one of its exemplars. The two commentaries at the end of the book by cultural theorist David Turnbull and sociologist Jens Lachmund reinforce this point at a more general level.

References

Canguilhem, G. (1966) *Le normal et le pathologique*, Paris: Presses Universitaires de France; English translation (1991) *The Normal and the Pathological*, New York: Zone Books.

Hutchins, E. (1995) *Cognition in the Wild*, Cambridge: The MIT Press.

Kohler, R. (1994) *The Lords of the Fly: Drosophila Genetics and the Experimental Life*, Chicago: The University of Chicago Press.

Toulmin, St (1953) *The Philosophy of Science: An Introduction*, London: Hutchinson's University Library.

Part I

Mendelian genetics and linkage mapping

1 Linkage before Mendelism?

Plant-breeding research in Central Europe, *c.*1880–1910

Jonathan Harwood

It is a commonplace that scientific concepts or theories are sometimes based, not on new observations but on those made by an earlier generation of workers from a related practical domain. In genetics, for example, the distinction between phenotype and genotype drew upon, and made sense of, the recognition among nineteenth-century breeders that not all variation was heritable. Similarly, the Mendelian analysis of the distribution of traits in several generations following a controlled cross built upon nineteenth-century breeders' observations in trying to combine traits from both parents via hybridization.

The concept of a "map" based on linkage patterns, as developed by the Morgan school from 1913, is another instance of the scientist imposing a particular conceptual meaning upon longstanding observations. For as I will show here, it was well known among nineteenth-century plant-breeders (as by animal-breeders earlier) that particular traits were usually inherited together (known as "correlations"), though occasional deviations from the pattern were also recognized. Significantly, the breeders were not simple empiricists interested only in useable rules of thumb, for they too advanced explanations for correlated traits, albeit of a very unMendelian kind. Comparing late nineteenth-century breeders' explanations of correlation with those advanced by early Mendelians suggests that the rediscovery of Mendelism was accompanied, at least in some quarters, by a fundamental shift in the underlying vision of the organism.

In the following section of the chapter I sketch how and why late-nineteenth-century academic plant-breeders began to work on correlations and how they made sense of them. In the section 'Early Mendelian views of correlation', I turn to the quite different approaches to correlation taken by Wilhelm Johannsen and Erich Tschermak, both of whom were addressing questions of plant-breeding from a Mendelian perspective. And in the Conclusion I consider what light this contrast might shed upon the new generation of Mendelians.

Nineteenth-century breeders' work on correlation

Animal-breeders appear to have recognized correlations relatively early. By the late eighteenth century, Robert Bakewell had concluded that it was impossible to breed sheep for both better wool and more mutton. And by the early nineteenth century, those breeding for high quality wool knew that it was not productive to select for both fine wool and long fibers (Wood and Orel 2001). But during the course of that century they also established important positive correlations; for example, certain morphological traits were useful indicators of milk yield (e.g. gleaming coat, large spaces between ribs, strength of the "milk vein") (Schindler 1893).

Plant-breeders recognized correlations rather later. In German-speaking Europe commercial plant-breeding was first undertaken in the beet-sugar industry. Although firms were manufacturing sugar from about 1800, it was only in mid-century that they began to select for beets with elevated sugar-content (taking up a practice developed by Vilmorin in France). Initially the method used for identifying sugar-rich variants involved checking the specific gravity of a standard-sized core removed from the beet. But this was a relatively labor-intensive method. Aware of the results obtained by animal-breeders, therefore, the beet-breeders were on the lookout for morphological traits that were associated with high sugar-content. Eventually they established that the size and form of the leaf, the size and shape of the beet, and the color of the beet were correlated with sugar-content. This was a valuable finding because it gave breeders a simple, if crude, criterion by which to reduce the number of beets that they would subsequently need to screen for sugar (Schindler 1893; Rümker 1894; Westermeier 1897).

Cereals growers began to take up breeding from the 1870s, and they too discovered correlations between the plant's external visible traits and its internal physiological ones. A small number of stems at the upper end of the plant, for example, correlated with higher yield while in rye green kernel-color was associated with high baking quality (Liebscher 1896; Tschermak 1907). But other correlations proved to be more hindrance than help. As German wheat growers became more interested during the 1870s in boosting yields, many of them imported the high-yielding British variety "Squarehead." But they soon found that Squarehead did not survive continental winters very well, nor did its flour make good bread. So German cereals breeders began to cross Squarehead with various native varieties, hoping to obtain hybrids which were both high-yielding *and* high quality. But they found it very difficult; yield and quality—whether one considered baking quality, disease-resistance, or winter-hardiness—appeared to be antagonistic traits (e.g. Remy 1907; Tschermak 1907; Edler 1914). These negative correlations were deemed to be exceedingly important since it meant that in order to get the best results, breeders must not focus narrowly upon any single trait but rather upon the plant as a whole, selecting for variants which *combined* a series of desired properties (e.g. Liebscher 1893; Steglich 1898; Rümker 1901). Private-sector breeders at the turn of the century were keen to see such correlations worked out, and a number of academic breeders into the 1920s were happy to oblige (Rimpau 1894; Beseler 1904; Rümker 1905; Hillmann 1910; Stephani 1911).

By all accounts the most important stimulus to the academic study of correlations was the collaborative work of Franz Schindler and Emanuel Proskowetz

(Rümker 1901; Fruwirth 1909a). Proskowetz was a Moravian estate-owner who took up barley breeding in the 1870s and developed a very successful new variety, the "Hanna-barley." More important for my story, however, is that in 1885 he joined with an academic (Adolf von Liebenberg) to found an Austrian agricultural association (Verein zur Foerderung des landwirtschaftlichen Versuchswesens in Österreich) whose members undertook systematic varietal-testing on barley and sugar-beets in order to identify the best varieties for the region. And in the course of this work Proskowetz became acquainted with the evidence for correlations (Liebenberg 1897; Proskowetz 1937). Following training in agronomy and plant-physiology, Schindler took up his first academic post in the mid-1880s and began to test wheat varieties, indigenous as well as imported, in the Hanna region of Moravia. During this work Schindler noticed that when Western European varieties were introduced into Moravia, several of their traits changed in concert. No trait, he concluded, could be understood in isolation; it was always linked to other constitutional features of the plant (Schindler 1891). He also became acquainted with Proskowetz, and the two began to publish collaboratively. In 1890 they jointly gave a paper at the International Congress for Agriculture and Forestry in Vienna ("What is the significance of correlations in wheat and sugar-beets for the theory and practice of plant-cultivation?") which was soon cited as a landmark in plant-breeding research (Schindler 1893; Proskowetz 1924).[1]

The substance of their argument was laid out in more detail a few years later in Schindler's book *The Relationship of Wheat to its Climate and the Law of Correlation: A Contribution to the Scientific Foundations of Agronomy* (Schindler 1893). Schindler pointed to work on correlation by various nineteenth-century biologists, not least by Darwin who had devoted considerable space to "correlative changes" and "correlations of growth" in *Variation of Animals and Plants under Domestication*, though Darwin's examples were mainly from animals and houseplants. Schindler found it remarkable, however, that although Darwin's book was well known among late-nineteenth-century plant-breeders and though the latter had often noticed correlations, no one had yet drawn attention to their *practical* significance.

In accord with his longstanding interest in plant-physiology, Schindler attempted to explain correlation in physiological terms.[2] His conception of correlation was a highly deterministic one: if one trait of a correlated set was altered, "the others also invariably change" according to "an inner law." Correlated traits "never change independently of one another" (Schindler 1893: 137, 158; see also 1891). He may have felt justified in referring to a "law" of correlation because Darwin had done so in *The Origin* and later works (Darwin 1968: 134–5, 1875 vol. 2: 311). But Darwin's concept of correlation was noticeably looser, allowing for occasional exceptions. In some cases, Darwin suggested, apparent correlation might actually be due merely to historical accident; for example all of the descendants of a particular species might inherit two characters that their ancestor happened to possess, though there was no internal connection between them (Darwin 1968: 182–8).

Morphological traits could be very useful indicators of physiological traits like yield or quality because structure and function were intimately connected

(Schindler 1893: 160, 166). Conversely, where traits were negatively correlated, Schindler attributed this to a process of "compensation" whereby nutritive substances consumed in large quantities for one set of processes would then not be available for others.[3] In deploying this concept, he may have been drawing upon some of Goethe's biological work from the 1790s or upon Etienne Geoffroy de St Hilaire's principle of "balancement organique" which stated that a normal or diseased organ never becomes unusually large unless another part of the same system suffers accordingly. And, in the 1830s Alphonse de Candolle had formulated a similar law for plants (Johannsen 1909: 242; Appel 1987).[4] For Schindler, at any rate, the nature of correlation had important implications for breeding method. It was doubtful, he thought, whether it would ever be possible to combine traits that were physiologically antagonistic through the use of hybridization (Schindler 1893: 157–8, see also 1891).

At the same time, however, Schindler recognized that there were many contradictory results on correlation in the literature. Correlations, which were often claimed to be invariant, did not seem to hold everywhere (*Korrelationsbrecher*). Proskowetz, for example, had found that the correlation routinely reported by German cereals breeders between yield and late-ripening simply did not hold in Moravia. There the high-yielding Hanna-barley, for example, ripened much *earlier* than low-yielding barleys (Liebenberg 1897; Proskowetz 1937).[5] How could such contradictions be accounted for if correlations were as law-like as Schindler claimed? Schindler's answer was again a physiological one: a plant's properties were determined not only by internal biological processes but also by environmental conditions. The key to understanding the contradictory findings concerning yield and late-ripening, for example, lay in the length of the vegetation period. The reason why so many observers had concluded that high yield and late-ripening were correlated was that their results were obtained in milder maritime climates as in Britain, Northern France or Northern Germany. There the climate permitted a long vegetation period so that the plants which ripened *latest*, were able to exploit this fact, assimilating over the longest period and thus building up the largest biomass or yield. But in harsher continental climates like the Hanna region of Moravia, spring came late and summers were very dry. In order for a plant to produce a high yield there, it had to ripen very *early*, exploiting the moisture still available at the beginning of the growing season before the onset of summer. And this was why imported Squarehead wheats, bred to have a long vegetation period, continued to give high yields in Brittany but not in Central Europe (cf. Liebenberg 1897).[6]

Within a few years of the appearance of Schindler's book Mendel's work was rediscovered, and some academic plant-breeders were hopeful that the new body of theory would provide a fuller understanding of correlation (Rümker 1905). Initially, however, attention shifted away from complex physiological traits to morphological ones whose inheritance was simpler to analyze, and the new Mendelians distanced themselves from the earlier claims, both practical and theoretical, made for correlations.

Early Mendelian views of correlation

As is well known, several of the early Mendelians turned to the study of heredity with substantial knowledge of plant-breeding, among them Wilhelm Johannsen and Erich von Tschermak. From 1892 until 1905 Johannsen was professor of plant-physiology at the Royal Agricultural College in Copenhagen where he worked on variation in barley. By the late 1890s he had become an enthusiast for Vilmorin's pedigree method of individual selection and was convinced of the importance of mutations in both breeding and evolution (Roll-Hansen 1978a). Tschermak obtained his doctorate in 1895 and worked for several years in commercial plant-breeding before taking up a post in agronomy at the Agricultural College in Vienna in 1902 (Tschermak 1958).

Working at an agricultural college, Johannsen was aware of the claims then being made for the practical utility of correlations, and in the early 1890s he began a series of experiments in order to test the common claim that yield and quality were inversely correlated. More particularly, he looked at the relationship between kernel-weight and protein-content in barley (Johannsen 1899).[7] In opposition to prevailing views, he found on the one hand that kernel-weight and protein-content were sometimes strongly positively correlated but, on the other, that the strength of the correlation varied considerably from one line to the next, and occasionally the two variables were even inversely correlated. Based on these findings (along with some results published by others), he developed a critique of the concept of correlation which was primarily directed at Schindler, whom he regarded as the main proponent of this view.

The conclusions which Johannsen drew from these findings were two-fold. First, he advanced a methodological critique of those statistical analyses of populations which attempted to infer causal relationships merely from correlational data (a critique which he was soon to use against the biometricians). Although it was well known, he conceded, that multiple desirable traits were rarely combined in a single variety, it did not follow that the reason for this was their "incompatibility"; each individual trait might arise only very rarely.[8] Moreover, another problem with statistical analyses was that the general relationships which they revealed could easily mask individual differences from one plant or line to the next, be they of genetic or environmental origin (Johannsen 1899: 618–21).[9] Second, Johannsen seems to have been uncomfortable with the general assumption of the organism as an integrated whole, upon which the argument for correlation was founded. We cannot simply assume, he argued, that the different functions or structure of the organism are correlated; it must be demonstrated in each case. With the principle of compensation, for example, one could readily imagine a machine whose work-output was limited, such that increasing its activity on one front would reduce what it could produce on another. But it was not always easy, he insisted, to decide to what extent similar conditions applied with organisms, especially where variation was concerned. It was not obvious, for example, why winter-hardiness in wheat should be incompatible with high yield, and until that was clarified, it would be incorrect to accept a general "law" that yield and quality were incompatible (Johannsen 1899: 600–1). Thus while Johannsen did not rule out the possibility that some alleged correlations might eventually be shown to have a real physiological basis (and he gave Schindler credit for at least searching for this), his overall stance was to chip away at the arguments for correlation from the standpoint of a tough-minded empiricist.

Erich Tschermak had been trying to improve plant-breeding methods when he stumbled upon Mendel's paper in 1900 (Harwood 2000). A few years after the rediscovery he published an extensive survey of the data on correlations in cereals (Tschermak 1907). After listing the commonly reported correlations, he drew attention to the numerous exceptions. To begin with, some traits appeared not to be correlated with anything, whether positively or negatively. But more importantly, where correlations existed, they were generally "incomplete" (i.e. partial). For example, the frequent claim that yield and winter-hardiness were antagonistic was flawed because, as Johannsen had showed, it was based upon average values for heterogeneous populations while ignoring individual plants which displayed both properties. Similarly, some common correlations did not hold in particular varieties. The only "true" correlations which he was prepared to acknowledge were those which persisted unchanged, despite mutation, crossing, or change of growing conditions.

As far as the causes of correlation were concerned, Tschermak seems to have been more interested in accounting for the exceptions than for the rules. The reason why correlations did not hold for all individuals within a population, he suggested, was due to mutation or recombination. Thus it was wrong to claim that negatively correlated traits could never be combined in the same plant. On the other hand, he seems not to have been particularly interested in accounting for those correlations that did exist ("strict" correlations, as he called them). Although citing the nineteenth-century theory of compensation as an attempt to explain antagonistic traits, he was unenthusiastic; it was misleading, he felt, to refer to "laws" of correlation because there were just too many exceptions. While conceding that even partial correlations were still useful to the breeder, Tschermak felt that the phenomenon of correlation had rather less theoretical significance than often claimed, and he made no attempt himself to advance an alternative explanation.

Why were Johannsen and Tschermak more skeptical of the evidence for correlations—and less concerned to explain them—than were pre-Mendelian breeders? In Tschermak's case I suspect that the answer lies in his enthusiasm for hybridization as a breeding method, dating from his first work in the 1890s. The rediscovery of Mendelism seems to have intensified this enthusiasm, for Tschermak—unlike Schindler—was convinced that hybridization could be made more efficient through the application of Mendelian principles (Harwood 2000). Given that conviction, along with the breeders' longstanding hope of combining quality and yield, it's not surprising that he would focus particularly upon the exceptions to commonly reported (inverse) correlations since these were crucial to breeding success. Clarifying the underlying basis of correlation was a subsidiary task of less practical significance.

Since he was employed in an agricultural college, one might have expected Johannsen to accept that "rough estimation" was actually a reasonable method for breeders to use, given the practical constraints under which they had to operate. But instead he insisted that breeders should select *directly* for desired physiological traits such as winter-hardiness, rather than selecting for morphological traits which were merely correlated with them (Johannsen 1909: 309–11), though this was scarcely practicable. More generally, in his discussion of correlation one notices his sense of irritation with the "doctrines" and "beliefs" of the breeders, and he complains of "loose talk" in the literature which ignored counter-evidence (Johannsen 1909: 287–8, 1911: 142–3). Though he recognized that the aims of the breeder and the biologist were different, he remained impatient nonetheless with the shortcuts taken by the former:

> the indirect assessment of one character by measuring the intensity of another is a poor indicator, unless one is content with a good deal of uncertainty. In exact work one must necessarily carry out *direct measurement of the character in question*. Anything else is more or less rough estimation [*lose Schätzung*].
>
> (Johannsen 1909: 299, emphasis in original)

For practical breeders, he noted, it may not matter whether one talks of a "law" of correlation or not, but from a biological standpoint it was important whether two characters always varied together or only under particular conditions. (In saying this, Johannsen was hardly doing justice to his opponents. Correlation was not just a breeders' tool but had been a concern to biologists like Geoffroy and de Candolle. And Schindler, though an academic breeder, had in fact emphasized that correlations did not hold under all growing conditions, as well as offering a physiological explanation for it.)

Conclusion

Assuming that this contrast between Tschermak and Johannsen versus Schindler *et al.* was typical of the new Mendelians versus late-nineteenth-century academic breeders, it raises the question whether Mendelism may have brought about a wholesale shift in thinking about the nature and meaning of correlation. The emergence of mapping by the eve of the First World War seems to point in this direction. And superficially it might appear as though academic breeders were also changing their minds. For in Germany several leading figures reckoned that Mendelism meant that the breeder must henceforth think of the plant, not as a whole, but as an aggregate of separate characters (Fruwirth 1909b: xii; Kiessling 1914: 10; Roemer 1914). In the United States, H.J. Webber made the same point:

> We no longer conceive the species, race or variety as a fixed ensemble of characters.... [but rather as] made up of a certain number of unit characters that are in large measure associated together by the accident of evolution or breeding and which are separable entities in inheritance.
>
> (Webber 1912: 30)

But for the breeders' attention to shift toward individual characters meant neither that *all* such characters were independently inherited, nor that even the independently inherited ones bore any physiological relation to one another. Indeed, it is clear that a number of academic breeders—some of them enthusiastic Mendelians—continued to regard correlation as of considerable practical importance right into the 1930s (Webber 1906; Fruwirth 1909b: vi; Kryzymowski 1913; Engledow 1925: 33; Baur 1932: 22).

A case in point was Carl Kraus, professor of agronomy at the Technische Hochschule in Munich. In his analysis of correlations in oats and barley in 1905 (Kraus 1905), to be sure, he underlined several of Johannsen's cautionary points: that individual plants often deviate markedly from the average correlation of the population, and that even where strong statistical correlation (even within purelines) exists, one cannot infer underlying causal connections between the characters in question. But unlike Tschermak or Johannsen, Kraus made no attempt to account for the numerous exceptions to correlation on grounds of mutation or recombination. Instead his explanations were physiological. Where an individual plant failed to display a correlation observed in the population, he argued, it was either because no underlying causal connection existed or because it did, but particular external conditions, along with internal compensatory relations between the parts, had combined to alter the usual relationship between the characters (an interpretation close to that of Schindler and Proskowetz a dozen years earlier). If breeding were to rest upon a scientific foundation, he concluded, it was essential to study the underlying causes of correlation.

But Mendelian biologists seem to have been less hesitant to discard the assumption of the integrated organism. The most extreme expression of this view was the concept of "unit characters" (in which each trait was determined by an independent Mendelian character) championed by Hugo de Vries (Spillman 1912; cf. Falk 1995). August Weismann evidently expressed similar views in 1902, and Lucien Cuenot's support for the concept was evident in his remark that Mendel was "worthy to take a place beside those who established the basis of atomic chemistry."[10] To be sure, not all Mendelians were immediately persuaded. As Hans-Jörg Rheinberger shows, Carl Correns was initially doubtful that the overall character of the organism could be reduced to independent factors, but he soon found a solution by shifting the responsibility for integration from Mendelian factors in the nucleus to an unknown structure in the cytoplasm (Rheinberger, Chapter 2). T.H. Morgan hesitated for nearly a decade. As various historians have suggested, it may have been Johannsen's distinction between genotype and phenotype which finally allowed Morgan to overcome his aversion—as an embryologist—to unit-characters (Allen 1985; Falk 1995).

Although I have not investigated this matter systematically, I would tentatively suggest that by the First World War many Mendelians had found a variety of ways to reinterpret the evidence for correlation, all of which allowed them to preserve an atomistic conception of the organism. For example, the incidence of genuine correlation on the phenotypic level was downplayed by ascribing it to a merely fortuitous association of independent genes in the chromosome (linkage).

Similarly, pleiotropy enabled Mendelians to ascribe apparent correlations, not to a complex relation between several traits, but merely to a single gene with multiple effects. Furthermore, by postulating lethal genes Mendelians could account for what looked like severely antagonistic relationships between traits (i.e. the absence of certain combinations), not in terms of physiological compensation, but rather in terms of an additional gene that killed the embryo at an early stage.

As is well known, the essentially reductionist nature of these stratagems did not satisfy all sections of the biological community. From a largely embryological perspective Jacques Loeb drew attention to the apparent contradiction between the "fact" of the organism as a "harmonious whole" and the Mendelian picture of the organism as "merely a mosaic of independent hereditary characters" (Loeb 1916: v, cf. chs 1 and 9). In order to resolve this tension without discarding his physico-chemical account of the organism, he proposed a division of hereditary labor. Mendelian genes, he suggested, only impressed intraspecific characters upon the developing embryo; its more fundamental characters derived from the structure of the egg cytoplasm. Many evolutionists, at least in the German-speaking world, harbored similar doubts about Mendelism as a general theory of heredity, and their preferred alternative was much like Loeb's (Harwood 1993: 104–10). While atomistic Mendelian genes on the chromosome determined relatively trivial traits which were subject to natural selection, they argued, another form of heredity—essentially holistic in structure—must exist outside the chromosomes. Only non-selectionist mechanisms acting upon such a structure, they reckoned, could account for the coordinated appearance of higher taxonomic differences during the evolutionary process. Despite Johannsen's embrace of Mendelism as well as his eventual acceptance of the chromosome theory, even he endorsed this model of evolution. Moreover, Johannsen was by no means the only geneticist, especially in Europe, who was disturbed by Mendelism's apparent irreconcilability with the integrity of the organism as seen in embryological and evolutionary phenomena (Burian *et al.* 1988; Harwood 1993).

So what does the story of correlation tell us? Most obviously, it is a concrete historical reminder of what we knew anyway on logical grounds: that the fact of correlation need not be interpreted in terms of a map. Where the Mendelian interpretation posited a random association of genetic factors in an arbitrary array (co-location), nineteenth-century breeders thought in terms of a physiological interdependence among traits. More significantly, however, the story demonstrates the ease with which early Mendelians challenged the evidence for correlation and abandoned a physiological understanding of the phenomenon. Plant-breeders' concern with the correlation of parts seems to have been brushed aside by (many) Mendelians in much the same way as embryologists' emphasis upon the development of an integrated whole and evolutionists' insistence upon the coordinated character of evolutionary change: it was shelved as a puzzling anomaly that might one day be resolved. But this was a task for plant physiology, embryology, or evolutionary theory since it was not deemed—at least by those of Morganian conviction—to be the responsibility of genetics. The history of correlation thus prompts us to ask once again what it was about the Mendelians' experience, circumstances, knowledge, or interests, which made them willing to embrace such a distinctive vision of the organism.

Notes

1 I have so far been unable to locate a copy of their 1890 paper.

2 In the 1890s agronomy in the German-speaking world was still dominated by approaches from agricultural chemistry, but Schindler is said to have been one of the first who sought to reconstruct agronomy on physiological foundations (Proskowetz 1924).

3 The agronomist, Carl Fruwirth, later invoked the same concept (Fruwirth 1909a: 171–6).

4 By the 1870s Darwin, at least, was attributing the concept to Geoffroy and Goethe (Darwin 1875 vol. 2: 335).

5 In wheat, too, the sheen on the kernel (*Glasigkeit*) and baking quality often correlated but not always (Edler 1898).

6 Others were subsequently to confirm the impact of environment upon correlation (e.g. Pearl 1911).

7 The protein-content of barley was practically important because high-protein varieties were good for animal feed but unsuitable for brewing.

8 Within a few years of the rediscovery of Mendelism, he was suggesting that apparent correlations could be broken down through hybridization or mutation (Johannsen 1909: 302, 398, 417ff, see also 1903: 65), and many others were probably due to the pleiotropic effects of single genes (Johannsen 1911: 148).

9 Four years later this idea would be central to his critique of the efficacy of selection upon pure-lines (Johannsen 1903).

10 Cuenot 1904, cited in Zallen and Burian (1992). (I thank Dick Burian for providing this source.) On Weismann see Roll-Hansen (1978b). Comparisons between the Mendelian analysis of traits and the resolution of chemical compounds into constituent atoms were not unusual: for example, Bateson (Paul and Kimmelman 1988: 286), Baur (Harwood 1993: 245), or Haldane (1927).

Bibliography

Allen, G. (1985) "T.H. Morgan and the Split between Embryology and Genetics, 1910–1935," in T.J. Horder, J.A. Witkowski, and C.C. Wylie (eds) *A History of Embryology*, Cambridge: Cambridge University Press, 113–46.

Appel, T. (1987) *The Cuvier-Geoffroy Debate: French Biology in the Decades before Darwin*, New York/Oxford: Oxford University Press.

Baur, E. (1932) "Konsequenzen der Vererbungslehre für die Pflanzenzüchtung," *Handbuch der Vererbungswissenschaft*, IIID: 1–30.

Beseler, O. (1904) "Über Pflanzenzucht und deren Ausnutzung durch die Praxis," *Fühlings Landwirtschaftliche Zeitung*, 53: 689–95.

Burian, R., Gayon, J., and Zallen, D. (1988) "The Singular Fate of Genetics in the History of French Biology, 1900–1940," *Journal of the History of Biology*, 21: 357–402.

Cuenot, L. (1904) "Les recherches experimentales sur l'hérédité mendelienne," *Revue generale des Sciences pures et appliquées*, 15: 303–10.

Darwin, C. (1968) *The Origin of Species by Means of Natural Selection*, 1st edn, London: Penguin.

—— (1875) *The Variation of Animals and Plants under Domestication*, 2nd edn, London: John Murray.

Edler, W. (1898) *Anbauversuche mit verschiedenen Sommer- und Winterweizensorten*, Berlin: Unger (= Arbeiten der Deutschen Landwirtschafts-Gesellschaft, 32).

—— (1914) "Über moderne Getreidezüchtung," *Fühlings Landwirtschaftliche Zeitung*, 63: 572–84.

Engledow, F. (1925) "The Economic Possibility of Plant-Breeding," in F.T. Brooks (ed.) *Report of the Proceedings of the Imperial Botanical Conference, 1924*, Cambridge: Cambridge University Press, 31–40.

Falk, R. (1995) "The Struggle of Genetics for Independence," *Journal of the History of Biology*, 28: 219–46.

Fruwirth, C. (1909a) *Die Züchtung der landwirtschaftlichen Kulturpflanzen, vol. I: Allgemeine Züchtungslehre*, 3rd edn, Berlin: Parey.

—— (1909b) "Tier- und Pflanzenzüchtung," *Jahrbuch für wissenschaftliche und praktische Tierzucht*, 4: i–xxvi.

Haldane, J.B.S. (1927) "Letter to the Editor," *Nature*, March 26: 456–7.

Harwood, J. (1993) *Styles of Scientific Thought: The German Genetics Community, 1900–1933*, Chicago: University of Chicago Press.

—— (2000) "The Rediscovery of Mendelism in Agricultural Context: Erich von Tschermak as Plant-Breeder," *Comptes rendus de l'Académie des Sciences, serie III: Sciences de la Vie*, 323: 1061–7.

Hillmann, P. (1910) *Die deutsche landwirtschaftliche Pflanzenzucht*, Berlin: Deutsche Landwirtschafts-Gesellschaft.

Johannsen, W. (1899) "Über die Abänderungen der Gerste mit besonderer Rücksicht auf das Verhältnis des Gewichtes der Körner zu ihrem Gehalt an stickstoffhaltigen Substanzen," *Zeitschrift für das gesammte Brauwesen*, 22: 487–91, 519–23, 540–2, 551–4, 566–9, 579–82, 599–604 and 617–22.

—— (1903) *Über Erblichkeit in Populationen und in reinen Linien: ein Beitrag zur Beleuchtung schwebender Selektionsfragen*, Jena: G. Fischer.

—— (1909) *Elemente der exakten Erblichkeitslehre*, Jena: G. Fischer.

—— (1911) "The Genotype Conception of Heredity," *American Naturalist*, 45: 129–59.

Kiessling, L. (1914) "Erfolge und Aufgaben der Pflanzenzucht mit bes. Berücksichtigung der bayerischen Verhältnisse," *Bericht über die 48. Wanderversammlung bayerischer Landwirte in Erlangen*, 1914.

Kraus, C. (1905) "Die Gliederung des Gersten- und Haferhalmes und deren Beziehungen zu den Fruchtständen," *Beiheft zur Naturwissenschaftlichen Zeitschrift für Landwirthschaft und Forstwissenschaft*, 1: 1–153.

Kryzymowski, R. (1913) "Beziehungen zwischen der Betriebsintensität und der Sortenfrage," *Jahrbuch der Deutschen Landwirtschafts-Gesellschaft*, 28: 456–67.

Liebenberg, A. von (1897) *Zur Naturgeschichte und Cultur der Braugerste*, Vienna: Frick.

Liebscher, G. (1893) "Fortschritte in der Pflanzenzüchtung," *Jahrbuch der Deutschen Landwirtschafts-Gesellschaft*, 8: 152–62.

—— (1896) "Die Getreidezüchtung, ein Mittel von grosser Bedeutung für die Rentabilität des Getreidebaues," *Deutsche Landwirtschaftliche Presse*, 23: 152.

Loeb, J. (1916) *The Organism as a Whole from a Physicochemical Viewpoint*, New York/London: G.P. Putnam's Sons.

Paul, D. and Kimmelman, B. (1988) "Mendel in America: Theory and Practice, 1900–1919," in R. Rainger, K. Benson, and J. Maienschein (eds) *The American Development of Biology*, Philadelphia: University of Pennsylvania Press, 281–310.

Pearl, R. (1911) "Some Recent Studies on Variation and Correlation in Agricultural Plants," *American Naturalist*, 45: 415–25.

Proskowetz, E. von (1924) "Vorwort," in *Beiträge zum landwirtschaftlichen Pflanzenbau, insbesondere Getreidebau: Festschrift zum 70. Geb. Prof. Franz Schindlers*, Berlin: Parey, III–XIII.

—— (1937) *Memorabilien, V.*, Praze: Czechoslovakian Academy of Agriculture.

Remy, T. (1907) "Einige Gedanken über die Gefahren und Nachteile des modernen Züchtungsbetriebes," *Deutsche Landwirtschaftliche Presse*, 34: 687–8.

Rimpau, W. (1894) "25 Jahre landwirtschaftliche Pflanzenzucht," *Deutsche Landwirtschaftliche Presse*, 21: 11.

Roemer, T. (1914) "Mendelismus und Bastardzüchtung," *Arbeiten der Deutschen Landwirtschafts-Gesellschaft*, 266: 1–102.

Roll-Hansen, N. (1978a) "The Genotype Theory of Wilhelm Johannsen and its Relation to Plant Breeding and the Study of Evolution," *Centaurus*, 22: 201–35.

—— (1978b) "Drosophila Genetics: A Reductionist Research Program," *Journal of the History of Biology*, 11: 159–210.

Rümker, K. von (1894) "Einiges über Zuckerrübenzüchtung," *Blätter für Zuckerrübenbau*, 1: 194–7.

—— (1901) "Zuckerrübenzüchtung," *Jahrbuch der Deutschen Landwirtschafts-Gesellschaft*, 16: 219–31.

—— (1905) "Korrelative Veränderungen bei der Züchtung des Roggens nach Kornfarbe," *Jahrbuch für landwirtschaftliche Pflanzen- und Tierzucht*, 2: 69–78.

Schindler, F. (1891) "Die sogenannten Korrelations-Erscheinungen in ihrer Bedeutung für den Pflanzenbau," *Deutsche Landwirtschaftliche Presse*, 18: 341–2.

—— (1893) *Der Weizen in seinen Beziehungen zum Klima und das Gesetz der Korrelation*, Berlin: Parey.

Spillman, W.J. (1912) "The Present Status of the Genetics Problem," *Science*, 35: 757–67.

Steglich, B. (1898) "Über die Züchtung des Pirnaer Roggens und Untersuchungen auf dem Gebiet der Roggenzüchtung im allgemeinen," *Jahrbuch der Deutschen Landwirtschafts-Gesellschaft*, 13: 198–210.

Stephani, W. (1911) "Die Pflanzenzuchtstation des landwirtschaftlichen Instituts an der Universität Halle," *Landwirtschaftliche Umschau*, 3: 1–4.

Tschermak, E. von (1907) "Korrelationsverhältnisse und Bastardierung der Getreidearten und Bastardierung der Zuckerrübe," in C. Fruwirth (ed.) *Die Züchtung der landwirtschaftlichen Kulturpflanzen*, vol. 4, Berlin: Parey.

—— (1958) *Leben und Wirken eines österreichischen Pflanzenzüchters*, Berlin/Hamburg: Parey.

Webber, H.J. (1906) "Correlation of Characters in Plant Breeding," *Proceedings of American Breeders' Association*, 2: 73–83.

—— (1912) "The Effect of Research in Genetics on the Art of Breeding," *American Breeders Magazine*, 3: 29–36, and 125–34.

Westermeier, N. (1897) "Korrelationserscheinungen bei Squarehead," *Fühlings Landwirtschaftliche Zeitung*, 46: 598–606.

Wood, R.J. and Orel, V. (2001) *Genetic Prehistory in Selective Breeding: A Prelude to Mendel*, Oxford: Oxford University Press.

Zallen, D. and Burian, R. (1992) "Lucien Cuenot and Mendelian Experimentation on Animals," paper given at the joint British–North American meeting in the History of Science, Toronto, July.

2 Carl Correns and the early history of genetic linkage

Hans-Jörg Rheinberger

Introduction

In a couple of recent papers (Rheinberger 2000a,b), I have attempted to reconstruct the experimental pathway that led Carl Correns to restate the Mendelian segregation ratios in 1900 and, after a few years of hesitation, to fully endorse the principle of the discreteness and the free recombinability of genetic factors during the process of fertilization. To be more precise, we have to distinguish two aspects of the problem: the first is the complete separation of paired factors from each other, in contrast to their blending; the second is the independent assortment of the different pairs themselves, the alternative being the coupling of characters.

With respect to the first problem, the possibility that in certain hybrids the characters do not split in later generations, Correns kept his choices open for years. He carefully retained in his mind Mendel's results with *Hieracium*, of which he might have learned from his teacher and Mendel's correspondent, Carl Naegeli. Even after the Danish botanists Christen Christiansen Raunkiaer and Carl Emil Ostenfeld had shown in 1903 (Hansen-Ostenfeld and Raunkiaer 1903) that *Hieracium* hybrids exhibit a peculiar form of parthenogenetic procreation and thus do not sexually reproduce in a regular fashion, Correns was not ready to completely drop the possibility of a "homoeogonic" behavior, which he opposed to the "schizogonic" behavior of the pea-type (Correns 1901c: [56]).[1] "A complete clarification of the conditions under which the characters split and do not split is only to be expected from the future," he declared in a 1905 paper read before the *Gesellschaft deutscher Naturforscher und Ärzte* (Correns 1905a: [481]). In later years, however, he repeatedly expressed his conviction that the pea-type of inheritance, the independent reassortment of paired factors, was the core of the new genetics; the rest were corollaries. In a paper on "The first twenty years of Mendelian inheritance," published in a *Festschrift* on the occasion of the tenth anniversary of the Kaiser Wilhelm Society in 1921, we read:

> The most essential of the new ideas is certainly that for the particular characters of organisms there exist individual, discrete, bodily *Anlagen*, "genes," "factors." They are independent of each other and remain completely

> unchanged if they come together with the *Anlagen* of another individual in the case of hybridization. During the formation of the gametes, they become again cleanly separated and distributed in the sexual cells according to the laws of probability.
>
> (Correns 1921: [1139])

My focus in this chapter is limited to the second problem, the independence of different character pairs with respect to each other. I would like to show how Correns came to deal with the phenomenon of coupled characters, and how he represented the phenomenon in the space of characters and the space of factors opened through the resurfacing of Mendel's laws around 1900. After being hit by the publication of Hugo de Vries' memoir in the *Comptes rendus de l'Académie des Sciences de Paris*, which de Vries sent him in April 1900 (de Vries 1900a), Correns rushed to publish his own results on peas, his paper coming out a few weeks later (Correns 1900a). There, he explicitly stated that two different pairs of opposing characters segregate independently from each other in the second hybrid generation and recombine according to the rules of probability, and he concluded in the words of Mendel: "With this it is demonstrated that the behavior of each of two differing character pairs in hybrid combination is independent of the otherwise existing differences in the two parent plants" (Correns 1900a: [16]). But just as he had pages before questioned, contra de Vries, the generality of the rule of the dominance of one character over its homologue, he also added a cautionary clause to this point. In a footnote to the proofs, we read: "This rule, too, does not hold generally; there are strains (*Sippen*) with coupled (*gekoppelten*) characters" (Correns 1900a: [16], footnote 2).

This kind of crosschecking activity, involving several experimental lines based on different organisms, became a hallmark of Correns' genetic work. His protocols show that over half-a-dozen genera, among them *Zea Mays*, *Pisum*, *Matthiola*, *Mirabilis*, and *Campanula*, had already become the subject of intense breeding studies between 1894 and 1899 (Rheinberger 2000b). I will come back to some epistemological characteristics connected to Correns' experimental style at the end of this chapter.

Experiments with *Matthiola*

Correns published another paper in 1900 wherein he elaborated on this preliminary note by reporting his experiments with different varieties of *Matthiola* (Correns 1900b). He had encountered the phenomenon of coupling in the course of a series of experiments involving the hybridization of variants of this garden plant that he had started in 1896 with the aim of shedding light on the question of xenia—that is, on the immediate appearance of traits of the pollen-giving plant on and around the seeds of the pollen-receiving plant. These experiments had been suggested by Trevor Clarke's 1866 report on a case of "something like" xenia for this genus (Clarke 1866; Correns 1900b: [27]).

One of the varieties that Correns used for his experiments had been cultivated in the Botanical Garden of the University of Tübingen; the others he had purchased from a seed dealer in Erfurt. They consisted of seven different strains, among them the "best English summer gillyflower, sulfur-yellow with varnished leaves [*Lackblatt*]."[2] Correns sowed them in April of 1896 and made the first artificial pollinations during that summer. For his experiments, he chose the Tübingen garden variety *annua* and, in addition, three of the purchased varieties with three different seed colors—yellow, yellow-brown, and blue—in accordance with his purpose to look for possible xenia. The paper states laconically that the hybridizations were "not always successful" (Correns 1900b: [28]). The protocols show that he had difficulties with the artificial fertilization of his plants: Good results were only obtained with a sulfur-yellow variety (*Matthiola glabra*) and the *annua* of the Botanical Garden (later renamed *Matthiola incana*), and then only in the case of *glabra* as mother plant and *incana* as pollen-giving plant, but not in the reciprocal cross. Correns sowed seeds resulting from this successful hybridization in 1897, but none of the growing plants flowered that year, so he had to await the summer of 1898 to get the record straight. For his future agenda he noted: "To conduct: a ♀ + sy ♂ !"—that is, the reciprocal cross between *annua* (a) and the sulfur-yellow variety (sy)—the reason being, still, "the color of the embryo!" and therefore the question of xenia. He also envisaged adding another round of "sy ♀ + a ♂," in order to be able to make backcrosses at a later stage.[3] Correns performed these additional crosses in 1898, and the backcrosses a year later in 1899. By the end of 1898 he knew that, as he subsequently stated in the paper, "the partial blue coloration of the seeds which occurs in races of gillyflowers with yellow seeds through pollination with pollen from races with blue seeds, as observed by Gaertner and Trevor Clarke, must *not* be regarded *as formation of xenia*, because it rests on the coloration of the *hybrid embryo*" (Correns 1900b: [29]). In 1899, when the reciprocal crosses of 1898 gave the first few flowers, he realized that in five of the eight different character pairs which he had chosen to observe (hairiness versus hairlessness of the green parts, form of the seed wings, pigmentation of the seed coat, simple versus double flowers, size of the plant), one character dominated over the other, whereas in the other three (coloration of the flowers, time of blooming, coloration of the epidermis of the seeds) the hybrids came to fall in between. Correns decided to call the dominant–recessive character pairs "heterodynamic" and the ones with intermediate features "homodynamic," because in the latter case the characters showed up "together" (Correns 1900b: [31]). This nomenclature, however, was not adopted by the genetics community.[4]

As I have shown in a detailed analysis of Correns' corn and pea experiments, Correns must have got an inkling of segregation regularities while studying the crosses of certain maize varieties during the winter of 1897/1898; he was thus prepared to see the consequences of these regularities in his experiments of 1898 and 1899, just at the time when he was ready to raise his second generation of *Matthiola* hybrids (Rheinberger 2000a). He had no problem obtaining them: the plants were perfectly fertile and self-pollinating. The seeds obtained in 1898 showed segregation under dominance: one quarter were perfectly yellow, three quarters were more-or-less blue. Only 15 of these seeds were sown in 1899. The majority, however—that is the impressive number of 525—were sown only in the spring of 1900. A first inspection of the plants gave Correns enough confidence to insert the note on the coupling of characters in *Matthiola* in the proofs to his *Pisum* paper in May 1900. The complete results were evaluated in the summer of 1900. It became clear that an independent reassortment of the eight different character pairs did not hold in the case of the genus *Matthiola.* Correns writes:

> The factual behavior requires of course the assumption that there is segregation, and that the products arise in equal numbers; but it also shows that instead of 256, only *two* different sexual nuclei arise, one part carrying *all* the Anlagen for the characters of the *incana* variety, the others *all* the Anlagen for those of the *glabra* variety.
>
> (Correns 1900b: [34])

Correns then went on with a differentiation in what he called the "separability" (*Trennbarkeit*) of characters. There was one class of characters which he called "hemi-identical" (Correns 1900b: [35]), shortly thereafter renamed as "semi-independent" characters (Correns 1901a: [78]). Such characters were not separable in the offspring because they resulted from one and the same *Anlage* through which they were both brought into being; for instance, the red color of the flower and the red spots in the pits of the leaves in peas. Thus, as a consequence, they always went together for reasons lying in the physiological function corresponding with or triggered by the *Anlage* itself. In this case, it was responsible for a pigment that colored different parts of the plant. Here, too, Correns' clumsy terminology did not stick (Bateson and Saunders 1910: 126).[5] Today, this phenomenon is referred to as pleiotropy. The other class of character inseparability was that of the *Matthiola* type just described. Here, the inseparability of characters could not be traced back to "a cause lying in the nature of the *Anlagen* of the characters themselves" (Correns 1900b: [35]). It had to do with the organization of the genetic material. For in certain varieties of *Matthiola*, as Correns stated by referring to his own experience and to that of others, these characters were perfectly separable, whereas in other varieties the very same characters were not. Correns decided to call them "conjugated" or, as he had done before, "coupled" characters. In another footnote he added that both cases fell under the rubric of what in earlier times had been discussed as the "correlation" of hereditary characters. Correns cautioned, however, that the two cases of semi-independence and conjugation certainly did not exhaust the wide range of correlation phenomena (Correns 1900b: [35–6]). The notion of correlation and its role in the history of heredity is further discussed in Jonathan Harwood's contribution to the present volume (Chapter 1).

Correns concluded from the behavior of *Matthiola* that two forms of splitting had to be distinguished. The first, as already mentioned at the beginning of the chapter, was the separation of the two components of an antagonistic (or identical) pair of *Anlagen.* Correns now called it "zygolytic" separation, indicating that it produced cells with a reduced content of germ plasm. The other was the separation of the different *Anlagen* pairs from each other, which Correns now called a "seirolytic" separation, indicating that their serial arrangement was affected, in fact was broken, split, or "lysed" (Correns 1900b: [36]). In the case of *Matthiola*, obviously, he observed zygolytic segregation, but not seirolytic splitting. For the time being, Correns had to leave open the question of whether, and if so, how these two separation processes might hang together or eventually collapse into one and the same mechanism. The problem was rendered even more complicated considering the fact that Mendel had not observed either type of segregation in his *Hieracium* crosses, which Correns cautiously kept in the back of his mind.

Correns' chromosome theory

Correns returned to the problem two years later in a paper responding to criticism from the noted plant cytologist, Eduard Strasburger (Correns 1902a). Strasburger (Strasburger 1900: 766–70; 1901) had challenged Correns' notions about a "qualitative reduction-division" occurring at a certain point during the formation of male and female germ cells (Correns 1900c: [21]; 1901a: [247–9]). Already in a 1901 review for the *German Botanical Society*, Correns, without going into further details, had remarked:

> It appears obvious enough to place the locus of the *Anlagen* in the nucleus, in a manner known, for instance, from O. Hertwig 1900,[6] more specifically in the chromosomes, and to have the segregation of the pairs happen in the course of a nuclear division.
>
> (Correns 1901b: [278])

Just as Correns had been pressed by de Vries to publish his experimental results on peas and corn, he now felt pressed by Strasburger to specify and release his theoretical assumptions about the time and mode of chromosomal separation in a more explicit fashion. Now he repeated more precisely: "We are inclined [...] to assume that the segregation of the *Anlagen* pairs results from a nuclear division, a hereditarily unequal division [*erbungleiche Theilung*], a qualitative reduction-division" (Correns 1902a: [303]).

He then went on to devise a mechanism that would account for both forms of lysis. However, he cautiously insisted on looking at the proposed mechanism as a mere "construction." "It is completely impossible to give anything else than a construction today," he stressed (Correns 1902a: [305–6]). The construction went as follows: Correns assumed that in one and the same chromosome the two antagonistic—or else identical—*Anlagen* of each character pair lie adjacent to each other so that the different pairs together form a linear row, and he illustrated this with the following drawing (Figure 2.1). During a regular cell division, according to Correns' model, the chromosome divided longitudinally—in the plane of the paper with respect to the drawing—so that each of the *Anlagen* was cut in half and each daughter cell received one half of the complete set of pairs. During formation of the germ cells, in contrast, the chromosome divided perpendicularly to the plane of the

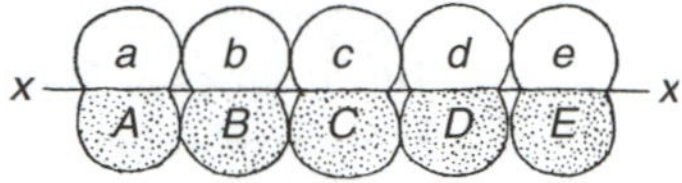

Figure 2.1 "Zygolytic" segregation of *Anlagen* in a coupled fashion (Correns 1902).

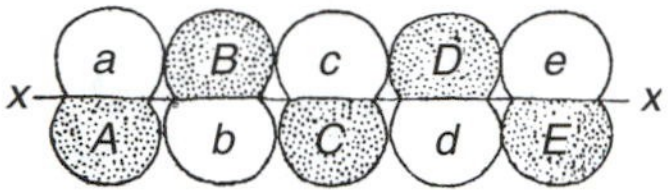

Figure 2.2 Segregation after "seirolytic" rearrangement of *Anlagen* pairs (Correns 1902).

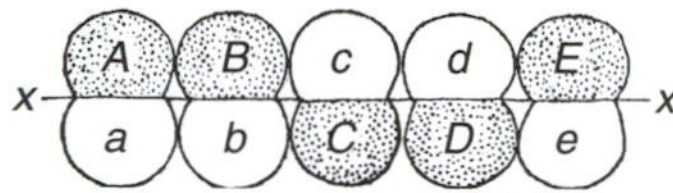

Figure 2.3 Another segregation pattern after "seirolytic" rearrangement of *Anlagen* pairs (Correns 1902).

paper, with the consequence that each daughter cell received only one of the two *Anlagen* of each pair. This model easily explained the transmission process in the case of a single character pair where each germ cell came to carry only one of the two *Anlagen.* At the same time it nicely explained why, as in the case of *Matthiola,* a whole set of characters could be passed on together in a coupled fashion with the same original combination of characters as received from the father and the mother, respectively. This was the "zygolytic" reduction-division. As to the independent assortment of characters derived from different pairs of *Anlagen*—as observed, for instance, in the case of peas—Correns went on assuming that, before the longitudinal reduction-division of the chromosomes, the coupling, or conjugation, between the adjacent character pairs loosened so that they could freely rotate independently from each other, as shown in Figures 2.2 and 2.3. The result was a statistical redistribution of the *Anlagen* on the different halves of the chromosomes, amounting to a recombination of the characters received from mother and father, respectively. This "seirolytic" splitting process was then followed by a longitudinal reduction-division in a plane perpendicular to the normal nuclear division, resulting in germ cells with all possible combinations of *Anlagen* for all possible combinations of characters in the offspring. The non-splitting of the *Hieracium* type required the additional assumption that the *Anlagen* could also rotate only by 90 degrees so that each germ cell qualitatively received everything. Although Correns clearly marked his ideas as a hypothesis, he pointed out that it was nonetheless based on "a certain correspondence with the cytological data" (Correns 1902a: [309]).

Two years earlier, while musing over the results of his pea experiments, Correns had jotted a note on a sheet of paper in which he stated that "for the manner of reduction, or halving, it is very important that the characters are independent of each other, that one of them can already have become constant, [while] the other is not [yet constant]." And since he could not imagine "*any* constant arrangement" that would do the job, he assumed that the *Anlagen* could become differently positioned during the process of fertilization: "One could imagine that the pairs of *Anlagen* are arranged in a *serial manner* and that during fertilization not all the Anlagen of A and those of B come to lie with one another." As a result, the rearrangement now termed "seirolytic" thus would already (or only, depending on the position one assumes in the reproductive cycle) have been effected in the zygote, as shown in the sketch (Figure 2.4).[7] As can be seen on the bottom of the

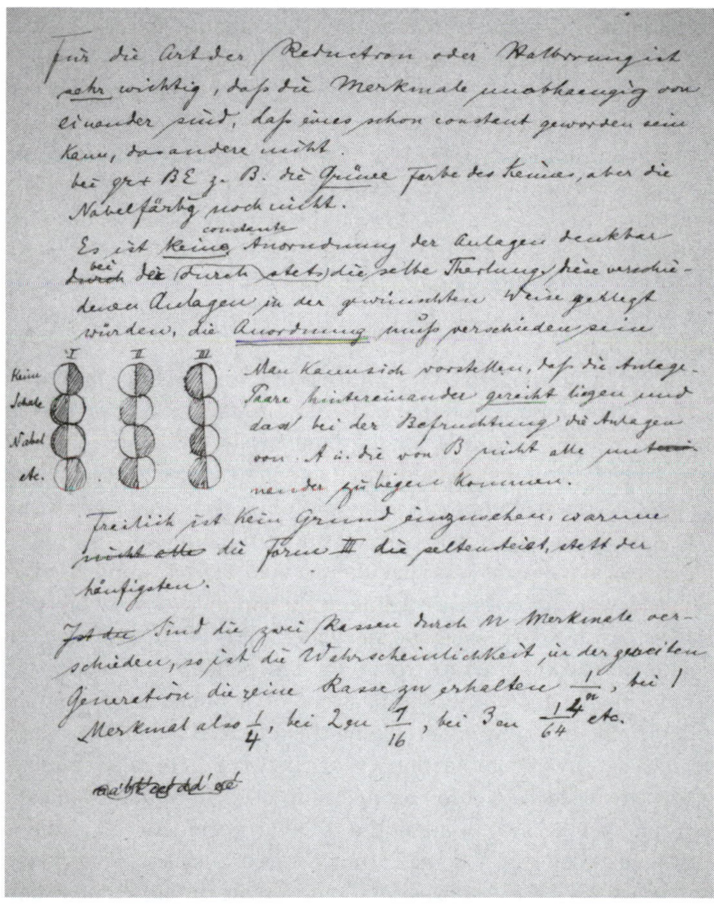
Für die Art der Reduction oder Halbirung ist sehr wichtig, daß die Merkmale unabhaengig von einander sind, daß eines schon constant geworden sein kann, das andere nicht.
bei gr+ BE z. B. die Grüne Farbe des Keimes, aber die Nabelfärbg noch nicht.
Es ist keine constante Anordnung der Anlagen denkbar bei Durch der stets die selbe Theilung, diese verschiedenen Anlagen in der gewünschten Weise gelegt würden, die Anordnung muß verschieden sein

Man kann sich vorstellen, daß die Anlage-Paare hintereinander gereiht liegen und daß bei der Befruchtung die Anlagen von A u. die von B nicht alle miteinander zu liegen kommen.
Freilich ist kein Grund einzusehen, warum nicht alle die Form III die seltenste ist, statt der häufigsten.
Sind die zwei Rassen durch n Merkmale verschieden, so ist die Wahrscheinlichkeit, in der zweiten Generation die reine Rasse zu erhalten $\frac{1}{4^n}$, bei 1 Merkmal also $\frac{1}{4}$, bei 2en $\frac{1}{16}$, bei 3en $\frac{1}{64}$ etc.

Figure 2.4 Early sketch of "serial" arrangement of *Anlagen*, undated (early 1900). Archive for the History of the Max Planck Society, Berlin—Dahlem, III. Abt, Rep. 17, Nr 115. (Reproduced with permission of the Archive for the History of the Max Planck Society.)

note, Correns tried another kind of rearrangement but obviously did not come to terms with it. In his 1902 paper, he took up this first sketch but gave it a different cytological interpretation. The arrays of circles now showed what can happen before the reduction-division—that is, before the formation of the germ cells—and not during or as a result of the process of fertilization.

Correns explicitly stated that he did not, with respect to his explanation, "misjudge the difficulty that lies in the *number* of chromosomes" (Correns 1902a: [306]). At this point, however, Correns did not take into consideration that he could have reached a similar result by assuming that different pairs of *Anlagen* could lie on qualitatively different chromosomes. With that assumption, he would have gotten around his hypothesis of a "seirolytic" splitting. We can only speculate about the deeper reason for the fact that Correns did not resort to this option. It may be connected to his observation that the very same character pairs accounting for the surface structure of the leaves (hairy/glabrous), the color of the flower, the seed color, or the height of the plant, which were "coupled" in his *incana* and *glabra* strains of *Matthiola*, were freely recombinable in other varieties of gillyflowers. That observation could have left him feeling the necessity to come up with an intrachromosomal instead of an interchromosomal solution. What resulted from his "construction" was the suggestion of a sort of free recombination, or exchange, of *Anlagen* at (as we would say today) homologous positions of the chromosome(s) of maternal and paternal origin. Correns was careful enough to stress at least in a footnote that his assumptions were "*not* inseparably connected with *any* definite conception about the division of chromosomes" (Correns 1902a: [302]).

In 1902, Correns thus operated with the assumption of a serial arrangement—that is, with a linear representation—of hereditary factors on the chromosomes. He further assumed two forms of longitudinal chromosomal division—a regular one in normal cell division and a reductive one in germ cell formation, the latter including the possibility of either a conjugation or a recombination of hereditary factors—and he did so in a very peculiar fashion. What he did not conceive of at this point, as we have seen, was that there could exist a number of coupling groups of *Anlagen* or characters according to the number of pairs of homologous chromosomes. As a consequence, he needed the assumption of a homologous recombination already in order to explain the independent segregation of factors, and not only for the more-or-less rare event of a breakage of coupling. This framework prevented him from developing the idea that the fact of coupling and the frequency of rare recombination events between generally coupled factors could be used to construct a chromosomal map of *Anlagen*; that is, to experimentally determine their relative position in a serial arrangement. This step was only taken several years later by Thomas Hunt Morgan and his group.[8] And it was only many years after the *Drosophila* mapping program had gained momentum that Correns appreciated the procedure as leading to a "*topography* of chromosomes." Doing so in 1921, after "the first twenty years of Mendelian inheritance," he rightly did not invoke his own paper on chromosome theory as a cornerstone in this development. He duly acknowledged instead Theodor Boveri as having been the first to adduce evidence, based on developmental physiological experiments, for the fact that the different chromosomes of one and the same nucleus were qualitatively different. He then went on to state:

> With that, a development was initiated which has led us already so far that it has become possible, with an especially favorable object, the fruitfly Drosophila, to determine even the *locus* of a particular hereditary *Anlage* on the chromosome, e.g. the color of the eye or the shape of the wing, i.e. that it has become possible to devise a *topography* of the chromosomes.
>
> (Correns 1921: [1143])

Concluding epistemological considerations

It was a question of choice of organism and style of work. First, Correns' own experimental material, the plants best suited for hybridization, did not easily lend themselves to an experimental program of gene mapping on the trivial grounds of their relatively complicated nuclear cytology and their long reproduction cycle. Second, whereas Morgan concentrated on one particular organism, the fruitfly, Correns went on to probe the scope of Mendelian inheritance by doing experiments with many different organisms and by analyzing rather complex and "anomalous" character patterns like those found in the variegation of leaves. Over a few years, from 1903 to 1907, he also came to demonstrate a case in plants where sex determination was inherited in a Mendelian fashion (Correns 1903, 1905b, 1907a,b; Rheinberger 2000b). The sometimes rather complicated sex determination in plants and, later on, the experimental manipulation of sex ratios, became his main scientific passions for over two decades. At the beginning of his hybridization studies, Correns stressed again and again that Mendel's rules could not claim general validity. In his early paper on *Gregor Mendel's 'Versuche über Pflanzen-Hybriden'* he remarked: "Mendel himself found that neither the rule of dominance nor the rule of segregation holds generally. It is therefore not recommendable to talk about laws ..." (Correns 1900c: [22]). As time went on, he became more and more convinced that many apparent exceptions—and many of those complicated cases which he himself had examined—could be accommodated to Mendel's framework. By 1920, his concern was no longer to claim a realm of heredity beyond Mendel, but to firmly approve the universality of Mendel's claims:

> I am convinced that the segregation of the progeny as conceived by Mendel accords to laws which we find everywhere in the organism [*sic*] where we encounter sexual procreation. In the end we will only have to explain the exceptions [from sexual reproduction].
>
> (Correns 1920: [1070])

The difference in the style of work is equally striking. Whereas Morgan not only assembled a whole group of *Drosophila* workers in his own laboratory, but managed to establish a *Drosophila* community distributed over the whole world (Kohler 1994), Correns remained a largely solitary experimental virtuoso whose results and conclusions rested on an intimate knowledge gained from experimentation with several hundred different plant species and varieties (Stein 1950), a knowledge which was hardly communicable and which he could profitably exploit only by doing the work himself.

There is another point that needs to be considered in this context. The phenomenon of "coupling" had a peculiar, by no means "statistical" meaning for Correns, a meaning which paradoxically both remained curiously continuous and changed subreptively over the three decades from 1900 until his death in 1933. In his paper on the gillyflower hybrids of 1900, Correns did not miss the chance to stress against his rival of those days, de Vries, that he viewed the existence of conjugated or coupled characters as evidence for the fact that the overall character of the species as a whole did not always recede into the background against its "composition from independent factors" (Correns 1900b: [36]; de Vries 1900b: 83–4), as maintained by the author of *Intracellular Pangenesis* (de Vries 1889). On the other hand, Correns himself had realized from rather early on in his transmission studies, at least since 1899, that the independent assortment of discrete hereditary factors based on the laws of probability was to become the very cornerstone of Mendelian inheritance as it was rapidly taking shape, not least under his own hands. It went together with a solidification of the categorical distinction between *Anlagen* and *Merkmale*, a distinction that resonated with the concepts of idioplasm and trophoplasm already conceived by Correns' teacher, Carl Naegeli. But if, as Correns had stated in his review of 1901, "we cannot uphold the idea of a *permanent fixation* [of the hereditary factors] in the germ plasm (*dauernd feste Bindung* [...] im Keimplasma)," as August Weismann as well as Naegeli had each assumed, and if chromosomal coupling was a possible, but not a ubiquitous and general, mechanism of inheritance, how then to explain the successive and regular physiological deployment of the *Anlagen* in the orderly development of the organism? To resolve this difficulty, Correns had come up with the following, as he put it, "heresy" in 1901:

> I propose to have the locus of the *Anlagen*, without permanent binding, in the nucleus, especially in the chromosomes. In addition I assume, outside the nucleus, in the protoplasm, a mechanism that cares for their deployment. Then the *Anlagen* can be mixed up as they may, like the colored little stones in a kaleidoscope; and yet they unfold at the right place.
>
> (Correns 1901b: [279])

In this way, Correns delimited a space of order, which we might call a physiological and developmental space, whose relations to the hereditary space remained to be elucidated. One might learn about the connection of both spaces through mapping parallel phenomena in both of them, and Correns gave the following example: Green peas could be induced to develop yellow seeds not only through hybridization with the dominant yellow variety, but they could also be induced to develop yellow seeds through the action of the larvae of a beetle. The latter event, according to Correns, was probably due to a "chemical influence" (*chemische Einwirkung*) (Correns 1901b: [281]). Instances like this might lead to an elucidation of the physiological conditions of action standing under the influence of hereditary factors. Twenty years later, in his *Festschrift* article of 1921, Correns stated succinctly:

> With the new results, the old controversy over the role of nucleus and cytoplasm in inheritance is solved in principle. The individual hereditary *Anlagen*, as demanded by the Mendelian transmission experiment, are located in the nucleus, that is in the chromosomes. [...] The hereditary *Anlagen* of the nucleus, if they fit, intervene in the processes of the cytoplasm, which must be different from taxon to taxon. Thus cytoplasm and nucleus work together.
> (Correns 1921: [1144])

In 1928, when he published his first review "On Non-Mendelian Inheritance," Correns had identified these mechanisms, or processes of the cytoplasm, with the "plasmon" of Fritz von Wettstein, which he accepted as the "specific," or even, in the words of Wettstein, "genetic element of the cytoplasm," although Correns continued to insist on dispensing with "plasma-genes" (Correns 1928: 154, 163). To follow the development of Correns' interest in cytoplasmic inheritance, however, would be another story. I would like to conclude this chapter by stating that Correns remained interested throughout his career, not in the formal, or material, structure of the chromosomes, but in the complex relations between the genetic factor space and the organismic character space, with its multiple phenomena of dominance, intermediacy, pleiotropy, polygeny, phylogenetic preponderances of certain characters over others, and the emergence of new characters through the hybridization of strains with known *Anlagen* (Correns 1905c, 1902b). Topography—or "mapping" for that matter—remained for him, more than anything else, a challenge of relating genotype and phenotype.

Acknowledgments

I thank Raphael Falk and Jean-Paul Gaudillière for valuable comments on a first draft of this chapter. For a German version of this chapter see Rheinberger 2002.

Notes

1 The page numbers in brackets of the Correns papers are quoted from Correns 1924.

2 Archive for the History of the Max Planck Society, III. Abt, Rep. 17, Nr 77, sheet dated 22/IV. 96.

3 Archive for the History of the Max Planck Society, III. Abt, Rep. 17, Nr 77, sheet dated 13/V. 98. ♀ stands for female, ♂ for male.

4 We can only speculate why. With respect to heterodynamy, Mendel's terminology of dominance and recessivity stuck. Instead of homodynamy, the obvious notion of intermediacy took over.

5 Bateson and Saunders rejected it without exactly understanding what Correns meant.
6 Correns' list of references quotes Hertwig 1898. There is, however, no entry for Hertwig 1900 as quoted in the text.
7 Archive for the History of the Max Planck Society, III. Abt, Rep. 17, Nr 115, folder "Pisum-Kreuzungen 1896–1900," undated sketch, presumably early in 1900.
8 Compare the contribution of Raphael Falk (Chapter 3) to this volume.

References

Bateson, W. and Saunders E.R. (1910) *Reports to the Evolution Committee of the Royal Society*, London: The Royal Society.

Clarke, Major T. (1866) "On a Certain Phenomenon of Hybridism Observed in the Genus Matthiola," *The Gardeners' Chronicle and Agricultural Gazette*, June 23, 588.

Correns, C. (1900a) "G. Mendel's Regel über das Verhalten der Nachkommenschaft der Rassenbastarde," *Berichte der Deutschen Botanischen Gesellschaft*, 18: 158–68.

—— (1900b) "Über Levkojenbastarde," *Botanisches Centralblatt*, 84: 97–113.

—— (1900c) "Gregor Mendel's 'Versuche über Pflanzen-Hybriden' und die Bestätigung ihrer Ergebnisse durch die neuesten Untersuchungen," *Botanische Zeitung* 58, Abt II, 229–35.

—— (1901a) *Bastarde zwischen Maisrassen. Mit besonderer Berücksichtigung der Xenien*, Stuttgart: Erwin Nägele.

—— (1901b) "Die Ergebnisse der neuesten Bastardforschungen für die Vererbungslehre," *Berichte der Deutschen Botanischen Gesellschaft*, 19: 71–94.

—— (1901c) "Ueber Bastarde zwischen Rassen von Zea Mays, nebst einer Bemerkung über die 'faux hybrides' Millardet's und die 'unechten Bastarde' de Vries'," *Berichte der Deutschen Botanischen Gesellschaft*, 19: 211–20.

—— (1902a) "Ueber den Modus und den Zeitpunkt der Spaltung der Anlagen bei den Bastarden vom Erbsen-Typus," *Botanische Zeitung*, 60: 65–82.

—— (1902b) "Ueber Bastardirungsversuche mit Mirabilis-Sippen," *Berichte der Deutschen Botanischen Gesellschaft*, 20: 594–608.

—— (1903) "Weitere Beiträge zur Kenntnis der dominierenden Merkmale und der Mosaikbildung der Bastarde," *Berichte der Deutschen Botanischen Gesellschaft*, 21: 195–201.

—— (1905a) "Über Vererbungsgesetze," *Verhandlungen der Gesellschaft deutscher Naturforscher und Ärzte*, Leipzig: Vogel, 201–21.

—— (1905b) "Weitere Untersuchungen über die Gynodioecie," *Berichte der Deutschen Botanischen Gesellschaft*, 23: 452–63.

—— (1905c) "Einige Bastardierungsversuche mit anomalen Sippen und ihre allgemeinen Ergebnisse," *Jahrbücher für wissenschaftliche Botanik*, 41: 458–84.

—— (1907a) "Die Bestimmung und Vererbung des Geschlechtes, nach Versuchen mit höheren Pflanzen," *Verhandlungen der Gesellschaft deutscher Naturforscher und Ärzte*, 794–802.

—— (1907b) *Die Bestimmung und Vererbung des Geschlechtes, nach neuen Versuchen mit höheren Pflanzen*, Berlin: Borntraeger.

—— (1920) "Pathologie und Vererbung bei Pflanzen und einige Schlüsse daraus für die vergleichende Pathologie," *Medizinische Klinik*, 16: 364–9.

—— (1921) "Die ersten zwanzig Jahre Mendel'scher Vererbungslehre," *Festschrift der Kaiser Wilhelm-Gesellschaft*, Berlin: Springer, 42–9.

—— (1924) *Gesammelte Abhandlungen zur Vererbungswissenschaft aus periodischen Schriften 1899–1924*, Berlin: Springer.

—— (1928) "Über nichtmendelnde Vererbung," *Zeitschrift für induktive Abstammungslehre*, Supplementband 1: 131–68.

Hansen-Ostenfeld, C.E. and Christiansen Raunkiaer, Ch. (1903) "Kastreringsforsøg med Hieracium og andre Cichorieae," *Botanisk Tidsskrift*, 25: 409–12.

Hertwig, O. (1898) *Die Zelle und die Gewebe*, II. Buch. Jena: Fischer.

Kohler, R. (1994) *Lords of the Fly. Drosophila Genetics and the Experimental Life*, Chicago: The University of Chicago Press.

Rheinberger, H.-J. (2000a) "Carl Correns' Experimente mit Pisum, 1896–1899," *History and Philosophy of the Life Sciences*, 22: 187–218.

—— (2000b) "Mendelian Inheritance in Germany between 1900–1910. The Case of Carl Correns (1864–1933)," *Comptes Rendus de l'Académie des Sciences Paris, Sciences de la Vie/Life Sciences*, 323: 1089–96.

—— (2002) "Carl Correns und die frühe Geschichte der genetischen Kopplung," in J. Schulz (ed.) *Fokus Biologiegeschichte. Zum 80. Geburtstag der Biologiehistorikerin Ilse Jahn*, Berlin: Akadras, 169–81.

Stein, E. (1950) "Dem Gedächtnis von Carl Erich Correns nach einem halben Jahrhundert der Vererbungswissenschaft," *Die Naturwissenschaften* 37: 457–63.

Strasburger, E. (1900) "Versuche mit diöcischen Pflanzen in Rücksicht auf Geschlechtsverteilung," *Biologisches Centralblatt*, 20: 657–65, 689–98, 721–31, 753–85.

—— (1901) "Ueber Befruchtung," *Botanische Zeitung* 59, Abt II, 353–68.

Vries, H. de (1889) *Intracellulare Pangenesis*, Jena: Fischer.

—— (1900a) "Sur la loi de disjonction des hybrides," *Comptes rendus de l'Académie des Sciences Paris*, 130: 845–7.

—— (1900b) "Das Spaltungsgesetz der Bastarde," Vorläufige Mittheilung, *Berichte der Deutschen Botanischen Gesellschaft*, 18: 83–90.

3 Applying and extending the notion of genetic linkage

The first fifty years

Raphael Falk

> Linkage was first discovered, in the sweet pea, by Bateson and Punnett in 1906. The interpretation they gave is now discredited; but in the same year Lock suggested that, if homologous chromosomes undergo exchanges of materials (as has been suggested by Correns in 1902 on dubious theoretical grounds), then failure of such interchange might account for linkage—*i.e.*, he postulated that linkage is due to genes lying in a single chromosome pair, and that crossing over is due to exchange of materials between homologs.
>
> Sturtevant and Beadle 1962 (1939): 360

Four major ideas have shaped modern genetic research: Mendel's conception of inheritance of discrete *Faktoren*, Johannsen's distinction between genotype and phenotype, Morgan's notion of genetic linkage, and Watson and Crick's model of DNA structure. In this chapter I deal with the third, less acknowledged, of these major epistemic breakthroughs: the interpretation of deviations from independent segregation of Mendelian factors as function of the location of genes along chromosomes. Contrary to Mendel's law of independent inheritance of *Faktoren*, correlated inheritance of traits was time and again observed. However, in the early days of Mendelism there was no clear distinction between multiple effects of the same factor and multiple factors each with a different effect. I propose that the notion of genetic linkage was conceived in the context of resolving such correlation between inherited traits by discriminating those due to the mechanics of inheritance of discrete genes from those due to multiple physiological effects of specific genes. Although linkage maps were only devices that presented results of genetic experiments they were believed to be at least collinear with the structures of the material chromosomes. In this sense, they were hypothetical constructs (MacCorquodale and Meehl 1948) or virtual maps of the chromosomes. But once established, linkage became a central methodological tool of genetic analysis. Here I examine how the virtual maps constructed from linkage data provided the instruments for the establishment of the chromosome theory of inheritance and of chromosomal mechanics as a hypothetical construct. Furthermore, I contend that linkage became also an experimental device for the examination of the integration of genetic functions in development and evolution. These include notions such as "position effect" changes of phenotypes, cordoned-off blocks of evolutionary co-adapted genes, or inadvertent sweepings of neighboring genes causing "linkage disequilibrium." With the transition of classical to molecular genetics new tools and methods were developed, but to a large extent many of the new concepts were elaborated on the background of established genetic concepts. The examination of homologies between organisms by *in vitro* hybrids of their DNA molecules, the location of genes on DNA restriction maps or by DNA walking are basically modern extensions of the notion of genetic linkage.

Compound unit-characters

De Vries, and in his footsteps Bateson and their colleagues believed organisms to be "built up of distinct units" (de Vries 1900). It was the inheritance of such "unit-characters" that Mendel's laws were supposed to explain. However, early on in their studies of the heredity of unit-characters, Bateson and his associates encountered "compound characters," such as the birds' comb, which appeared in four "antagonistic" forms that segregated according to Mendel's rule of independent units. They first suggested the inheritance to be one of "resolution"—"the breaking up of the compound allelomorphs of the original parent" in the gametes (Bateson *et al.* 1905). Also other cases of "outward or zygotic characters"—what we will call today adult phenotypes—were interpreted as gametically compound, "being represented in the gametes by more than one factor" (Hurst 1906). Red flower color in sweet peas, the red color of "Fireball" tomatoes, the yellow-gray coat color of the "Belgian Hare," "all are really compound characters, each being represented in the gametes by more than one factor" (Hurst 1906: 114). As it turned out, the criteria for entities of structural or functional characteristics would not necessarily correspond to those of the unit-characters of inheritance (Schwartz 2002). Matters became, however, more complicated when experimental coupling or repulsion between the gametic components of the unit-characters turned out to be partial and at specific proportions that deviated from the expected Mendelian ratios (Figure 3.1). When Bateson detected cases of two or more unit-characters in which "the proportions do not accord with Mendel's assumption of random segregation" (Morgan 1911) he interpreted these along his 1891 "Theory of Repetition of Parts," of symmetry and segmentation in organisms with repetitive patterns. As he explained the theory in a letter to his sister: "You see, an eight-petalled form stands to a four-petalled form as a note does to the lower octave" (Hutchinson and Rachootin 1979: xi). Such a transcendental physico-chemical morphological principle became the central thesis of Bateson's work in his major opus *Materials for the Study of Variation* (Bateson 1894). It was now applied to the coupling and repulsion interpretation of the non-random segregation of unit-characters (Coleman 1970). Bateson's reduplication model suggested differential repeated duplications of cells with different genetic contents.

Such a preformationist notion of unit-character was unacceptable to Morgan. As an experimental embryologist he struggled against the preformation notion of

	Gametic series				Number of gametes in series	Number of zygotes formed	Nature of zygotic series			
	AB	*Ab*	*aB*	*ab*			*AB*	*Ab*	*aB*	*ab*
Partial repulsion from zygote of form $Ab \times aB$	1	$(n-1)$	$(n-1)$	1	$2n$	$4n^2$	$2n^2+1$	n^2-1	n^2-1	1
	1	31	31	1	64	4096	2049	1023	1023	1
	1	15	15	1	32	1024	513	255	255	1
	1	7	7	1	16	256	129	63	63	1
	1	3	3	1	8	64	33	15	15	1
	1	1	1	1	4	16	9	3	3	1
Partial coupling from zygote of form $AB \times ab$	3	1	1	3	8	64	41	7	7	9
	7	1	1	7	16	258	177	15	15	49
	15	1	1	15	32	1024	737	31	31	225
	31	1	1	31	64	4096	3009	63	63	961
	63	1	1	63	128	16384	12161	127	127	3969
	$(n-1)$	1	1	$(n-1)$	$2n$	$4n^2$	$3n^2-(2n-1)$	$2n-1$	$2n-1$	$n^2-(2n-1)$

Figure 3.1 Table of series of partial gametic repulsion and coupling and the corresponding proportions of resulting F_2 zygotes, as expected by Bateson and Punnett's (1911) model of differential reduplication of gametes. (Reproduced with permission from Bateson, W. and Punnett, R.C. (1911) "On Gametic Series Involving Reduplication of Certain Terms," *Journal of Genetics*, 1(4), 293–302, published by Indian Academy of Sciences, Bangalore, India.)

heredity as he identified it in E.B. Wilson's interpretation of Weismann's distinction between the germ and the soma lines (Griesemer 2000: 264). From the inception of his studies in heredity Morgan emphasized the many-to-many relationships between Mendelian factors and traits (see, e.g. Morgan 1910a: 451, 461; also: Allen 1985: 120; Falk and Schwartz 1993). He was bothered by the one-factor—one-trait notion immanent in Bateson's interpretation of unit-characters (see Falk 2001: 293). However, Johannsen's (1911) differentiation between the genotype and the phenotype allowed him to come to term with Mendelian apparent preformation (Allen 1985; Falk and Schwartz 1993), and consequently, with the notion that the chromosomes were the material sites of the Mendelian factors (Morgan 1913). Morgan put forward an interpretation that overcame Bateson's confounding the *mechanics of the inheritance* of the Mendelian factors and their *physiological effects on development.*[1] He contrasted Bateson's hypothesis of unit-characters with his own hypothesis that discriminated correlation between transmissions of genotypic units from correlation between phenotypic effects of such units (Morgan 1911). "Coupling and repulsion" were not just cases of "compound characters" that were differentially repeated during gametogenesis. They were of a different kind.

Chromosomes constrain independent segregation

During the first decade of the twentieth century, there was increasing evidence, mainly contributed by Wilson and his students, to the involvement of chromosomes in heredity. Morgan resolved the difficulty of compound unit traits that "do not accord with Mendel's assumption of random segregation" without renouncing the many-to-many developmental alternatives of factors and traits, by relegating non-random segregating factors (obviously factors or genes were recognizable only by following phenotypic effects) to the chromosomes:

> I venture to suggest a comparatively simple explanation based on results of inheritance of eye color, body color, wing mutations and the sex factor for femaleness in *Drosophila.* If the materials that represent these factors are contained in the chromosomes, and if those factor that "couple" be near together in a linear series, then when the parental pairs (in the heterozygote) conjugate like regions will stand opposed... [W]hen the chromosomes separate (split)... the original material will, for short distances, be more likely to fall on the same side of the split, while remoter regions will be as likely to fall on the same side as the last, as on the opposite side.
>
> (Morgan 1911)

Morgan's concern for the need to distinguish between the notion of developmental pleiotropy, the production of apparently unrelated and often variable manifold phenotypes of a gene, and that of genotypic "linkage," the constantly frequent co-inheritance of distinct factors, which were confounded in the concept of unit-character, is exposed in Sturtevant's description of the "moment of insight" many years later, in his *A History of Genetics*:

> In 1909 Castle published diagrams to show the interrelations of genes affecting the color of rabbits. It seems possible now that these diagrams were intended to represent developmental interactions, but they were taken (at Columbia) as an attempt to show the spatial relations in the nucleus. In the latter part of 1911, in conversation with Morgan about this attempt—which we agreed had nothing in its favor—I suddenly realized that the variations in strength of linkage, already attributed by Morgan to differences in the spatial separation of the genes, offered the possibility of determining sequences in the linear dimension of a chromosome.
>
> (Sturtevant 1965: 47)

Edgar Altenburg is of course right in emphasizing "that no one man is to be credited with the chromosome theory." Just as in the development of the atomic theory of physics, "so the chromosome theory was the result of the growth of biology" (Altenburg 1945: 76). Still, the insight that *partial linkage* relationships could be translated into topological relationships, that is, into linear maps of the chromosomes as bearers of the genetic factors, although attributed to Sturtevant, was already explicated in Morgan's original paper:

> [W]e find coupling in certain characters, and little or no evidence at all of coupling in other characters; the difference depending on the *linear distance* apart of the chromosomal materials that represent the factors... The results

> are a simple mechanical result of the location of the materials in the chromosomes, . . . and the proportions that result are not so much the expression of a numerical system as of the *relative location* of the factors in the chromosomes.
>
> (Morgan 1911, emphasis added)

Thus, the idea of linkage was conceived to resolve the problems of two or more characters that segregate in proportions that did not accord with Mendel's assumption of random segregation. Sturtevant's great contribution was the empirical transformation of linkage data into the one-dimensional maps of the chromosomes (Sturtevant 1913). He turned the phenomenon of linkage into a quantitative empirical tool for the elucidation of the organization of the factors of heredity, independently of their developmental and physiological effects. This was not a *conceptual segregation* of problems of heredity and development, as has been claimed by many to occur in the early years of genetics, but rather a *methodological distinction.*

Linkage as an analytic tool

The science of genetics was from its inception a discipline with strict reductionist aspirations. Mendel provided the general framework for the reduction of inheritance to *Faktoren* of discrete traits; Johannsen provided the insight that these factors for discrete traits should be reduced to *Etwas* that is deeper than the traits themselves.[2] Morgan and Sturtevant in their concept of linkage accepted this reductionist framework. Yet, they, together with Muller and Bridges, set this abstract reductionist notion in a comprehensive context of relevance. Linkage provided *genetic* analysis with a tool to investigate relationships beyond the discrete independent Mendelian entity, such as that of the chromosomes, and eventually the whole genome. Eric Lander and Robert Weinberg (2000) in their "Journey to the center of biology," celebrating the completion of the draft of the sequence of the entire human genome, maintain "arguably, the greatest insights came from Alfred Sturtevant." Sturtevant realized that his experimental results "could be explained by a simple model in which genes were arrayed along a linear 'linkage map', . . . Gene mapping rapidly became a powerful tool of genetics," the impact of which extends to the revolution in biology at the turn of the millennium.

As a tool linkage endowed the conceptual framework of genetics with a wide array of insights. It contributed directly to the theories of the structural as well as functional organization of genes. Contrary to early notions of independent genes, arranged along the chromosomes like beads on a string, attention was directed to functional interactions of linked mutant sites, such as "position-effects" (Goldschmidt 1955). Similarly, differentiating the effect of two closely linked mutations on the same homologue (*cis*) from the same mutations each on the other homologue (*trans*) (Lewis 1951) provided the key to the fine structure analysis of the genes. The structural organization of functionally co-regulated linked genes established the operon conception (Jacob and Monod 1961). The concept of linkage also promoted theories of evolution and selection, such as the notions of evolution of the complexity of differentiation by adjacent gene-duplications

(Ohno 1970) and the concept of linkage-disequilibrium when selection pressure or migration affected gene frequencies of linked genes, irrespective of the neighbors' own adaptive values (Lewontin and Kojima 1960). Even notions of developmental genetics, such as fate mapping of the embryonic primordia of *Drosophila* by the frequency of concordance of the adult organs' phenotype in genetic mosaics, is a direct extension of genic linkage maps (Hotta and Benzer 1972).[3] It contributed to the understanding of the mechanics of inheritance at the molecular level not less than at the cytological level. It was the first step toward the science of *genomics.*

It must, however, be kept in mind that although linkage maps were mere virtual, paper presentation of breeding data, the inspiration for Morgan's chromosomal interpretation of linkage was explicitly material, namely Janssens observations of spermatogenesis in the Slender Salamander *Batrachoseps attenuatus* (Morgan 1910a, 1911). In 1909, Janssens published his "chiasmatype theory" based on cytological observations (Figure 3.2). As described by Muller:

> A great bulk of evidence has accumulated to show that during the period of [meiotic] synapsis, homologous chromosomes come into contact, and in many cases chromosomes can be seen to be twisted around each other during one stage or another of synapsis. The essential point postulated by the chiasmatype theory is that, as the paired chromosomes draw apart again,

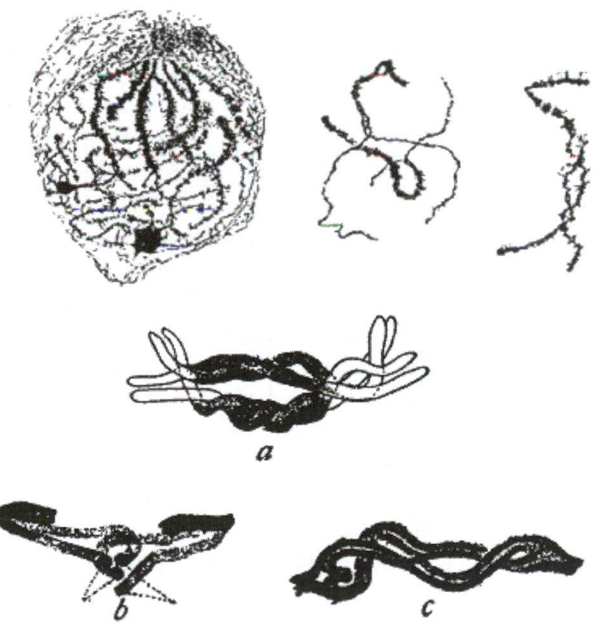

Figure 3.2 Early meiosis and schematic drawing of chromosome-pairs that show one to three chiasmata at various stages of meiosis in males of *Batrachoseps attenuatus* (after Janssens 1909).

> they do not always untwist completely, but may break at some points where they are crossed... in this way a recombination of parts is accomplished.
> (Muller 1916: 198)

This emphatically physical interpretation of crossing-over of linked genetic factors as consequence of their location on homologous chromosomes that twist around each other until they break, and the rejoining of the "sticky ends" after relaxation of the tension, dominated genetic thought for many years, to the exclusion of any other approach. For most of the next two decades there were, however, no adequate experimental systems in which integrated cytological-chromosomal and genetic-linkage studies could be carried out.

Two major papers, published in 1916 by Morgan's students, established the theory of chromosomal inheritance with the genes assuming physical sites at specific loci along. One was Bridges' proof of the correlation between the cytologically observed X-chromosome non-disjunction, that is, failure of the segregation of the chromosomes at meiosis, and the empirically observed deviation from the expected segregation of sex linked markers of Drosophila (Bridges 1916). The other was Muller's analysis of "The mechanism of crossing over" in which he experimented with coincidence and interference of crossing-over in multiply linked genetic markers of Drosophila flies (Muller 1916). From early on Muller was the most explicitly committed materialist in Morgan's group regarding the nature of genes (see Falk 1986). Muller demonstrated that "factors behave as though they are joined in a chain; when interchange takes place, the factors stick together in sections according to their place in line and are not interchanged singly" (Muller 1916: 366). Thus, linkage is a phenomenon revealed when exchange occurs between *blocks* or segments of entities along which genes are arranged at fixed loci. Such entities are the chromosomes that pair at meiotic prophase when they also seem to exchange segments. Muller's further discovery of the fourth linkage group of Drosophila, expected on the basis of the fly's chromosome number, filled "the chief gap yet remaining in the series of genetic phenomena that form a parallel to the known cytological facts in *Drosophila ampelophila*" (Muller 1914). These studies strongly supported the material theory of chromosomal inheritance, but did not prove it.[4] Neither did they reveal any information on the mechanism of crossing-over, with one exception: Bridges found that "very rarely a female which is heterozygous for a recessive sex-linked gene produces an exceptional daughter which is pure recessive." Such an exceptional daughter got both X-chromosomes from her mother; she is thus the product of X-chromosome non-disjunction, yet she is homozygous for a recessive marker for which her mother was heterozygous. "The very remarkable case is thus presented of an exceptional daughter, one of whose X chromosomes has undergone crossing over while the other has not!" (Bridges 1916: 120–1)

> It is impossible to obtain exceptions of this type from an XX or XXY oocyte unless the crossing over has taken place at a four strand stage. Therefore the proof that these exceptions have arisen from such oocytes will

> at the same time be proof that crossing over takes place during a four strand stage, to which Janssens has given the name chiasmatype.
>
> (Bridges 1916: 122)

Bridges was, however, careful in his interpretation that crossing over occurred between two of the four chromatids present at the time of exchange, since he could not exclude the possibility that the oocytes that produced these exceptional females were not accidental triploids. Only several years later did L.V. Morgan prove in her study of the progeny of (cytologically discernable) attached-X Drosophila females that daughters homozygous for maternal heterozygous markers were due to crossing over taking place between only two of the four chromatids (Morgan 1922).[5] The frequency of homozygotization of the markers in the progeny of such females was expected to be proportional to their distance from the centromere. This allowed not only to check the linear arrangement of the genes on the sex chromosome obtained by the standard mapping method, but also to place the centromere in relation to the markers (and indeed, it was placed in the opposite end of the sex chromosome of Drosophila than previously believed). This was confirmed by studies of segregation and crossing over in triploid flies. These studies also established that only two of the three-paired chromosomes synapse to produce recombinants at each site (Bridges and Anderson 1925; Bonnier 1943).

Recombination mechanics: chiasmatype or else?

As noted, although Bridges and Muller claimed that their studies both proved the chromosomal theory of inheritance and confirmed Jannsens' chiasmatype theory, these studies were merely consistent with the notion that linkage reflected some crossing over that occurred at the meiotic prophase. Thus, even though the experiments suggested that gene replication may be differentiated from chromosome exchange, they did not relate at all to the mechanism of exchange of markers.

Castle accepted that Morgan "beyond doubt established the fact that the genes within a linkage system have a very definite and constant relation to each other," but claimed "[t]hat the arrangement of the genes within a linkage system is strictly linear seems for a variety of reasons doubtful." As far as a physical connotation is ascribed to such maps, he doubted "whether the elaborate organic molecule ever has a simple string-like form" (Castle 1919). Castle was especially concerned that

> [i]n reality it has been found that the distances experimentally determined between genes remote from each other are in general less than the distances calculated by summation of supposedly intermediate distances, and the discrepancy increases with increase in the number of known intermediate genes. To account for this discrepancy Morgan has adopted certain subsidiary hypotheses, of "interference," "double crossing over," etc.
>
> (Castle 1919: 26)

Finding this method unsatisfactory, Castle resorted to reconstruction in three dimensions. In his "alternative to the hypothesis of linear arrangement" the arrangement is "rather in the form of a roughly crescentic plate longer than it is wide, and wider than it is thick" (the "rat-trap" or "wire-cage" model). Castle accepted the "fundamental assumption that the genes lie in the chromosomes and have a definite orderly arrangement," but rejected as an *ad hoc* assumption that "the arrangement of the genes within the chromosome is linear." Indeed, he agreed "the experimental data show that double-crossing-over *must occur*, if the arrangement of the genes is linear." However, double-crossing-over was an "unproven secondary hypothesis" (Castle 1919: 28–30). Castle put his finger here on a crucial point: Muller's 1916 evidence of the chromosomal theory of inheritance hinges on the chiasmatype theory and the interpretation of data as inevitable consequences of *mechanical* interference to double-cross-over of *linear blocks* of genes. Castle concluded "if the genes are not arranged in a single linear chain, the chiasmatype theory will need to be reexamined." He did not hide his predilection for a chemical reaction of "the replacement of one chemical radicle [*sic*!] with another within a complex organic molecule" (Castle 1919: 32), rather than a mechanical, brute force mechanism of recombination.

Muller's reaction to Castle's inability to perceive the metaphoric notion of the linear map[6] claimed, rather arrogantly, innocence: Nobody claimed that the linkage map represents any physical reality. The maps are merely graphically convenient presentations of the data.

> [I]t has never been claimed, in the theory of linear linkage, that the per cents of crossing over are actually proportional to the map distances: what has been stated is that the per cents of crossing over are calculable from the map distances... Whether or not we regard the factors as lying in an actual material thread, it must on the basis of these findings be admitted that the forces holding them linked together—be they physical, "dynamic" or transcendental—are of such nature that each factor is directly bound, in segregation, with only two others—so that the whole group, dynamically considered, is a chain... no implication as to the physical arrangement of the genes is intended when the terms "linear series," "distance," etc., are used.
>
> (Muller 1920: 98–101)

Despite the caveat in the final sentence, Muller continued to hold on to the chiasmatype model. He pointed out that "when the various conditions which have to be fulfilled at segregation are taken into consideration, any other explanation for these peculiarly linear linkage findings than an arrangement of the genes in the spatial, physical line proves to be hazardously fanciful" (Muller 1920: 101).

Yet, models other than that of the mechanical twisting of the chromosomes at meiosis were put forward. Belling who initially proposed "a working hypothesis for segmental interchange between homologous chromosomes" along the lines of Jannsen's chiasmatype theory (Belling 1928), later proposed a model of novel attachments of chromatids that are formed during replication between the newly duplicated factors next to the parental twisted chromatids (Belling 1933). This "copy choice" model was based on observations in favorable cytological material. Belling claimed that cytological observations in various plant species did not support breakage and rejoining of the chromosomal threads at early meiosis. Whereas Belling's model suggested a different mechanism, for recombination it maintained the notion that linkage reflected the topology of genes on the chromosomes. Other suggestions of crossing over were based on more general physiological considerations and did not demand necessarily a correlation between the frequencies of recombination and the physical topology of the chromosomes. Richard Goldschmidt noted already in 1917 that Morgan merely proved that some forces were involved, and that their proportional effects "may be represented geometrically as distances on a straight line" (Goldschmidt 1917: 83). Exchange of markers between chromosomes might be related to chromosome replication, and the process of crossing over could be used to unravel "the real nature of these forces," rather than the location of the genes along the physical map. He provided a model where "individual genes are assembled to the chromosome after the manner of antigen–antibody fixation, with a variable force providing for the numerical rules" (Goldschmidt 1955: 24). Winkler elaborated another theory, of direct change of individual alleles into each other, or a theory of "gene conversion" (Winkler 1930). As a matter of fact, such models had been refuted already in 1916 by Muller's evidence "that not single genes but whole blocks of genes are involved" in crossing over (Muller 1920: 114).

Notwithstanding possible alternative interpretations, J.B.S. Haldane noted that as late as 1954 most geneticists believed in crossing over as the breakage of two chromosomes at homologous points followed by exchange. "This process has generally been thought of in mechanical terms." Yet, he pointed out, "it is at least equally fruitful to think of it in chemical terms" (Haldane 1954: 110). He too suggested a model that linked chromosome duplication and exchanges that was, again, a kind of copy-choice mechanism.

> The genes and the whole chromosome are "copied" into a completely different structure, the relation being, perhaps, like that of antigen and antibody. This "template" or "negative" is again copied, giving *two* new positives . . . The close agreement of the distances between neighbouring units in protein and nucleic acid chain molecules renders this speculation attractive . . . Any account of the copying process must explain what happens in meiosis . . . the large diplotene chromosomes of Triturus oocytes are protein threads . . . containing little or no DNA, . . . If we assume that along each of them two threads of nucleic acid are laid down, but at a junction such threads sometimes exchange partners, we have the necessary conditions for "crossing over."
>
> (Haldane 1954: 108–9)

But the mechanistic breakage–exchange model prevailed. It is of special significance that Muller, who put great emphasis on the chemical properties of genetic factors

(Kamrat-Lang 1993), had decided that physics, rather than chemistry, was most relevant to understanding recombination.

> [t]he regularity of the mathematical relations observed in linear linkage, with its corollary, interference, proves that the disunion of parts of the chromatin structure from each other (in crossing over) is determined by geometrical and physical factors and not chemical bonds or affinities of a sort that would differ from point to point according to the atomic configurations within the gene material.
>
> (Muller 1929, cited in Muller 1962: 191)

Toward the end of the 1920s, when it was possible to induce major chromosomal aberrations and to detect them cytologically, special stocks with both cytological and genetic markers were constructed to verify that crossing over involved physical exchange of chromatids (Creighton and McClintock 1931; Stern 1931). These certainly excluded interpretations such as Winkler's suggestion of recombination by an inductive process of gene-conversion, but hardly challenged the chiasmatype conception of mechanical twist-and-break, versus, say, enzymatic reaction such as suggested by some copy-choice models. Simplistic models of copy-choice were, however, excluded by the fact that all four chromatids participated in multiple crossing-over events, rather than the expected two recombinant and two non-recombinant chromatids.

The notion of physical crossing over of linearly arranged sites was successfully extended by Pontecorvo and by Benzer to the fine structure analysis of genes in fungi and bacteria and in their viruses (see Holmes 2000), defying Muller's claim that the genes were "the smallest portion of protoplasm, separable by chromosome interchange" (Muller 1929: 189). However, the physical conception of recombination faced mounting difficulties with the increasing resolution power of the experimental systems. Fine structure analysis revealed increasing *negative interference*, that is, a high probability of adjacent recombination events for very close markers. Tetrad analysis in yeast and other fungi[7] revealed *gene conversion* (Lindegren 1953), or deviations from 1 : 1 recovery of alleles in meiotic tetrads, especially in the regions of exchange.

Quite a number of years were needed to overcome the *ad hoc* interpretations that were consistent with the old mechanistic notion of crossing over, such as negative interference being an artifact of localization of "normal" recombination to short specific segments of the chromosomes (with no recombination in the long stretches in-between). Eventually it was realized that at the molecular level of resolution crossing over need not be a point-event at exactly the same site in the participating chromatids, as had been considered to be the case at the level of the resolution power of the old genetic experiments. In 1963, Whitehouse still proposed a model based on breakage and rejoining of chromatids. He envisioned that recombination occurred at several points within "effective pairing regions," by lateral association of homologous regions, to give *hybrid DNA* segments (Whitehouse 1963). Shortly thereafter this model was elaborated by Holliday who suggested that a break in only one strand of the double helix led to the formation of a "heteroduplex" region, a region in which two single strands belonging to different double helix molecules were paired (Holliday 1964). Such a heteroduplex, if repaired could end up with the "wrong" connection, leading to chromatid exchange, whereas a "wrong" repair of a mismatch in the heteroduplex segment would lead to "gene-conversion." These models were finally elaborated into recombination procedures that were controlled by enzymatic reactions. The mechanistic models were superseded, and soon recombinase genes were identified.

Linkage maps

Genetic linkage maps are an odd concept. Maps, as a rule, are abstractions of some physical reality: A map of the streets of a city, a map of the ocean's shoreline, or a map of the countryside. Physical reality precedes its representation in maps. A road map is a way to represent a reality known to us. Genetic mapping applied the concept in the reverse. It started with an abstract notion and provided a map that gave this notion a virtual reality, of how we inferred reality to be. Linkage maps preceded the demonstration of physical, chromosomal reality. It was only later that these virtual maps were proven to have physical counterparts. Also contrary to most other maps, a genetic map is one-dimensional, a linear image of a notion, rather than the two-dimensional projection maps of spatial realities.[8]

Largely independent of the details of the mechanics of the phenomenon of recombination, Sturtevant's classic paper of "The linear arrangement of six sex-linked factors in *Drosophila*, as shown by their mode of association" (Sturtevant 1913) initiated a tradition of increasingly sophisticated mapping procedures in many plant and animal species. Bateson and associates' procedure of following deviations from the expected 9 : 3 : 3 : 1 segregation in the F_2 progeny of a mating made the calculation of "genetic distances" extremely cumbersome. The preferred technique became to produce, where possible, heterozygotes for two or more (usually recessive) markers in one sex (usually the female) and mate them to homozygotes for the recessive alleles of the other sex ("test-crosses") (Figure 3.3). There are four possible pairs of progeny of a test-cross of a heterozygote for the markers *ABC*/*abc*, namely, *ABC* & *abc*, *Abc* & *aBC*, *ABc* & *abC*, and *AbC* & *aBc*. If the markers are linked the pairs will be recovered in unequal frequencies. The least frequent combination (say *ABc* & *abC*) is assumed to be the one due to double cross-over, thus determining the sequential ordering of the triplet (to be *A*-*C*-*B* in the example) (Figure 3.4). Drosophila was found to be especially suitable for these studies, since it turned out that there is no crossing over in males (in many other species, there is less crossing over in males than in females). This allowed the direct location of genes to the same chromosome (synteny) in multiply-heterozygous males even for markers too far apart on the same chromosome to show linkage in the heterozygous females (Figure 3.5).

The introduction of tetrad analysis, examining (at least two of) the four products of the same meiotic event, in *Neurospora* and other species of fungi[9]

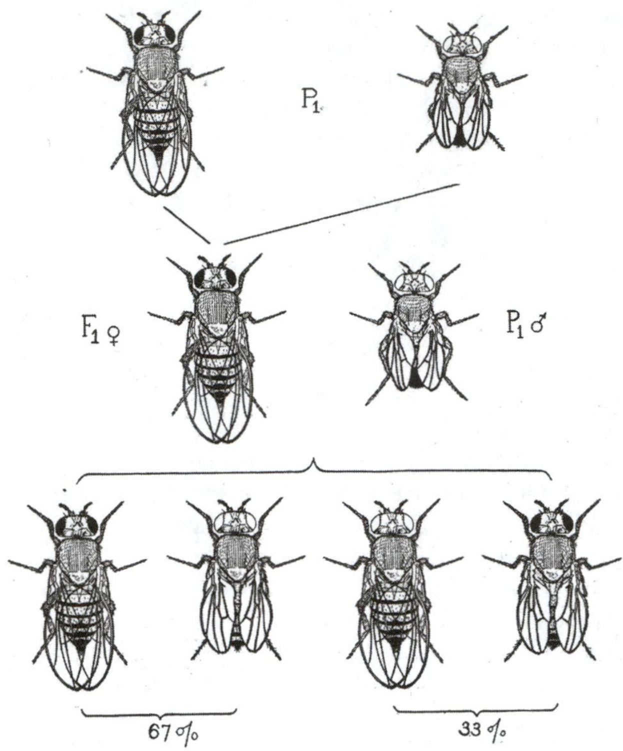

Figure 3.3 Morgan's (1926) presentation of inheritance of two characters, white eyes and miniature wings in *Drosophila* flies by mating a doubly mutant male to a wild type female (P_1) and back-crossing the F_1 female to a double mutant male. The genes are linked, since only a third of the F_2 progeny are recombinants.

allowed the inclusion of the centromere as a marker in the mapping procedure. Special methods were adapted for linkage studies in specific experimental systems, such as humans, where linkage could not be deduced directly from designed mating experiments. Already in the 1930s, linkage frequencies for genes mapped on the human X-chromosome (such as hemophilia and color-blindness) were determined by Haldane and others, thanks to the fact that matings of doubly heterozygous females to hemizygous[10] males were operationally equivalent to "test crosses." But for other than sex-chromosome (autosomal) markers in humans there was no way to decide whether the markers in the doubly heterozygote parent were in "coupling" or in "repulsion" (in *cis* or in *trans*, *AB/ab* or *Ab/aB*). If families of heterozygotes for two genes in which the alleles are in coupling are equally frequent as those in repulsion, any study that pools families will necessarily turn out to give a pattern of non-linkage. The sequential Lod (logarithm odds) scores method signified how to overcome this difficulty (Morton 1955). It asks what the

(a) $\frac{+\ ct\ +}{cv\ +\ v}$ X *cv ct v.*

(b) Progeny obtained in F2

Non-crossovers	+	*ct*	+	759
	cv	+	*v*	766
Crossovers region I (7.7 per cent)	+	+	*v*	73
	cv	*ct*	+	80
Crossovers region 2 (15.0 per cent)	+	*ct*	*v*	140
	cv	+	+	158
(0.2 per cent)	+	+	+	2
	cv	*ct*	*v*	2

(c) *cv* — *ct* — *v*

7.9 15.2

Figure 3.4 (a) Scheme of back-crossing *Drosophila* females heterozygous for the mutants cut-wings (*ct*) and cross-veinless wings (*cv*) and vermilion eyes (*v*) to *ct cv v* males. (b) The progeny obtained in F_2. (c) The genetic linkage map. The sequence is determined by the minority classes of +++ and *ct cv v* flies; these are assumed to be products of double cross-over. Hence the correct linkage arrangement is *cv ct v*. Of the total 1980 progeny (73 + 80 + 2 + 2) are recombinants between *cv* and *ct*, comprising 7.9% or 7.9 a "distance" of *centimorgans* and (140 + 158 + 2 + 2) between *ct* an *v*, locating these genes 15.3 *centimorgan* apart. Note the interference to double exchanges: the incidence of such exchanges is 0.2%, that is, only 16.7% of that expected if recombination events in the two intervals were independent of each other (after Sturtevant and Beadle 1962 (1939): 97–8).

relative odds are that markers' distribution in a given sibship came from linked loci with a certain percentage of crossing over (θ) as compared to the probability that this sibship would have been produced by unlinked loci. The data are examined for a range of linkage probabilities of θ. For each value the sum of the logarithms on the hypothesis of linkage are divided by the sum of logarithms on the hypothesis that the loci are unlinked, giving its "lod score" in that sibship. Lod scores of three or more, indicating that the probability of linkage at the rate θ between the markers is 1,000 or more times higher than that of independent segregation, were considered significant evidence for markers being linked. Eventually, in the late 1960s, the limitations of genetic mapping in humans were partly overcome by techniques of *in vitro* "parasexual hybridization" of somatic cells of humans with those of other mammalian species. In a parasexual hybridization different genetic systems are confronted by means other than fertilization and subsequent meiosis. The recruitment of parasexual hybridization techniques (such as heterokaryon formation in fungi, transformation and transduction in bacteria) had already proven to be most efficient for constructing linkage maps in prokaryotic systems. *In vitro* hybrid cells of mouse and human origins tend to loose

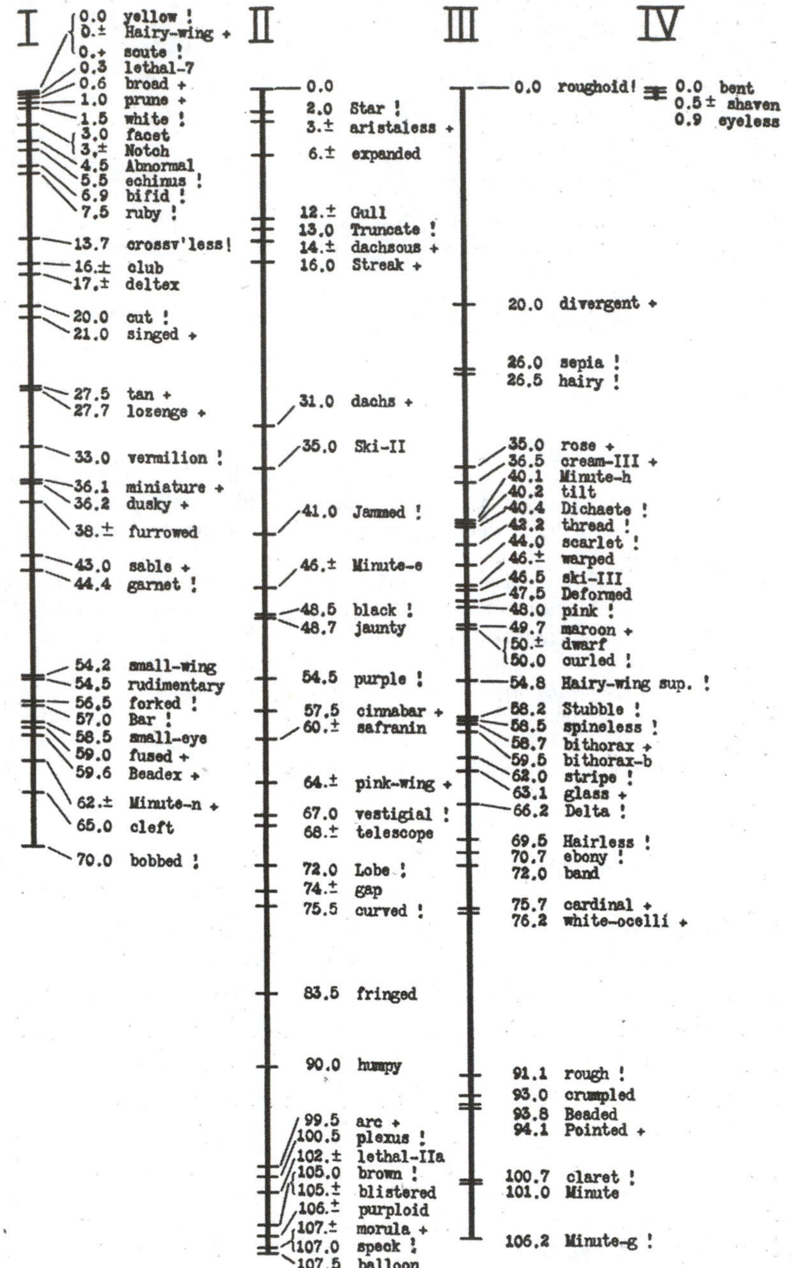

Figure 3.5 Linkage map of the four linkage groups of *Drosophila melanogaster* (Morgan 1926: 23).

the human chromosomes or fragments of them. The loss of a cellular trait that correlates with the loss of a specific chromosome or part of it is utilized to map the gene related to that trait to the lost chromosome.

The cytological link

Support for the linear map as representing the topology of the genes on the chromosomes came from Bridges' study of a dominant sex-linked mutation (*Notch*) in *Drosophila* that produces females with notched margin of the wings whereas no notched males survive (Bridges 1917). Notched females mated to white-eye males or to facet-eye males (*w* and *fa*, two mutations in different but closely linked genes) produced notched-white and notched-facet females, respectively. Bridges interpreted these results as the *Notch* mutation being a "deficiency" of a short segment of the chromosome, including the loci of *w* and *fa*. Corroboration for the deficiency notion was Mohr's finding that the frequency of crossing over between genes lying to the left and right of *Notch* (and of *w* and *fa*) was significantly reduced in females in the presence of the "deficiency" (Mohr 1924). However, no cytological confirmation was available for this virtual deficiency.

Things started to change toward the end of the 1920s, after Muller demonstrated the mutagenic effects of X-rays (Muller 1927). Major chromosomal aberrations could be observed microscopically in mitotic and meiotic metaphase plates, and their inheritance, often in correlation with that of marker genes, could be followed. This allowed the localization of the genes whose linkage relationships were changed to the rearranged chromosome segments, not only in organisms with relatively large chromosomes, like maize, but even in those with small chromosomes like *Drosophila*.

> In all cases so far found in which the cytological picture has disclosed that a section of a chromosome has become broken off from its original connection, and either lost or attached elsewhere, and in which at the same time the genetic analysis has been made, it has been found not only that certain genes have lost their original linkage relations with others in one of the linkage groups, in fact, in that particular linkage group which is ordinarily taken as corresponding with the chromosome here seen to be broken, but also that the genes involved form a "block," that is, *they constitute a coherent section of the linkage map*... There is no escape, then, from the conclusion that the previously constructed genetic map represented the genes as correctly distributed with respect to the two sides of the breakage point,...
>
> There can, therefore, no longer be room for doubt that the arrangement (that is, the order, but not necessarily the relative distance) of the genes as given in the linkage maps is the same as their actual, physical arrangement.
>
> In view of this, it follows too that the interchange which occurs between homologous groups of genes prior to segregation is an interchange of entire morphological sections of the homologous chromosomes... But to say this is to say that the so-called "mechanical theory of crossing over" is correct—the theory

> which holds that the chromosomes, in their normal process of interchange, become broken at one or a few points, and reattached in their sequels of the previously homologous members.
>
> (Muller and Painter 1929: 197–9)

The virtual chromosomes of linkage data were finally bolstered by physical reality.

A further dramatic change was still to come in the early 1930s. Balbiani recorded the existence of large banded strands in the salivary gland nuclei of Chironomus larvae already in 1881. A similar condition was found in the Malpighian tubules and other tissues of the larvae. The usual interpretation was that the strands formed a continuous "spireme," with only two free ends (Sturtevant 1965: 75). In July 1930, however, the Bulgarian geneticist Dontcho Kostoff called attention to the "Discoid structure of the spireme" in *Drosophila melanogaster*. He pointed out that "[t]he linear arrangement of the genes necessitates the assumption that the chromosomes are made up of chemically different components. The discoid structure of the chromosomes . . . indicates the existence of such chemical differences in the varying capacity to absorb haematoxylin." Kostoff noted further that "[t]hese discs may represent the actual packets in which inherited characters are passed from generation to generation" (Kostoff 1930). In January 1933, Heitz and Bauer showed that the spireme in the Malpighian tubules of the fly-like dipteran *Bibio hortulanus* was indeed a discontinuous structure, the number of components of which corresponded to the haploid number of chromosomes (Heitz and Bauer 1933; Painter 1934a: 176). Independently, and unaware of the latter's work, Painter, in looking for new material for the study of chromosomes, found it "quite natural" to investigate "the possibilities of the large structures found in the salivary gland of *D. melanogaster*." Work began in the early fall of 1932 (Painter 1933, 1934b).

> It has been found that the chromosomes in the salivary glands have a definite and . . . a constant morphology which enables one to recognize the same element in any cell . . . Needless to say, this places in our hands a method of studying translocations and plotting cytological maps which is a vast improvement over the study of metaphase plates heretofore used. But what is of far greater importance is the discovery, wholly unexpected, that in the salivary glands of old larvae the chromosomes may undergo somatic synapsis. As a result, homologues pair line for line, band for band, and unite into one apparent element. If, however, one of the homologues has an inverted section, we get typical inversion figures, such as may be seen in meiosis of corn, and by the bands and other landmarks we can tell, cytologically, just where the inversion occurred.
>
> (Painter 1934a: 175)

Likewise, the genetics of deletions and translocations could be checked and confirmed cytologically by following the band patterns of the polytenic chromosomes of heterozygotes for these aberrations (Figure 3.6). In the following years

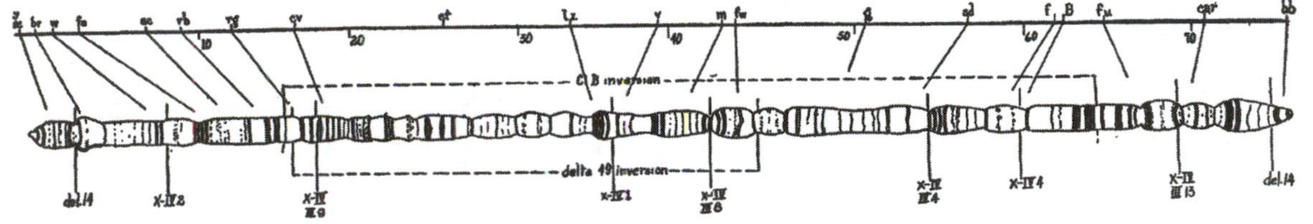

Figure 3.6 Painter's (1933) map of the X-chromosome from salivary gland cells of *Drosophila melanogaster*. Note the juxtaposition of the linkage map (with genetic markers and distances in *centi-morgans*) above the cytological map. Break points of chromosomal aberrations (*del*14 for a deletion of most of the X-chromosome, *X-Y*2 for a reciprocal translocation between the X and Y chromosomes, *ClB* inversion, etc.) are indicated on the cytological map. (Reprinted with permission from Painter T.S. "A New Method for the Study of Chromosome Rearrangements and the Plotting of Chromosome Maps," *Science*, 78(2034): 585–86. Copyright 1933 American Association for the Advancement of Science.)

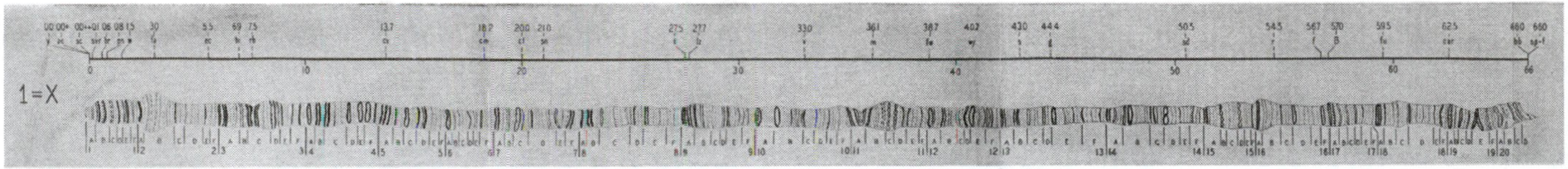

Figure 3.7 Bridges' alignment of the cytological map of the polytenic sex chromosome of *Drosophila melanogaster* with the linkage map. Note the division of the cytological map into sections (detail of part of the X-chromosome). (Source from Sinnott *et al.* 1950) (Reproduced here with permission of Oxford University Press.)

increasingly detailed cytological maps of the salivary gland chromosomes of *D. melanogaster* were presented, mainly by Calvin Bridges (Bridges 1935, 1938; Bridges and Bridges 1939). Polytene chromosome maps of other Drosophila and dipteran species, like that of the fly *Sciara* (Metz 1935), were also published. The maps of *D. melanogaster* were, however, unique in the detailed genetic data superimposed on them (Figure 3.7). Such data were obtained from changes of linkage relations correlated to the location of the breakage points of major aberrations. Bridges inferred from such data that "the structures seen in the salivary chromosomes" each "corresponds to one locus with 8 maternal and 8 paternal sister genes" (Bridges 1935: 63). More detailed fine positioning of the cytological sites of genes, were determined by following the common missing band of the polytenic chromosomes of series of partially overlapping deletions, like that of the white eyed *Drosophila* females heterozygotes for various aberrations of the X-chromosome (Demerec and Hoover 1936).

By the end of the 1930s, genetic linkage and cytological mapping were accepted as mutually complementary tools of genetic analysis. The culture of mapping dominated genetic research, from that of the dynamics of natural populations (Dobzhansky 1937) to the mapping of functions to individual genes (Beadle and Tatum 1941). Starting in the 1950s, it was extended to prokaryotes and to the molecular level. Here the rationale was greatly extended and elaborated, to the point that the old rationale of the mapping culture is often nearly completely obscured.

Conclusions: the impact of the linkage concept on genetic analysis

The idea that deviations from the Mendelian ratios in dihybrids could be due to the physical relationships between the genetic factors, distinct from physiological interactions in gene functions, proved to be most fruitful in shaping genetic research. Although initially stimulated by cytological observations, genetic linkage maps were intervening variables that presented the experimental data in the form of virtual maps. In the beginning it was largely the intuitive insistence of the researchers that considered the maps to be hypothetical constructs, maintaining and eventually bolstering the physical, cytological reality behind these linkage maps. Whereas in the early years the mapping culture contributed mainly to the mechanics of transmission genetics, its impact on all other aspects of genetic research became more conspicuous with time. It is not too far fetched to claim that molecular sequencing, from chromosome walking two decades ago, to modern ultra-mechanized DNA sequencing methods are direct extensions of Sturtevant's virtual genetic linkage maps of the 1910s or of Bridges' material cytological linkage maps of the 1930s. The central role that DNA sequencing plays in genomics, and nowadays also that of amino-acid spacing in phenomics, are significant extensions of Morgan's and his students' epistemology of genetic mapping.

It would not be an exaggerated assertion that in our age of all invasive molecular biology the only indicator that still uniquely differentiates genetic research is the application of linkage mapping techniques.

Notes

1 Note that in the first presentations of his linkage theory Morgan (1910b, 1911) related to "sex-limited" traits. Later on he discerned between "sex-linked" traits that were due to the mechanics of inheritance, and "sex-limited" traits that were associated with the physiology of development.

2 Johannsen's reduction of the phenotype to genotype was, of course, not the first attempt of biologists to distinguish between overt traits and their hereditary transmission. Weismann's germ plasm and somatic plasm, and Nägeli's idioplasm and trophoplasm were earlier attempts of such a reduction (I am grateful to Hans-Jörg Rheinberger for emphasizing this to me).

3 Benzer called the units of such fate maps "sturts" in honor of Sturtevant who first conceived of this fate mapping method, just as the distance along genic linkage maps are measured in "centi-morgans."

4 For example, chromosomes could be the phenotypic *manifestation* of genes. Thus their segregation according to the Mendelian rules would be a *consequence* of (abstract) gene action, like any of the seven traits of peas that Mendel followed, rather than providing the (material) *causal* basis for that segregation.

5 Normally a fly obtains one of its two sex chromosomes (two Xs in females, and an X and a Y in male progeny) from each parent. Hence, only one of the four products (tetrad) of a meiotic event is recovered in each progeny. In attached-X *Drosophila* the two sex chromosomes are attached to one centromere, instead of each chromosome being attached to its own centromere. Females with attached-X breed and in the stock obtained, daughters regularly get *both* their (attached) sex chromosomes from the *same meiotic event* during gametogenesis in their mothers. Thus, with respect to the sex chromosomes, in such a stock, two of the products of a meiotic event (half a tetrad) are recovered in each daughter. Only if crossing over between a female's X-chromosomes occurs among *two of four* strands may attached-X daughters carry one of their X's being crossover and the other being non-crossover.

6 Castle actually accepted that the linear model might be metaphoric: "Does it show the actual shape of the chromosome, or . . . is it only a symbolical representation of molecular forces? These questions we can not at present answer" (Castle 1919: 30). See also Falk (1995).

7 In yeast and many fungi species all four products of the same meiotic division are recovered together in a "bag" or *ascus*. This provides for analysis of all products of specific meiotic events, or "tetrad analysis." In some species the arrangement of the meiotic cells in the ascus allows also discrimination of the products of the first meiotic division from those of the second one. See also note 5.

8 These, however, are standard procedures of analytic geometry. As noted by Richard Goldschmidt, "*Es ist aber doch klar, dass man jede Proportion geometrisch als Entfernungen auf einer Geraden darstellen kann*" (Goldschmidt 1917: 83). Today we have extensive one-dimensional maps of two- and three-dimensional arrays in the form of sequences of digital data of computerized maps.

9 And of half-tetrad analysis in *Drosophila* attached-X females. See notes 5 and 7.

10 Males that carry only one X-chromosome and a partner Y-chromosome that, however, has no complementary genes to those of the X-chromosome are hemizygous for the genes of the single X-chromosome.

References

Allen, G.E. (1985) "T.H. Morgan and the Split between Embryology and Genetics, 1910–35," in T.J. Horder, J.A. Witkowski, and C.C. Wylie (eds) *A History of Embryology* (*The Eighth Symposium of the British Society for Developmental Biology*), Cambridge: Cambridge University Press, 113–46.

Altenburg, E. (1945) *Genetics*, New York: Henry Holt and Company.

Bateson, W. (1894) *Materials for the Study of Variation*, London: Macmillan.

Bateson, W. and Punnett, R.C. (1911) "On Gametic Series Involving Reduplication of Certain Terms," *Journal of Genetics*, 1(4), 293–302.

Bateson, W., Saunders, E.R., Punnett, R.C., and Hurst, C.C. (1905) "Report II.—Experimental Studies in the Physiology of Heredity & Experiments with Poultry," *Reports to the Evolutionary Committee of the Royal Society*, London: Royal Society.

Beadle, G.W. and Tatum, E.L. (1941) "Genetic Control of Biochemical Reaction in *Neurospora*," *Proceedings of the National Academy of Science, Washington*, 27: 499–506.

Belling, J. (1928) "A Working Hypothesis for Segmental Interchange between Homologous Chromosomes in Flowering Plants," *University of California Publications in Botany*, 14(8): 283–91.

—— (1933) "Crossing-over and Gene Rearrangement in Flowering Plants," *Genetics*, 18: 388–413.

Bonnier, G. (1943) "The Separation of Chromosomes in Triploids," *Hereditas*, 29: 62–4.

Bridges, C.B. (1916) "Non-disjunction as Proof of the Chromosome Theory of Heredity," *Genetics*, 1: 1–52, 107–63.

—— (1917) "Deficiency," *Genetics*, 2: 445–65.

—— (1935) "Salivary Chromosome Maps," *The Journal of Heredity*, 26: 60–4.

—— (1938) "A Revised Map of the Salivary Gland X-Chromosome," *The Journal of Heredity*, 29: 11–13.

Bridges, C.B. and Anderson, E.G. (1925) "Crossing over in the X Chromosome of Triploid Females of *Drosophila melanogaster*," *Genetics*, 10: 418–41.

Bridges, C.B. and Bridges, P.N. (1939) "A New Map of the Second Chromosome," *The Journal of Heredity*, 30: 475–7.

Castle, W.E. (1919) "Is the Arrangement of the Genes in the Chromosome Linear?" *Proceedings of the National Academy of Science, Washington*, 5(2): 25–32.

Coleman, W. (1970) "Bateson and Chromosomes: Conservative Thought in Science," *Centaurus*, 15(3–4): 228–314.

Creighton, H.B. and McClintock, B. (1931) "A Correlation of Cytological and Genetical Crossing-over in *Zea Mays*," *Proceedings of the National Academy of Science, Washington*, 17: 485–97.

Demerec, M. and Hoover, M.E. (1936) "Three Related X-Chromosome Deficiencies in Drosophila," *The Journal of Heredity*, 27: 206–12.

Dobzhansky, T. (1937) *Genetics and the Origin of Species*, New York: Columbia University Press.

Falk, R. (1986) "What Is a Gene?" *Studies in the History and Philosophy of Science*, 17(2): 133–73.

—— (1995) "The Manifest and the Scientific," in S. Maasen, E. Mendelsohn, and P. Weingart (eds) *Biology as Society, Society as Biology: Metaphors*, Dordrecht, Holland: Kluwer Academic Publishers, 57–79.

—— (2001) "The Rise and Fall of Dominance," *Biology & Philosophy*, 16(3): 285–323.

Falk, R. and Schwartz, S. (1993) "Morgan's Hypothesis of the Genetic Control of Development," *Genetics*, 134: 671–4.

Goldschmidt, R. (1917) "Crossing over ohne Chiasmatypie?" *Genetics*, 2: 82–95.

—— (1955) *Theoretical Genetics*, Berkeley and Los Angeles: University of California Press.

Griesemer, J.R. (2000) "Reproduction and Reduction of Genetics," in P.J. Beurton, R. Falk, and H.-J. Rheinberger (eds) *The Concept of the Gene in Development and Evolution*, Cambridge: Cambridge University Press, 240–85.

Haldane, J.B.S. (1954) *The Biochemistry of Genetics*, London: George Allen & Unwin.

Heitz, E. and Bauer, H. (1933) "Beweise für die Chromosomennatur der Kernschleifen in den Knäuelkernen von *Bibio hortulanus*," *Zeitschrift für Zellforschung und mikroskopische Anatomie*, 17: 76–82.

Holliday, R. (1964) "A Mechanism for Gene Conversion in fungi," *Genetical Research*, 3: 472–86.

Holmes, F.L. (2000) "Seymour Benzer and the Definition of the Gene," in P.J. Beurton, R. Falk, and H.-J. Rheinberger (eds) *The Concept of the Gene in Development and Evolution*, Cambridge: Cambridge University Press, 115–55.

Hotta, Y. and Benzer, S. (1972) "Mapping of Behavior in *Drosophila melanogaster*," *Nature*, 240: 527–35.

Hurst, C.C. (1906) "Mendelian Characters in Plants and Animals," *Report of the Third International Conference on Genetics*, London: Royal Horticultural Society, 114–29.

Hutchinson, G.E. and Rachootin, S. (1979) "Historical Introduction" to the re-edition of *William Bateson: Problems of Genetics*, New Haven and London: Yale University Press.

Jacob, F. and Monod, J. (1961) "Genetic Regulatory Mechanisms in the Synthesis of Proteins," *Journal of Molecular Biology*, 3: 318–56.

Janssens, F.A. (1909) "La Théorie de la chiasmatypie. Nouvelle interprétation des cinèses de maturation," *La Cellule*, 25: 389–411.

Johannsen, W. (1911) "The Genotype Conception of Heredity," *The American Naturalist*, 45(531): 129–59.

Kamrat-Lang, D. (1993) *Genetics Humanized: H.J. Muller between Science and Politics 1915–1932*, Unpublished PhD Dissertation, The Hebrew University, Jerusalem.

Kostoff, D. (1930) "Discoid Structure of the Spireme," *The Journal of Heredity*, 21(7): 323–4.

Lander, E.S. and Weinberg, R.A. (2000) "Journey to the Center of Biology," *Science*, 287(5459): 1777–82.

Lewis, E.B. (1951) "Pseudoallelism and Gene Evolution," *Cold Spring Harbor Symposia on Quantitative Biology*, 16: 159–72.

Lewontin, R.C. and Kojima, K.-I. (1960) "The Evolutionary Dynamics of Complex Polymorphism," *Evolution*, 14(4): 458–72.

Lindegren, C.C. (1953) "Gene Conversion in *Saccharomyces*," *Journal of Genetics*, 51: 625–37.

MacCorquodale, K. and Meehl, P.E. (1948) "On Distinction between Hypothetical Constructs and Intervening Variables," *Psychological Review*, 55: 95–107.

Metz, C.W. (1935) "Structure of the Salivary Gland Chromosomes in *Sciara*," *The Journal of Heredity*, 26: 177–88.

Mohr, O.L. (1924) "A Genetic and Cytological Analysis of a Section Deficiency Involving Four Units of the X-Chromosome in *Drosophila melanogaster*," *Zeitschrift für induktive Abstammungs- und Vererbungslehre*, 32: 108–232.

Morgan, L.V. (1922) "Non-criss-cross Inheritance in *Drosophila melanogaster*," *Biological Bulletin, Woods Hole*, 42: 267–74.

Morgan, T.H. (1910a) "Chromosomes and Heredity," *The American Naturalist*, 44: 449–98.

—— (1910b) "Sex Limited Inheritance in *Drosophila*," *Science*, 32: 120–2.

—— (1911) "Random Segregation versus Coupling in Mendelian Inheritance," *Science*, 34(873): 384.

—— (1913) "Factors and Unit Characters in Mendelian Heredity," *The American Naturalist*, 47(553): 5–15.

—— (1926) *The Theory of the Gene*, New Haven: Yale University Press.

Morton, N.E. (1955) "Sequential Tests for the Detection of Linkage," *American Journal of Human Genetics*, 7: 277–318.

Muller, H.J. (1914) "A Gene for the Fourth Chromosome of *Drosophila*," *The Journal of Experimental Zoology*, 17: 325–36.

—— (1916) "The Mechanism of Crossing over," *The American Naturalist*, 50(592–595): 193–221, 284–305, 351–66, 421–34.

—— (1920) "Are the Factors of Heredity Arranged in a Line?" *The American Naturalist*, 54(631): 97–121.

—— (1927) "Artificial Transmutation of the Gene," *Science*, 66: 84–7.

—— (1929) "The Gene as the Basis of Life," *Proceedings of the International Congress of Plant Sciences* 1: 897–921.

—— (1962) *Studies in Genetics: The Selected Papers of H.J. Muller*, Bloomington: Indiana University Press.

Muller, H.J. and Painter, T.S. (1929) "The Cytological Expression of Changes in Gene Alignment Produced by X-Rays in Drosophila," *The American Naturalist*, 63(686): 193–200.

Ohno, S. (1970) *Evolution by Gene Duplication*, Berlin: Springer.

Painter, T.S. (1933) "A New Method for the Study of Chromosome Rearrangements and the Plotting of Chromosome Maps," *Science*, 78(2034): 585–6.

—— (1934a) "A New Method for the Study of Chromosome Aberrations and the Potting of Chromosome Maps in *Drosophila melanogaster*," *Genetics*, 19: 175–88.

—— (1934b) "Salivary Chromosomes and the Attack on the Gene," *The Journal of Heredity*, 25: 465–76.

Schwartz, S. (2002) "Characters as Units and the Case of the Presence and Absence Hypothesis," *Biology & Philosophy*, 17(3): 369–88.

Sinnott, E.W., Dunn, L.C. and Dobzhansky, Th. (1950) *Principles of Genetics* (4th ed.), New York: McGraw-Hill.

Stern, C. (1931) "Zytologisch-genetische Untersuchungen als Beweise für die Morgansche Theorie des Faktorenaustauschs," *Biologisches Zentralblatt*, 51(10): 547–87.

Sturtevant, A.H. (1913) "The Linear Arrangement of Six Sex-Linked Factors in Drosophila, As Shown by Their Mode of Association," *Journal of Experimental Zoology*, 14: 43–59.

—— (1965) *A History of Genetics*, New York: Harper & Row.

Sturtevant, A.H. and Beadle, G.W. (1962 (1939)) *An Introduction to Genetics*, New York: Dover.

Vries, H. de (1900) "Das Spaltungsgesetz der Bastarde," *Berichte der deutschen botanischen Gesellschaft*, 18: 83–90.

Whitehouse, H.L.K. (1963) "A Theory of Crossing-over by Means of Hybrid Deoxyribonucleic Acid," *Nature*, 199: 1034–40.

Winkler, H. (1930) *Die Konversion der Gene*, Jena: Fischer.

4 Classical genetics and the geography of genes

Lisa Gannett and James R. Griesemer

Introduction

When we talk about mapping genes these days, we tend to think mostly about the mapping that takes place in molecular genetics. Associated with the Human Genome Project, for example, are: genetic maps that use hypervariable sites in the genome as markers to situate genes on chromosomes by relative distance ("genetic distance"); physical maps that locate genes on chromosomes by absolute distance (in units of DNA nucleotides); and the map that identifies each individual nucleotide of a standard genome, sometimes called the "ultimate map." These kinds of maps have their historical antecedents in mapping techniques developed in *Drosophila melanogaster*—the genetic linkage maps invented by Alfred Sturtevant in 1913 and the chromosomal maps made possible by T.S. Painter's discoveries of 1933–34.

Remarked upon less often is that geographical maps—maps that represent the geographical distribution of allelic or chromosomal variants across a species range—share these same historical antecedents, having arisen from an extension of mapping practices from classical laboratory genetics to the geography of genes in field populations. Early geographical maps of genes in populations are found in research papers authored jointly in the mid-1930s by Alfred Sturtevant and Theodosius Dobzhansky, two members of the T.H. Morgan lab, first at Columbia University and then at Caltech. These papers immediately predated the launching of the "Genetics of Natural Populations" research program that was carried out by Dobzhansky and collaborators between spring of 1937 and Dobzhansky's death in December 1975.

In this preliminary reflection on the nature of genetic mapping, we describe a historiographic framework within which to trace and interpret changes in mapping practices in relation to theoretical interests. The history of gene mapping and the Morgan school is familiar and already well told (Allen 1978; Provine 1981; Kohler 1994). It is not our purpose to contribute new historical data or substantially alter the story. Rather, our goal is to highlight continuities among experimental systems supporting the changing problems and practices to complement previous historiographies of discontinuities. It is only through continuity that experimental systems can be reproduced and therefore extended into new problem domains and worked according to changing theoretical interests.

We begin with genetic mapping practices around 1913 and identify several transformations in mapping technologies leading up to the GNP research program: "pure" genetic linkage mapping, comparative linkage mapping of inversions, cytological inversion mapping, phylogenetic mapping, geographical inversion mapping, and geographical frequency mapping. Using maps as indicators of changes in theoretical preferences, as well as transformations in mapping practices, we proceed to compare the Drosophila research carried out, first, by Sturtevant and Dobzhansky together and then by Sturtevant and Dobzhansky individually, and identify several divergences in theoretical interests. Though both Sturtevant and Dobzhansky were interested in evolutionary questions, Sturtevant was more concerned with classification and systematics and Dobzhansky with dynamic evolutionary change. Also, over the course of Dobzhansky's own GNP research, as his theoretical presuppositions changed, so did his maps.

Historiography of genetic mapping

Historiographically, we regard published genetic maps in two ways: as indicators of changing practices and theoretical interests on the one hand and as scientific products on the other hand. Maps, like other forms of visualization, are useful tools for analysts of science as well as significant historical products of scientific activity worthy of attention in their own right (Griesemer and Wimsatt 1989).

The history that concerns us centers on the origin and development of the GNP research program because it serves as an important reminder that genetic mapping concerns not only the representation of spatial (and temporal) order within chromosomes, but also the representation of spatial (and temporal) geographical order. While this point is already clear from the literature cited, there is a tendency in histories of the extension of classical laboratory genetics to the geography of genes in field populations to focus on discontinuities or "breaks" primarily of theoretical interests. We favor the view that pragmatic theoretical interests typically *deflect* the working of a mostly continuous experimental system. Our contribution is to note that changes in mapping practice mark such deflections in interesting and useful ways.

The history of the GNP research program has been amply documented by Provine (1981, 1986, 1991). The extension of experimental work on *Drosophila pseudoobscura* to genetics of natural populations is further discussed in Kohler (1991, 1994). Provine interpreted the GNP series as resulting, in part, from Dobzhansky's merger of his antecedent interest in a theory of evolution *in nature* with the Morgan group's experimental system for genetic studies, together with Dobzhansky's personal falling-out with Sturtevant and the latter's turn toward other problems after 1936. Dobzhansky learned the Drosophila trade after joining the group in 1927, but he brought naturalist's and evolutionist's interests with him from Russia. Thus, a prominent focus of Provine's work is to account for the discontinuity between Dobzhansky's GNP program and the very different purposes for which the experimental system that sustained it was originally constructed.

Sturtevant and other founders of the Morgan school who were responsible for the construction of the *D. melanogaster* experimental system displayed a substantial interest in evolutionary patterns, processes, and mechanisms. However, Dobzhansky was more prominent and successful in extending the Morgan school's system from its original laboratory context and model organism to the study of natural populations in the field. Provine identified the personal falling-out between Sturtevant and Dobzhansky as a turning point historically, a sort of "psychological break," coming several years after Sturtevant had formulated, in a 1936 letter to Sewall Wright, a program of comparative, phylogenetic, and genetic research on the A and B races of *D. pseudoobscura* expanding upon his collaborative work with Dobzhansky (e.g. Sturtevant and Dobzhansky 1936a,b; Dobzhansky and Sturtevant 1938). Provine finds in this early statement the "seeds of the GNP series: chromosomal and genic variability, use of the variability to deduce population parameters, or to discriminate between the hypotheses of theoretical population geneticists" (Provine 1981: 45). As their friendship fell apart, differences of theoretical outlook, problem interests, and most importantly, methodological preferences were amplified. Kohler attributes the falling out, in part, to a broader breakdown of the "moral economy" of the Caltech group. He links this breakdown to the decline of *melanogaster* as the dominant experimental system: Beadle had shifted to *Neurospora*, Dobzhansky to *D. pseudoobscura*, and Bridges, who sustained the *melanogaster* breeding program, died in 1938 (Kohler 1994: 253). Although there appears to be a real breakdown signaled by these events, there are also important continuities between the *melanogaster* system constructed by Morgan's original group and the *simulans* and *pseudoobscura* systems deflected from the *melanogaster* exemplar by Sturtevant and Dobzhansky. The experimental system of the Morgan school is best characterized in terms of the husbandry practices, breeding methods, and representational strategies Morgan and his group developed from about 1910 to 1920. The system was first developed using *D. melanogaster*, but was soon extended to other species. Here we focus on Sturtevant's extension to *Drosophila simulans* and his and Dobzhansky's work with *D. pseudoobscura* and *D. persimilis*.

The differences Provine notes between Sturtevant's 1936 formulation in his letter to Wright of the "*Drosophila pseudoobscura* Analysis" and Dobzhansky's series of GNP papers from 1938 to 1975 are that in the former, Sturtevant assumed "The stocks of *D. pseudoobscura* already collected are considered adequate, and no mention is made of either comparisons of variability in local populations or of such population dynamics as seasonal changes of genes or inversions" (Provine 1981: 45). The latter are the sorts of problems relevant to Dobzhansky's views on the evolutionary process, newly and thoroughly influenced by Sewall Wright and expressed in his 1937 book, *Genetics and the Origin of Species*, that he and his collaborators took up when they went to the field to collect from numerous localities.

Sturtevant's evolutionary interest in their joint work of the mid-1930s centered on reconstructing phylogenetic relationships of chromosomal inversion patterns, while Dobzhansky's interest moved increasingly toward patterns of variation within and among natural populations that were to be explained by forces and processes of evolution, as articulated by Wright. These theoretical differences are indeed reflected in the kinds of genetic maps Sturtevant and Dobzhansky produced, but the emergence of new kinds of maps depends on continuity of experimental system as well as discontinuity of theoretical interest for an adequate historical explanation.

To stories of psychological, moral economic, and theoretical breakdown must be added the story of the underlying continuity of the Drosophila experimental system. Fundamental to all of its variations are core activities of breeding, crossing, and mapping genes, which were established in the Morgan school as the basic technical means by which scientific questions would be rigorously and productively pursued.

Our consideration of the history of genetic mapping thus aims to trace continuities less emphasized by historiographic attention to *theories* of evolution (e.g. Fisher and mass selection versus Wright and selection within and among subdivided populations). By tracking changes in genetic mapping, we hope to show that Dobzhansky "reproduced," in his geographical mapping work with *pseudoobscura*, the *melanogaster* experimental system of the Morgan school, though in a new way, as Kohler emphasizes (1994, ch. 8), that is suited to his different theoretical interests.

In referring to the "reproduction" of an experimental system, which includes the Morgan school's extensions to *simulans, pseudoobscura, persimilis*, and other species, as well as more radical extensions to new kinds of things (such as geographical distributions), we follow the lead of Hans-Jörg Rheinberger:

> every system of material entities, and therefore every system of actions concerning such entities that can be said to possess reproductive qualities, may also be said to possess its own intrinsic time. Internal time is not simply a parameter of the system's existence in space and time. It characterizes a sequence of states of a system insofar as it undergoes continuing cycles of nonidentical reproduction. Research systems, with which I am here concerned, are characterized by a kind of differential reproduction by which the generation of previously unknown things through unprecedented events becomes the reproductive driving force of the whole machinery.
>
> (Rheinberger 1997: 180)

Genetic maps are ticks of intrinsic time in the Drosophila experimental system. Changes in maps mark the deflected continuity through reproductive changes as the system generates previously unknown epistemic things. These changes are manifested through technical innovations and recombinations of theoretical interests.[1]

Hybrids all the way down (and up): problems, protocols, and maps

"Pure" genetic linkage mapping

Linkage mapping began with Sturtevant (1913), based on Morgan's interpretation of Janssens' chiasmatype hypothesis. The 1913 paper exemplifies the core activity of mapping and its published inscriptions. Since we are mainly concerned with Sturtevant's activities in relation to the GNP series, we will not consider the history of linkage mapping *per se*, but rather focus on Sturtevant's exemplary map. Sturtevant begins with a description of the ingredients of his study: six factors in *D. melanogaster* that co-segregate with the X chromosome. The paper as a whole describes a "method used for calculating the gametic ratios" that he needed to produce a measure of relative distance between linked factors, using the convention that 1% crossing over is one map unit.

The familiar protocol is to cross parents that are homozygous for two (and later, more) co-segregating recessive (mutant) traits with parents carrying the homozygous dominant (wild type) alleles. Then, the F1 hybrids are backcrossed to the double recessive parents. The numbers of progeny in the F2 generation are counted. These fall into the two parental classes (double recessive and wild type), plus two new classes of recombinants—flies having one or the other but not both of the parental traits. (The method is nicely described in Kohler 1994: 65–71.) The proportion of the recombinant types ×100 gives the percentage "crossing over" between the factors, that is, the frequency with which the factors are exchanged. On the chiasmatype theory, crossing over of factors is the result of physical exchange of chromosome pieces due to breaks between the physical locations of the factors on homologous chromosomes and rejoining of pieces of homologues. Thus, hybridizing parents results in the hybridization of chromosomes.

When pairwise crosses are performed for a number of co-segregating factors, and linkage relations are assumed to reflect spatial order, the collection of crossing over relationships determines the spatial order of factors in the chromosome and relative distances between factors can be interpreted as a function of crossover frequencies. Distances between outlying factors can, for example, be predicted or calculated as the sum of the distances connecting intervening factors.[2]

We shall see that this experimental system is also "differentially reproductive" in Rheinberger's sense: it could be used to generate previously unknown things, such as inversions, through unprecedented types of hybridization events. The extension of the system in this reproductive way depended on novel technical innovations to new modes of hybridization.

Sturtevant was careful to point out that his mapping method does not determine whether percentage crossing over represents actual spatial distances in chromosomes. That would require a further assumption of "uniform strength" (resistance to breaking and recombining) along the length of the chromosome. He also pointed out that the most accurate results will obtain in crosses between factors that are close together, to avoid the possibility of double crossing over that would give the same proportions among offspring classes as no recombination, thus undercounting the number of crossovers and therefore underestimating distance.

The culmination of the paper is a single diagram (Figure 4.1), a linear linkage map representing the order relationships and relative distances among the factors studied.

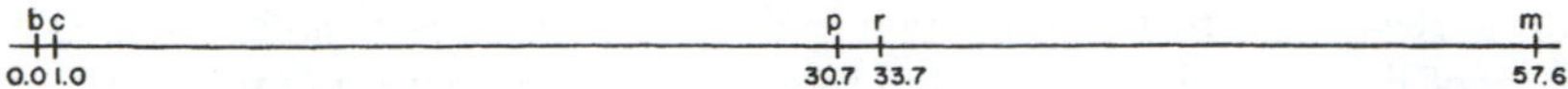

Figure 4.1 Sturtevant (1913), linear linkage map, representing the order relationships and relative distances among the factors studied by recombination analysis. The line represents a chromosome; symbols indicate the names of factors; numbers indicate relative distance as measured by recombination frequency. (Reprinted from Sturtevant, A.H. "The Linear Arrangement of Six Sex-linked Factors in Drosophila, as shown by their Mode of Association," *Journal of Experimental Zoology*, © 1913, by permission of Wiley-Liss Inc. a subsidiary of John Wiley & Sons Inc.)

The rest of Sturtevant's paper considers potential complications due to double- and higher-order crossing over as well as discrepancies in distances measured among the same factors by other studies.

Comparative linkage mapping of inversions

In 1920, Sturtevant reported on the genetics of *D. simulans*, a species he named in 1919. The experimental breeding and mapping system for genetic analysis that was developed in *D. melanogaster* was extended to *D. simulans* in a very literal sense in the 1920 paper: Sturtevant hybridized the two species by crossing female *melanogaster* to male *simulans*. All previous attempts to hybridize Drosophila species had failed.

Although the material content of the experimental system was hybridized in a new way—species hybrids rather than strain hybrids within species—the form of the experimental protocol was conserved in this new work as far as the material permitted. Hybridization between species would be the basis for extending genetic analysis to problems of species differences, speciation, and some aspects of evolution, just as hybridization between pure trait lines within species had been the basis of the Mendelian methodology at the center of the Morgan school's *melanogaster*-based experimental system.

However, the resulting offspring in Sturtevant's *melanogaster* × *simulans* crosses were all female and all sterile. According to Provine, this was "a sadness" to Sturtevant because it represented a limit to the extension of the *melanogaster* experimental system to trans-species evolutionary problems (Provine 1991: 2).[3] No backcross of these sterile flies could be made to parental types, so conventional mapping could not be carried to completion. As Sturtevant wrote:

> It had been hoped, had the hybrids been fertile, that the genetic make-up of *simulans* could be studied through the hybrids. This hope disappeared when the hybrids were found to be sterile, so the problem had to be attacked in another way,—namely, by studying the genetics of pure *simulans*.
>
> (Sturtevant 1921a: 43; quoted in Provine 1991: 2)

The reciprocal cross as well as crosses involving non-disjunction XXY females of either species produced a variety of "regular" and "exceptional" male and female offspring. Exceptional offspring are those that receive sex-linked genes from other than the usual parent (daughters getting all, rather than half, their sex-linked genes from their mother; sons getting all their sex-linked genes from their father, rather than their mother).

The sterility of trans-species hybrids together with the sex-ratio bias among progeny led Sturtevant to speculate about, and then plan more experiments to explore the causes of, his results (e.g. incompatibility of *melanogaster* X chromosomes and *simulans* cytoplasm) as well as mechanisms that might prevent such hybridization from occurring in the first place ("sexual selection" or mating preferences).

In 1921, Sturtevant reported on the comparative gene arrangements of *melanogaster* and *simulans*, using his newly identified alternative means of attack through the linkage mapping of "pure" *simulans*, that is, hybridizing among *simulans* lines within that species. He mapped several similar genes in both species and used hybrids between the species to determine whether the genes from each were allelic or not. The mutant factors "dachs" and "deltoid" in *simulans* resembled factors in *melanogaster*, for example, but were not allelic because they occur in different chromosomes. Deltoid, however, resembles delta in *melanogaster* and each is lethal when homozygous recessive. Because hybrid offspring in crosses of delta *melanogaster* with deltoid *simulans* do not develop, Sturtevant inferred that *simulans* deltoid is allelic to *melanogaster* delta. By similar sorts of trans-species hybrid tests of allelism, combined with linkage mapping in each pure species, Sturtevant was able to produce linkage maps for allelic loci in both species. He found that the same three loci do not occur in the same order in the two species. Three *simulans* genes occur in the order: scarlet, deltoid, peach, while the same genes in *melanogaster* occur in the order: scarlet, peach, delta. Sturtevant explained the difference as the result of an "inversion" of the segment of chromosomes carrying the genes (1921b: 235–7).

The *pair* of linkage maps thus maps an inversion between the two species by means of *comparison* (Figure 4.2).

Sturtevant studied many inversions by means of "comparison genetics," deflecting the *melanogaster* experimental system to the study of hybrid sterility by

0.0	dachs	0.0	roughoid
14.2	scarlet		
39.0	deltoid	41.5	scarlet
		44.5	peach
76.5	peach	63.5	delta
		101.0	minute-23

Figure 4.2 Sturtevant (1921), two-species linkage comparison map between *D. melanogaster* and *D. simulans*, the first documentation of a chromosomal inversion.

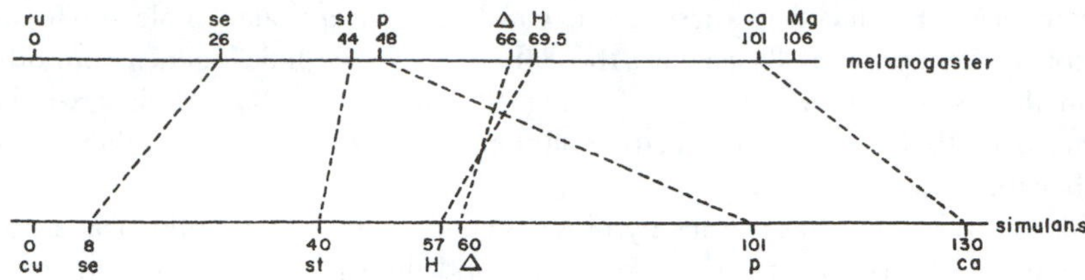

Figure 4.3 Sturtevant and Plunkett (1926), comparison map, showing a chromosomal inversion hybrid by means of crossing dotted lines that connect loci between hybridized chromosomes. (Originally published in *The Biological Bulletin.*)

mapping inversion hybrids, for example, this one (Figure 4.3) from Sturtevant and Plunkett (1926).

The core hybridization protocols remain the same as in "pure" linkage mapping, although the "strains" separately husbanded now come from distinct species and the comparison of pure linkage maps and hybrid tests of allelism replace single linkage maps produced from the backcross hybrids. Comparative inversion mapping is the result of a new way of using the Drosophila experimental system; the generation of previously unknown things—inversions—can become the driving reproductive force of the deflected system *because* of its fundamental continuity with the undeflected experimental system.

Cytological inversion maps

In 1933 and 1934, Painter (Figure 4.4) described a new method of genetic mapping in *D. melanogaster*: cytological mapping of stained chromatin bands from chromosomes of the salivary gland cells.[4] We will not here go into detail about the cytological methods involved in visualizing these chromosome banding patterns. Most interesting for our purposes is Painter's mapping of the correspondence between factors in the genetic linkage map and bands in the cytological map for the X chromosome.

Because the cytological technique is fairly simple compared to the breeding methods required to do a linkage analysis of a whole chromosome, a scientist primarily interested in inversion patterns might prefer the quicker and visually quite accurate cytological methods, provided the correspondence with the linkage map was adequately established. This seems to have been Dobzhansky's preference. In his 1936 paper with Sturtevant on the association of a "sex-ratio" gene with an inversion in the A and B races of *D. pseudoobscura*, complex linkage studies of hybridizations between the races as well as cytological studies were performed. A whole series of linkage maps are presented along with the claim that cytological studies confirmed the existence and position of the inversion (Sturtevant and Dobzhansky 1936a).

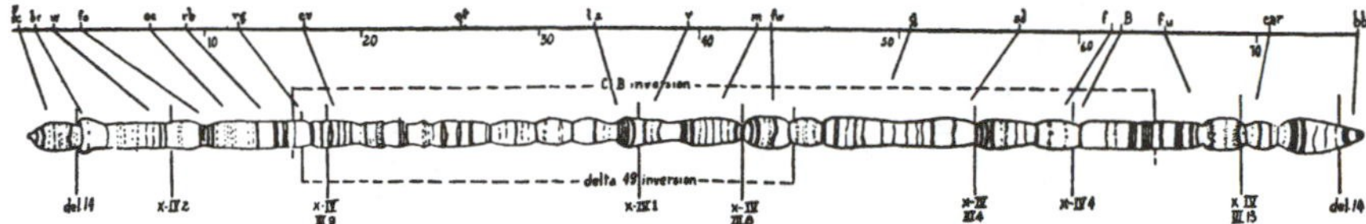

Figure 4.4 Painter (1933), cytological map of the X chromosome in *D. melanogaster* produced by staining chromatin bands of chromosomes of the salivary gland cells. Slanting vertical lines show correspondences between the genetic linkage map (above) and cytological banding map (below). (Reprinted with permission from Painter, T.S. "A New Method for the Study of Chromosome Rearrangements and Plotting of Chromosome Maps," *Science*, 78: 585–586, © 1933 American Association for the Advancement of Science.)

This seems to be the last time Dobzhansky published a paper in which the production of new linkage maps played a substantial role in his thinking. Once the correspondence between the two kinds of maps was established, direct study of cytological maps was much faster and afforded the possibility of characterizing the large number of population and species hybrids needed for investigating the evolutionary genetics of natural populations. There are no linkage maps in Dobzhansky's 1937 book, *Genetics and the Origin of Species*, although there are cytological maps. It is noteworthy that Dobzhansky's cytological maps are maps of inversion hybrids (in this case repeating a diagram from a 1936 paper coauthored with Tan (Figure 4.5)).

Cytological inversion hybrid maps initially did the same work for Dobzhansky that the genetic linkage data for detecting inversion hybrids had done. They revealed genetic variation within and among species. The possibility of rapid assessment of inversion hybrids was important for the establishment of the GNP series because linkage mapping could not have provided enough data fast enough to sustain an acceptable rate of production. The existing methods using the original experimental system ("pure" genetic linkage mapping) or its deflected hybrid (comparative linkage mapping) required, for each comparison, either fertile hybrids (to make backcrosses) or two series of linkage studies (one for each strain, race or species) plus hybrid tests for alleleism (for comparative genetics).

Perhaps more important still is that the relaxation of these particular demands of linkage mapping led to new mapping possibilities envisioned for the cytological work by Sturtevant in his letter to Wright and in the joint papers of 1936 and 1938 (from work performed in 1936). Provine (1981, 1991) emphasizes the limitation Sturtevant felt in studying *melanogaster* × *simulans* hybrids because the F1 offspring were sterile. We have seen that he got around this limitation with comparative genetic mapping. When cytological mapping entered the picture, a new possibility was generated because of the cytological method's ability to detect complex patterns of inversion quickly, easily, and accurately: if multiple inversions overlap one another, then it is possible to construct a historical scenario for the

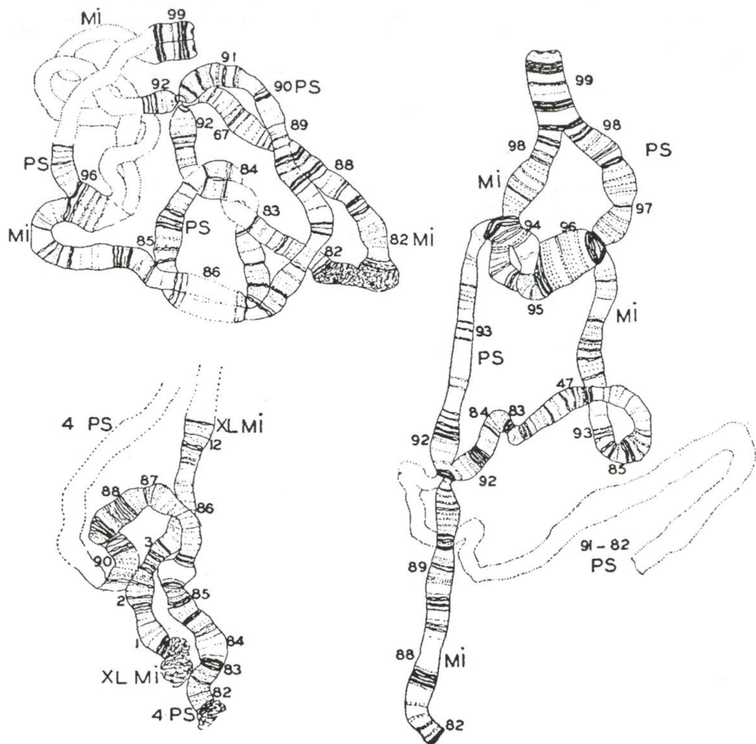

Figure 4.5 Dobzhansky (1937), inversion hybrid cytological maps of *D. pseudoobscura* crossed with *D. miranda*. (Reprinted from *Genetics and the Origin of Species* by T. Dobzhansky, © 1937 Columbia University Press, with permission of the publisher.)

temporal sequence of inversions. In their move to extend the Drosophila experimental system to *pseudoobscura*, Sturtevant and Dobzhansky exploited a novel feature of *pseudoobscura*: the large number of inversions in chromosome III of *pseudoobscura* compared to other species of Drosophila and compared to other chromosomes of *pseudoobscura*. Moreover, several inversion sequences may occur in a given locality. The prospects were vast for hybridization studies, the core technique for analyzing variation using a genetic experimental system, and which could be analyzed cytologically. Thus, the deflection of the Drosophila system to study inversion hybrids by cytological methods in *pseudoobscura* generated still more unknown things.

Phylogenetic maps

Different chromosomal inversions detected by cytological methods and found to occur on the same chromosome in the species, for example, on the third chromosome in *D. pseudoobscura*, may or may not be overlapping. Where inversions do overlap, it is possible to make inferences about the degree to which the chromosomes are genealogically related. That is, temporal relations can be inferred on the basis of patterns of spatial relations, and phylogenetic maps constructed as a result. Dobzhansky and Sturtevant worked together during 1935–36, examining the hybrids produced by crossing A and B races of *D. pseudoobscura* in order to establish phylogenies for the species. Results of this phylogenetic research were first published in 1936, in a paper coauthored by Sturtevant and Dobzhansky titled "Inversions in the Third Chromosome of Wild Races of *Drosophila pseudoobscura*, and Their Use in the Study of the History of the Species" (Sturtevant and Dobzhansky 1936b).

The pedigrees of overlapping inversion patterns detectable in hybrids of third chromosomes in *D. pseudoobscura* gave, in Sturtevant's words, "... the possibility of constructing an honest-to-God air-tight phylogeny" (quoted in Provine 1981: 43). His confidence stems from features of the cytological preparations of salivary gland chromosomes and the nature of inversions: homologous chromosomes in progeny that are heterozygous for an inversion will produce a characteristic "loop-like" configuration in salivary gland cell preparations rather than the linear banding patterns (Dobzhansky and Sturtevant 1938: 29; see also Dobzhansky 1937).

The upper part of Figure 4.6 shows a conventional coordinate system and cytological map. There is no corresponding linkage map provided. None is needed for the new kind of work. The lower part of the figure shows various cytological inversion maps in hybrids from various pairs of localities. All show the loop structure characteristic of inversion heterozygotes.

Dobzhansky and Sturtevant then establish the continuity of the new method they are about to describe with the comparative genetics that Sturtevant developed in his deflection of genetic linkage to the *melanogaster* × *simulans* experimental system: "This chromosome pairing furnishes an easy and accurate method for comparison of the gene arrangements in different strains of the same species, or in different species if these can be crossed" (Dobzhansky and Sturtevant 1938: 29).

They then go on to summarize the method for producing the data needed for addressing this historical question of phylogeny:

> A strain is selected the gene arrangement in which is arbitrarily chosen as a standard. Strains to be tested are crossed to the standard one, and the chromosomes are examined in the salivary glands of the larvae of the first generation hybrids. If the strains crossed are identical with respect to gene arrangement, all the chromosomes in the hybrids are represented by paired strands radiating from the chromocenter. If the gene arrangements are different in any respect, some of the chromosomes in the hybrids show abnormal pairing configurations, from the appearance of which the precise nature of the difference can be deduced.
>
> (Dobzhansky and Sturtevant 1938: 29)

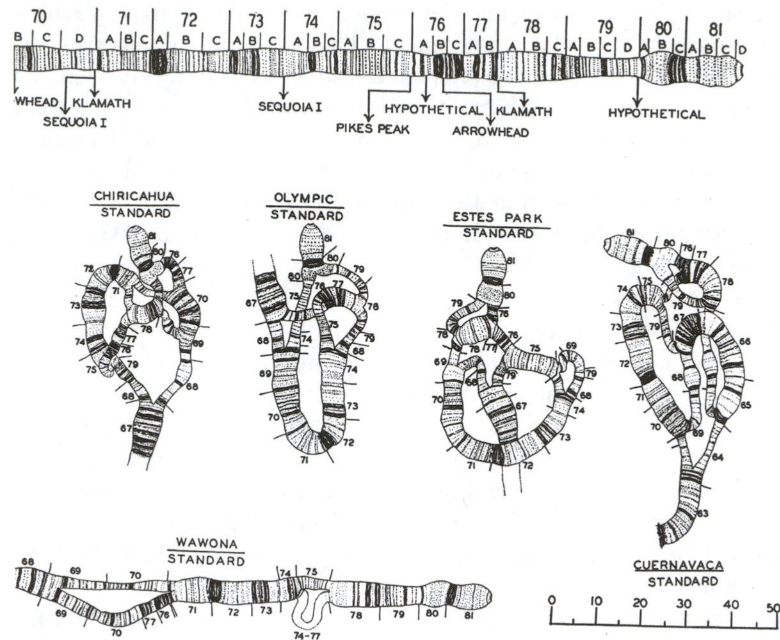

Figure 4.6 Dobzhansky and Sturtevant (1938), cytological inversion hybrid maps of *D. pseudoobscura* third chromosomes showing a conventional coordinate system and cytological map (above) and cytological inversion maps in hybrids from various pairs of localities (below). Note the recombination frequency key in the lower right of the figure, analogous to a distance key in a traditional geographic map. (Reprinted with permission of the Genetics Society of America.)

As Sturtevant pointed out in the 1936 letter to Wright, one could not tell "where one is to start the pedigree" because the method outlined here takes some arrangement arbitrarily as a standard of comparison. However, using a parsimony argument (1938: 32–3), multiple sets of relationships can yield fairly robust conclusions about the temporal order of occurrence of new gene arrangements (e.g. inversion patterns) as well as about pairwise temporal relationships in pairwise hybridizations. They describe a hypothetical set of three arrangements related by the occurrence of inversions:

> [I]f the three arrangements, ABCDEFGHI, AFEDCBGHI, and AFEHGBCDI, are all observed to occur in nature, the probability of the direct origin of the first from the third, or vice versa, becomes almost nil. Indeed, this would involve the assumption that due to a mere coincidence the chromosome has been broken at exactly the same two places on at least two separate occasions. . . . It follows, then, that the phylogenetic relationships of the three gene arrangements represented above must be 1 → 2 → 3, or 3 → 2 → 1, or

> 1 ← 2 → 3, but not 1 ↔ 3. In other words, although we can not determine directly which of the three arrangements is the ancestral and which are the derived ones, if any one is selected as the original then the course of the evolution is thereby fixed.
>
> (Dobzhansky and Sturtevant 1938: 29)

The phylogeny Dobzhansky and Sturtevant produce for gene arrangements in the third chromosome of *D. pseudoobscura* (also printed in Dobzhansky 1937: 93, fig. 7) includes double-headed arrows between gene arrangements which the collective evidence provides no parsimonious way to decide is ancestral. Other arrangements are inferred not to be ancestral because they would necessitate more "steps" to produce the rest of the arrangements. These are related to others by single-headed arrows (Figure 4.7).

It is important to note several continuities as well as discontinuities between this kind of map and previous ones. First, the phylogeny maps temporal relationship (two-headed arrows) and temporal order (one-headed arrows) rather than spatial order as in linkage maps. Also, there is no measure of relative temporal distance between arrangements as there is for relative spatial distance. On the other hand, many linkage maps show only spatial order rather than relative distance, especially when different linkage studies confirmed a given order but found statistically

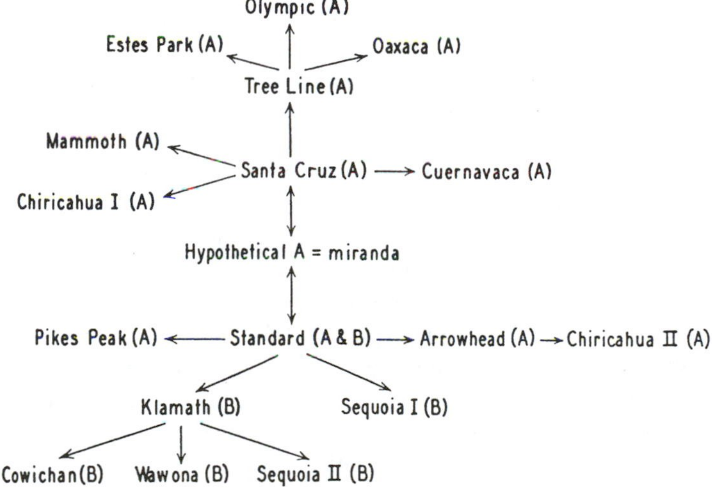

Figure 4.7 Dobzhansky and Sturtevant (1938), phylogeny map of gene arrangements in the third chromosome of *D. pseudoobscura*. Single-headed arrows indicate the direction from ancestral to descendant arrangements, based on the assumption that evolution proceeds parsimoniously: rearrangements requiring fewer inversion steps would be more likely than those requiring more steps. Double-headed arrows imply that there is no parsimonious way, based on the evidence, to decide which arrangement is ancestral. (Reprinted with permission of the Genetics Society of America.)

significant differences in crossover frequencies. Most relevant to our claims about continuities among experimental systems, chromosome inversion phylogenies are built out of hybridization and detection of inversions, even if these are via cytological mapping rather than linkage mapping. They nevertheless depend on building an aggregate map from a series of pairwise hybridizations. It is the new notion that hybridized gene *arrangements*, detectable in salivary gland cytological preparations, are the genetic entities in the *pseudoobscura* system that make this system a deflection of the previous ones.

As pointed out earlier, one motivation for using *pseudoobscura* was the abundant variation of inversion patterns within and among localities and populations as well as among chromosomes, strains, races, and species. Perhaps this heterogeneity of "genetic entities" is what allowed Dobzhansky and Sturtevant to collaborate for a time in the use of this system. Sturtevant was clearly interested in reconstructing phylogenies in a way that Dobzhansky was not (Provine 1981). Dobzhansky had been interested in variation in nature and found a way to exploit the *pseudoobscura* experimental system to those ends in the GNP series.

Geographical inversion maps

Genuine geographical maps, on which are marked the localities from which the flies bearing particular gene arrangements were collected, appear in publications by Sturtevant and Dobzhansky during this same period. These geographical distribution maps at first present only simple "locality" data—the presence of an arrangement at a place.

Maps representing the geographical distribution of gene arrangements in races A and B of *D. pseudoobscura* appear in Dobzhansky's 1937 *Genetics and the Origin of Species* and in the 1938 paper, "Inversions in the Chromosomes of *Drosophila pseudobscura*," coauthored by Dobzhansky and Sturtevant (Figure 4.8). It is possible to discern the geographical ranges of the various chromosomal types from these maps, but there is no indication of the frequencies with which these types occur at given locations. Observations of even a single case of a particular gene arrangement are included. Thus, the geographical variability that is mapped is qualitative, not quantitative. Similarly, the 1937 paper by Sturtevant and Dobzhansky, "Observations on the Species related to New Forms of *Drosophila affinis*, with Descriptions of Seven," contains a geographical map that represents the North American distribution of species and subspecies related to *D. affinis* and *D. pseudoobscura* without indicating the relative frequencies with which species and subspecies types are found.

These geographical inversion maps that depict qualitative patterns of variability in gene arrangements across the geographical range of *D. pseudoobscura* become juxtaposed in interesting ways with the phylogenetic maps constructed from overlapping chromosomal inversions. The 1938 paper coauthored by Dobzhansky and Sturtevant combines the phylogenetic and geographical distribution maps in order to draw a "working hypothesis" concerning the likely evolutionary history of *D. pseudoobscura*. Connections are made between the phylogenetic relations

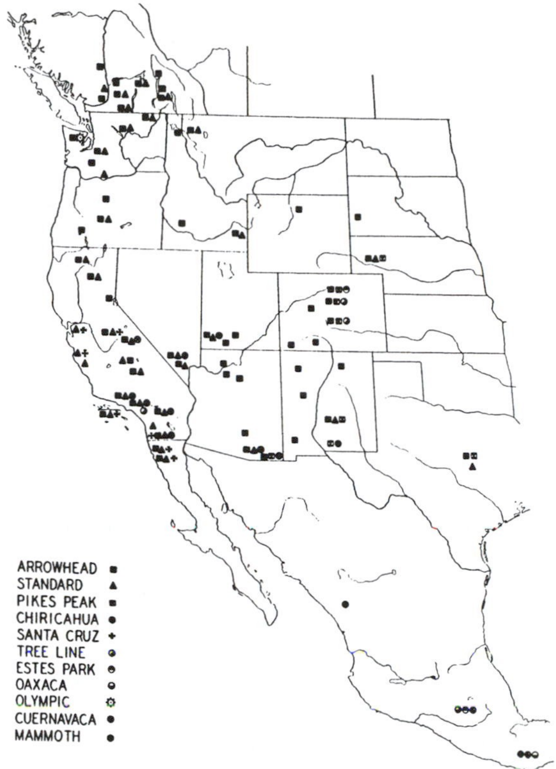

Figure 4.8 Dobzhansky and Sturtevant (1938), geographical map of gene arrangements in race A of *D. pseudoobscura*. The map indicates geographical localities and, implicitly, ranges, but there is no indication of the frequencies with which these types occur at given locations. Observations of even a single case of a particular gene arrangement are included. (Reprinted with permission of the Genetics Society of America.)

among various chromosomal inversion types and their present-day patterns of geographical distribution in an attempt to discover the site of origin for each chromosomal type and to reconstruct migration histories. For example, the "guiding hypothesis" accepted by the authors is that the geographical origin of the *pseudoobscura* group is the Pacific Coast Region since all three of the likely "original forms" of third chromosomes (Santa Cruz, Hypothetical, and Standard) are found there. Race B is supposed to have originated in the southern part of its range (mid- to southern California) and spread northward because Standard, the postulated ancestral sequence for B, is most prevalent there and Sequoia I, the only sequence derived directly from Standard, is found just there. A section of the 1938 paper titled "The relative frequencies of different gene arrangements within a region" indicates that quantitative data were being collected so that the proportions of the different inversions at each location could be discerned. Preliminary results from data collected in central and southern California between April 1936 and April 1937 appear in a chart. A number of ways of mapping these inversion frequencies are developed in Dobzhansky's subsequent publications.

Geographical frequency maps

In the papers of the GNP series, and in Dobzhansky's work with GNP contributors (e.g. Dobzhansky and Epling 1944), a variant type of geographical map appears. These include not just locality data, but *frequencies* of the various gene arrangements present at that locality. A prototype of the geographical frequency map appears in the 1936 Sturtevant–Dobzhansky paper on "sex-ratio" (Sturtevant and Dobzhansky 1936a).

The map (Figure 4.9) shows numbers of tested chromosomes sampled from various localities either carrying, or not carrying, the sex-ratio gene mentioned. Frequencies could be inferred from the data presented in the map. It is not clear whether Sturtevant or Dobzhansky provided the impetus for including this data in the published map. A particularly clear form of geographical frequency map appears in Dobzhansky (1944), the second essay in the monograph by Dobzhansky and Epling. In this kind of map, frequencies are represented in a histogram and linked to localities on the map (Figure 4.10).

To obtain frequency data for chromosomal inversion types in different populations, the chromosomal inversion mapping system had to be exploited in a new way. The limitations of the methods Sturtevant and Dobzhansky were using in the mid-1930s in furnishing a quantitative analysis of the variability in natural populations is discussed in the coauthored 1938 paper. Laboratory strains of *pseudoobscura* had been derived from single wild females with several strains isolated in most locations. This provides qualitative information but only "rough" quantitative data. One particular concern expressed was that "the variety of gene arrangements originally present in a given strain may be decreased if this strain is kept in the laboratory for many generations" (Dobzhansky and Sturtevant 1938: 30). An alternative technique for quantitative analysis was suggested: that the chromosomal makeup of captured males and male offspring of captured females be studied by outcrossing with a female of a known laboratory strain. This made it possible to screen large numbers of flies from the same population.

The papers of the GNP series include many geographical locality maps, more in fact than there are geographical frequency maps. There are even more frequency tables associating localities with frequencies of gene arrangements. Frequency data were clearly of critical importance to tracing, interpreting, using, and testing the implications of Sewall Wright's mathematical theory of evolutionary population genetics. However, data tables are a different kind of visual objects than maps and outside the scope of our story. As we will see in the next section of the chapter, Dobzhansky introduced a variety of geographical frequency maps in support of different hypotheses concerning evolutionary mechanisms, especially, as time went on, natural selection.

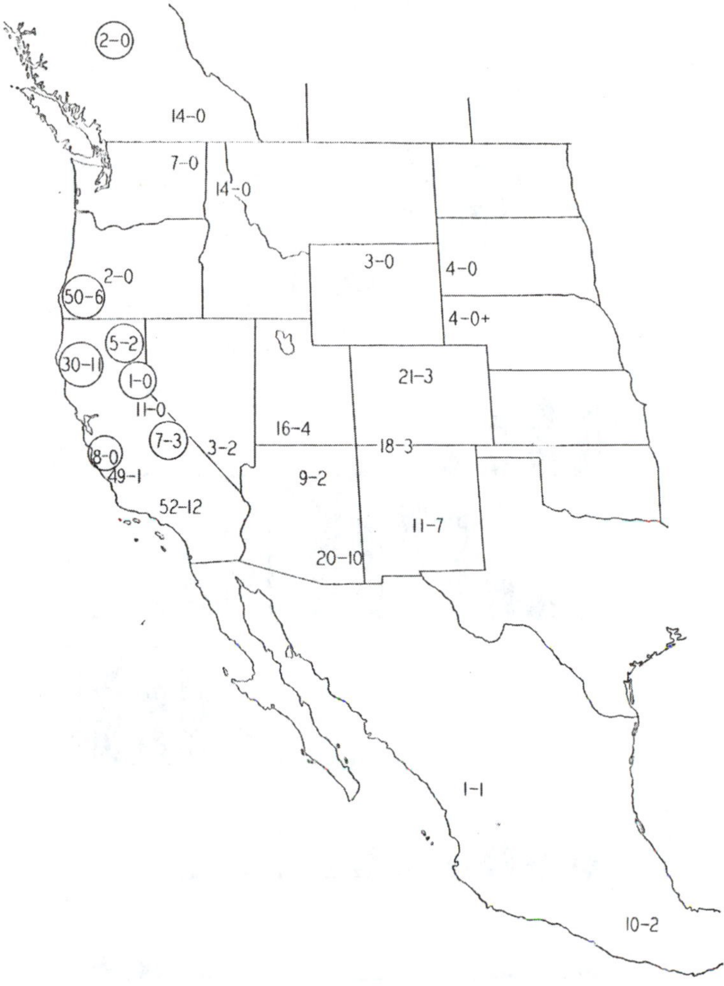

Figure 4.9 Sturtevant and Dobzhansky (1936), proto-geographical frequency map, showing the distribution of a "sex-ratio" gene in races A and B of *D. pseudoobscura*. Gene frequencies can be inferred from the data presented. (Reprinted with permission of the Genetics Society of America.)

Pragmatic aspects of geographical maps

Pragmatists recognize that scientific content is shaped by aims, interests, and values embedded in particular contexts of explanation. Some of those who are skeptical about a pragmatic account of scientific explanation may admit that such aims, interests, and values creep in when humans are objects of knowledge, but not

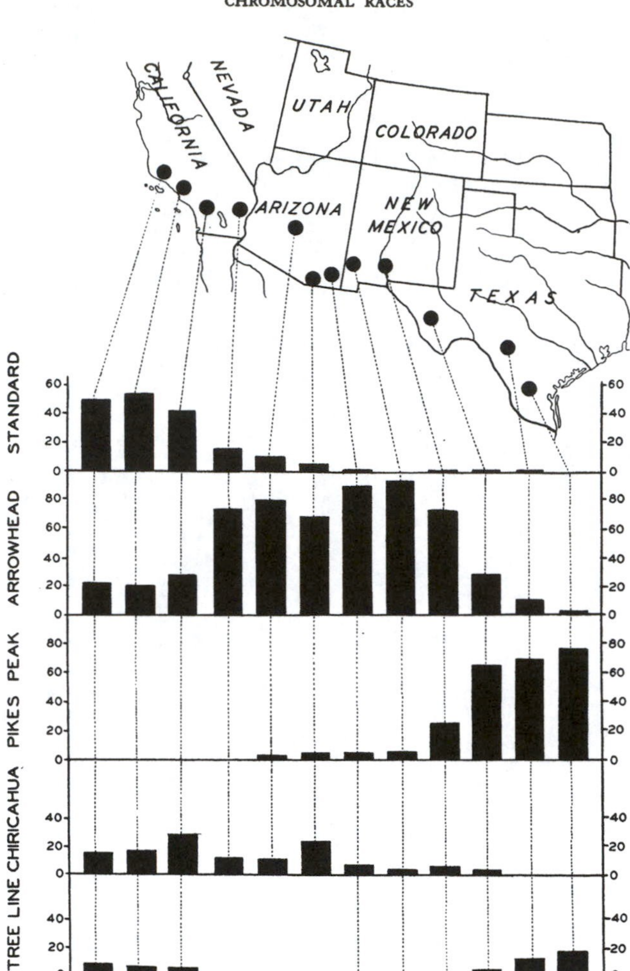

Figure 4.10 Dobzhansky and Epling (1944), geographical frequency map, with frequencies indicated by histogram bars linked to corresponding localities by dotted lines. (Reprinted with permission of the Carnegie Institution of Washington Publications.)

otherwise. However, published geographical maps arising in the course of the research into the genetics of natural populations of *D. pseudoobscura* that was undertaken, first by Sturtevant and Dobzhansky jointly and subsequently by Dobzhansky and collaborators other than Sturtevant, indicate how divergences in theoretical preferences are associated with diverse ways of ordering genes (or chromosomal types) in space and in time.

It is not surprising that maps would serve as reliable indicators of changes in theoretical interests. It seems incontestable that in so far as we regard maps as representations, we have to understand them as pragmatically constituted. Maps are not pictorial representations of the world; they are not photographs. Maps are abstractions that privilege some features of the world and ignore others. Maps are perspectival—what gets included on a map and what gets left off of a map depends on the aims, needs, interests, and conventions associated with specific incidences of map-making. One assumes that maps are accurate representations if the particular spatial (or temporal) relations chosen for depiction are indeed so ordered in the world. But this recommends the map as good or bad only relative to a given context. This pragmatic character of maps—their context-dependence and contingent privileging of some features of the world over others—makes them valuable tools for helping us to find our way around the terrain of population genetics research.

In 1913, when Sturtevant invented linkage mapping, theoretical interests in the Morgan lab at Columbia University were focused on structure–function relations. Mutant flies were laboratory tools that provided the means of identifying physiologically important genes and uncovering the basic mechanisms of heredity that determine how traits are passed from parents to offspring. This treats mapping relations as if they are invariant across space and time. Variation in the species is a necessary condition for the discovery of any structure–function relations, and yet regions of the chromosome are ascribed functions relative to a presumed homogeneity of chromosome, cell, organism, and species. Since linkage maps represent *the* chromosomal arrangement of genes for the species, they establish a species-invariant norm. Comparative linkage inversion maps, cytological inversion maps, phylogenetic maps, geographical inversion (distribution) maps, and geographical frequency maps reflect a different set of theoretical interests, that is, interests in the problems of evolutionary biology. Geographical maps recognize the genetic heterogeneity of species explicitly; they are products of the realization that this heterogeneity is not just fodder for structure–function studies in the laboratory but merits investigation in its own right out in the field.

Sturtevant and Dobzhansky came to their collaborative work on the natural populations of *D. pseudoobscura* with research interests that were similar in many ways. Both were interested in taxonomy. Dobzhansky worked on ladybird beetles in Russia before coming to the United States to do postdoctoral research in Columbia University's famous "fly room." Sturtevant was a taxonomist of Drosophila species since his student days, collecting wild Drosophila for this purpose on his travels (Provine 1991). Both were keenly interested in evolution and the mechanisms of speciation, in particular in identifying the genes responsible for the development of interspecific sterility. These complementary interests facilitated their joint study of chromosomal inversions in natural populations of *D. pseudoobscura* and their efforts to extend the experimental system from laboratory to field. However, the collaboration was short-lived. The geographical maps that were associated with their collaborative research, and the ways in which

Sturtevant and Dobzhansky each made use of these maps, are indicative of the diverging pathways their theoretical interests came to take.

The most extensive reports on Sturtevant's and Dobzhansky's collaborative efforts studying *D. pseudoobscura* appeared in Dobzhansky's 1937 *Genetics and the Origin of Species* and in a coauthored 1938 article in *Genetics* titled "Inversions in the Chromosomes of *Drosophila pseudoobscura*." A phylogenetic map of gene arrangements in the third chromosome of *D. pseudoobscura* and a map representing the distribution of gene arrangements in race A of *D. pseudoobscura* are found in both publications; a map of the geographical distribution of gene arrangements in race B is found only in the 1938 article. The 1938 paper closely combines information provided by the phylogenetic and geographical inversion maps, moving from one to the other to propose a "working hypothesis" concerning the likely evolutionary history of *D. pseudoobscura*. Emphasis is on the geographical origins of different chromosomal inversion types found in races A and B and how migration from these sites of origin explains current distribution patterns. There are three gene arrangements (two actual and one hypothetical) viewed as contenders for the species' ancestral or "original form." The Pacific Coast region, where they are found, is proposed as the geographical origin of the group. Because Drosophila species most closely related to *pseudoobscura* are found in Europe and not the eastern United States, the recommendation is made that additional research be carried out on Drosophila in northern Asia in order to be able to estimate the time and direction of migrations between Europe and North America.

Interestingly, in *Genetics and the Origin of Species*, Dobzhansky mentions none of these hypotheses concerning the evolutionary history of *D. pseudoobscura*. The maps appear there, but they are not combined in this way. In the section on "Inversion and racial differentiation" where the phylogenetic and geographical maps for *D. pseudoobscura* appear, Dobzhansky draws attention to the geographical map of gene arrangements in race A to emphasize the "almost bewildering amount of variation in the gene arrangement within the species" (Dobzhansky 1937: 92) and the presence of

> all the intermediates...between the condition where a gene arrangement may be described as an 'individual variation' in flies coming from a definite locality, and one where a definite chromosome structure becomes an established racial characteristic for a certain fraction of the species.
>
> (Dobzhansky 1937: 94–5)

In the chapter on "Selection," Dobzhansky correlates distribution regions of races A and B with selection due to temperature differences. In other words, geographical patterns of chromosomal diversity are important for what they say about race formation and causes of evolution generally, and not origins and historical migrations in *pseudoobscura* specifically.

It is safe to say that phylogenetic maps reflect life-long interests of Sturtevant's. As a young student, he traced the pedigree of his family's horses; in his later years, he charted intellectual pedigrees in a book on the history of genetics (Lewis 1995).

Dobzhansky became interested in phylogenetics only while working with Sturtevant in 1935–36. As he wrote in a letter to Miloslav Demerec:

> Sttt and myself are spending the whole time studying the inversions in the third chromosome in geographical strains of pseudoobscura. We are constructing phylogenies of these strains, believe it or not. This is the first time in my life that I believe in constructing phylogenies, and I have to eat some of my previous words in this connection.
>
> (Demerec correspondence [B/D 394]: Feb. 17, 1936 letter from Dobzhansky; underline in original)

The project outline Sturtevant sent to Wright in March 1936 refers to the need to construct both phylogenetic and geographical inversion maps. It mentions the goal to construct "an honest-to-God air-tight phylogeny" by means of overlapping chromosomal inversions. Geographical distribution maps (for third chromosome inversions, variant Y-chromosomal types, and modifiers) are deemed important specifically for what they will contribute to the solution of "historical problems." As we have seen, Provine considers this outline to be the foundation for the research Dobzhansky later carried out, the "seeds of the GNP series" (Provine 1981: 45). But it is important not to overestimate such continuities: already, in 1936, Dobzhansky's theoretical interests were diverging from Sturtevant's. As just mentioned, geographical distribution maps are not used at all for "historical problems" by Dobzhansky in *Genetics and the Origin of Species*, and this book is based on the Jesup lectures he gave at Columbia University in the fall of 1936.

In *Genetics and the Origin of Species*, Dobzhansky uses geographical distribution maps as qualitative representations of causal mechanisms of evolution in natural populations: how individual genetic or chromosomal differences are compounded into racial and species differences and the effects of temperature differences on natural selection. In the opening chapter, Dobzhansky makes his theoretical preferences—and the direction evolutionary geneticists should take—quite clear. He refers favorably to Darwin as unique among nineteenth-century biologists for his focus on "the causal rather than the historical problem" (Dobzhansky 1937: 8). Dobzhansky characterizes genetics, like physiology, as a "nomothetic" (law-creating) science. He urges evolutionary biologists to adopt an experimental approach that focuses on such mechanisms, to investigate "the common properties of living things" (Dobzhansky 1937: 6). Evolutionary biologists should no longer seek to describe the past using phylogenies for these pertain only to "the peculiarities of separate species" (Dobzhansky 1937: 6). In other words, *D. pseudoobscura* is interesting to the geneticist because of what it says about the mechanisms of evolution in all species, and not because of its own evolutionary history. Dobzhansky wanted to understand evolution as "a process of change or movement" and not as "a cross section of phylogenetic lines" (Dobzhansky 1937: 12).

Subsequent variations in geographical mapping strategies continue to be useful indicators of changes in Dobzhansky's theoretical preferences. During the late

1930s and early 1940s, influenced by Wright's shifting balance theory, Dobzhansky focused on genetic changes in populations due to random drift and how drift operates as a significant evolutionary factor only in small, fairly isolated populations. So we find in GNP I (coauthored with Queal) and GNP III (authored by Koller) efforts to determine breeding population size. The maps that appear in these articles are topographical maps with collecting sites marked on them. Possible geographical barriers to gene exchange that subdivide populations into smaller breeding units are marked: the desert valleys that separate the mountain ranges east of the Sierras into "island-like mountain forests" in GNP I and the canyons of a single mountain range, the Panamint Range, in GNP III (Dobzhansky and Queal 1938; Koller 1939) (Figures 4.11 and 4.12).

GNP IV (Dobzhansky 1939) provides geographical distribution maps of third chromosomal inversion and Y-chromosomal types, as in the 1938 paper but for Mexico and Guatemala. Although he refers to the phylogenetic map published

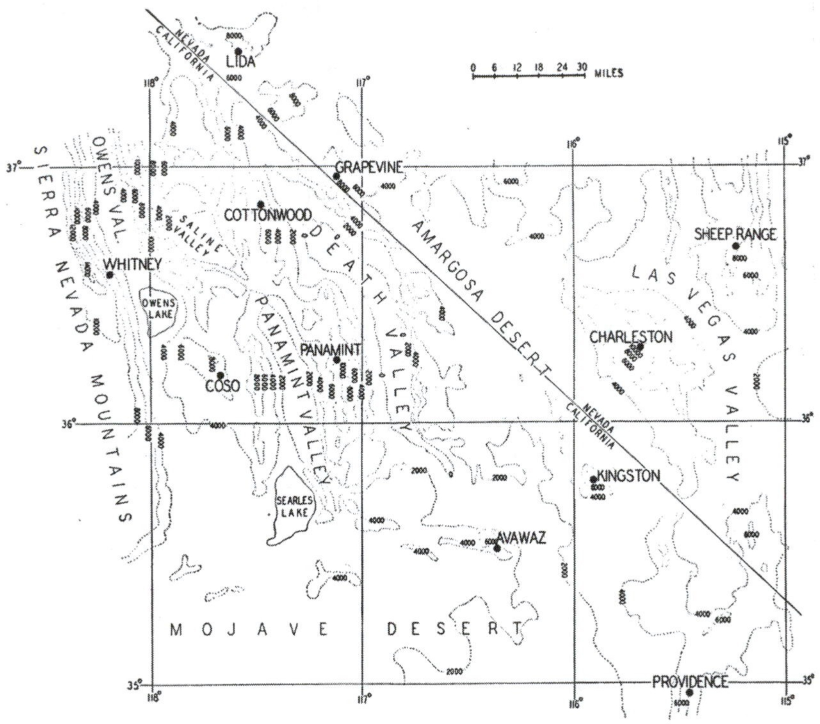

Figure 4.11 Dobzhansky and Queal (1938), GNP I topographic collection map. Collecting sites near the Mojave Desert, California, are marked on a topographical map and possible geographical barriers to gene exchange that subdivide populations into smaller breeding units are indicated. (Reprinted with permission of the Genetics Society of America.)

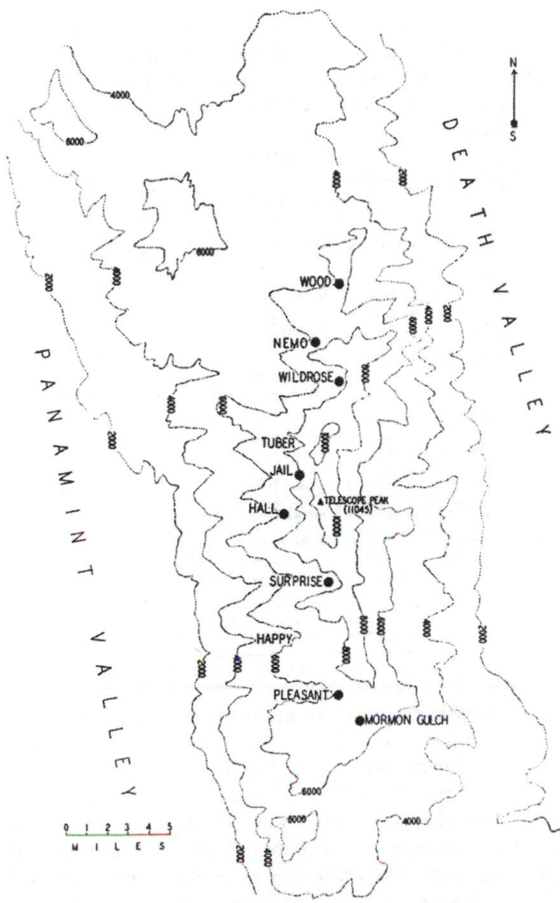

Figure 4.12 Koller (1939), GNP III topographic collection map in the Panamint Range near Death Valley, California. (Reprinted with permission of the Genetics Society of America.)

in 1938, Dobzhansky makes no "historical" use of it. Instead, he focuses on distribution patterns of the chromosomal types, attending especially to discontinuities. The discontinuous distribution of Y-chromosomal types points to the Isthmus of Tehuantepec as a boundary between Mexican and Guatemalan populations (Figure 4.13).

Qualitative and quantitative differences in third chromosomal inversions suggest a division between populations of east-central Mexico and of west-central Mexico and Guatemala. For the species as a whole, its range extending north to British Columbia, Dobzhansky divides third chromosomes into "northern types" and "southern types," noting that there are no chromosomal types common to the

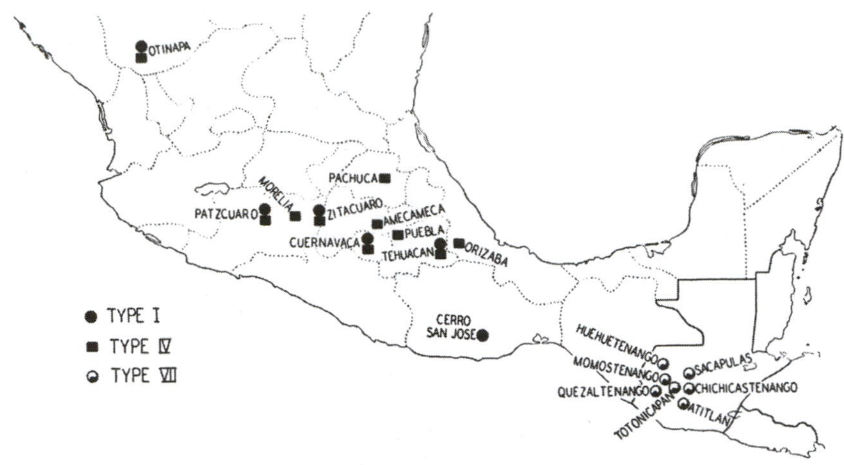

Figure 4.13 Dobzhansky (1939), GNP IV geographical distribution map of Y-chromosome arrangements in Mexico and Guatemala, showing their discontinuous distribution. (Reprinted with permission of the Genetics Society of America.)

northern and southern limits of the distribution. He represents intervening areas as a "mixture" of the two types, "northern" and "southern."

However, from the mid-1940s on, Dobzhansky began to favor natural selection as the predominant mechanism of evolutionary change. Geographical maps no longer point to discontinuities in chromosomal types, population boundaries, and barriers to gene exchange but to temporal changes in inversion type frequencies and relationships between these frequencies and selective features of the environment. The appearance of geographical frequency maps marks this change in Dobzhansky's theoretical preferences. In GNP XVI (Dobzhansky 1948), collecting sites are marked on an ordinary map of the Yosemite Park region accompanied by a graph that shows horizontal and vertical distances between these sites. Also included are graphs of the relative frequencies of three chromosomal types at different elevations and at different times of the year. (These images are superimposed in Figure 4.14.)

The temporal dimension is also incorporated in geographical frequency maps that track frequencies in chromosomal types at regular intervals over a number of years, ultimately over three decades (GNP XXVII [Dobzhansky 1958], GNP XXXV [Dobzhansky *et al.* 1964], GNP XXXVIII [Dobzhansky *et al.* 1966], and GNP XLII [Anderson *et al.* 1975]). Dobzhansky continued throughout his career to be interested in causal mechanisms, not "historical problems." Although the GNP XLII (Anderson *et al.* 1975) paper includes a revised phylogenetic chart (with race B renamed *D. persimilis*), no use is made of it. Not only was Dobzhansky uninterested in historical migrations, he was also extremely dismissive of migration *per se* as a causal explanation of patterns of genetic variation. He argued against

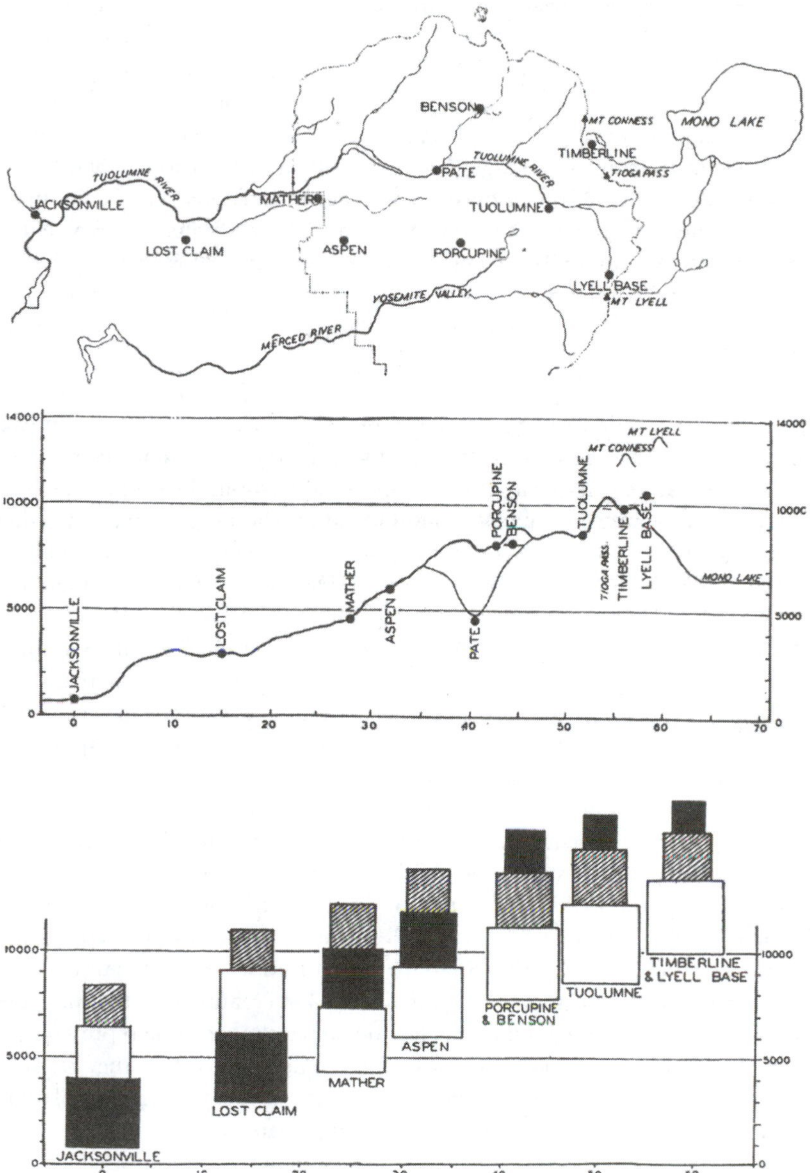

Figure 4.14 Dobzhansky (1948), GNP XVI geographical, topographical, and frequency distribution maps of *D. pseudoobscura* chromosomal arrangements in California. Dobzhansky's figure 1 and figure 3 are juxtaposed. (Reprinted with permission of the Genetics Society of America.)

the possibility that, in *pseudoobscura*, migration from neighboring populations could be responsible for seasonal fluctuations in inversion frequencies (GNP XVI) or for the changes in inversion frequencies that were tracked in Californian populations over many years (GNP XXVII, XXXV, XXXVIII, XLII). In GNP XXVI (Dobzhansky 1957), a paper on *D. willistoni*, Dobzhansky admits that observations that genetic polymorphism gradually decreases moving from the South American continent to larger/closer islands and then to smaller/farther islands can be explained by assuming that *willistoni* originated on the continent and then spread gradually to islands off the coast. But he prefers an explanation that does not appeal to "chance" and "historical factors." This is that polymorphism is an adaptive response to environmental diversity and will be more pronounced where greater variety in ecological niches exists—on the mainland more than islands, on larger more than smaller islands.

These geographical maps, then, are indicators of theoretical interests that point to divergences between Sturtevant and Dobzhansky and changing preferences in Dobzhansky's own work. Sturtevant was interested in using geographical maps in combination with phylogenetic maps to understand the evolutionary history of *D. pseudoobscura*. Dobzhansky found geographical maps valuable for their qualitative representations of causal mechanisms in evolution more generally, focusing initially on drift and then on selection. Diverging interests led these theorists to situate themselves and their investigations differently with respect to space and time and determined whether it was spatial and temporal continuities or discontinuities that would be privileged. To construct phylogenetic maps, one must attend to the spatial continuities of chromosomes—homologies or, in the case of *pseudoobscura*, the extent to which chromosomal inversions overlap. For the study of drift and isolation as mechanisms of evolutionary change, it is necessary to find spatial discontinuities—in the geographical distribution of alleles (or chromosomal types) and in geographical features as potential barriers to migration and gene exchange. At the same time, this bounds populations to render them discrete spatio-temporal objects. The study of natural selection as a mechanism of evolutionary change requires focus on patterns of gene (or chromosomal) variation in space and over time. Spatial discontinuities are de-emphasized. Geographical differences are important if involved in creating selection pressures (e.g. different temperatures at different elevations) but these can be represented as "patchy." Geographical barriers become conceived in terms of how they might be overcome for the spread of adaptive gene complexes to occur among populations. Population boundaries are not so important to delineate.

From a pragmatic perspective, one sees how genic and chromosomal variability is divvied up differently in time and in space because of differences in aims, interests, and values associated with particular explanatory contexts. Different theoretical preferences led Sturtevant and Dobzhansky, and then Dobzhansky over the course of the GNP series, to differ in whether temporal and spatial continuities or discontinuities were privileged. This provides an alternate historical analysis. Other accounts have portrayed the split between Sturtevant and

Dobzhansky, Dobzhansky's development of a new experimental system, and Dobzhansky's ultimate success as consequences of Sturtevant's "typological thinking" and Dobzhansky's "population thinking."

Mayr and Kohler rely on the typological-population distinction in this way. In a letter Mayr wrote to Dobzhansky at the time of the Conference on the Evolutionary Synthesis, he asks Dobzhansky to comment for the historical record on Sturtevant's views on natural populations and suggests:

> What is [*sic*] really boils down to is the fact that you as a naturalist were interested in population problems and Sturtevant, who had been trained much more along the lines of a rather old fashioned, typological taxonomy, was not. If one is a typologist, one simply has no need of or interest in populations.
>
> (Mayr correspondence, papers on Evolutionary Synthesis Conference [B/M451]: April 17, 1975 letter to Dobzhansky)

In a subsequent letter to Dobzhansky, Mayr continues along these lines:

> There is one matter I always wanted to know more about. Sturtevant always prided himself in being an ant specialist. Did his studies on ants ever contribute anything that added to our understanding of evolution? How can you explain that Sturtevant maintained such a strictly typological species concept when working with such extremely variable creatures as ants?
>
> (Mayr correspondence, papers on Evolutionary Synthesis Conference [B/M451]: May 1, 1975 letter to Dobzhansky)

Kohler, relying on correspondence between Mayr and Provine, provides a similar analysis:

> Sturtevant's late work dramatizes how differently he and Dobzhansky saw and used wild flies. Sturtevant had a highly typological concept of species, and treated different species in the laboratory as if each one were genetically homozygous. To put it a little differently, Sturtevant treated undomesticated species precisely as if they were standardized, domesticated *melanogaster*. His traditional view of species reflected his traditional laboratory practices.
>
> (Kohler 1991: 363)

Kohler suggests that Dobzhansky was open to the empirical evidence of how truly variable species are, evidence to which Sturtevant seemed blind. Describing Dobzhansky's movement from collecting from geographically separated populations in 1936 to more localized populations in 1937, Kohler writes: "This experience in the recesses of the Panamint Mountains was what finally caused Dobzhansky to abandon the last vestiges of the typological view of species, which had informed his work with Sturtevant and to which Sturtevant remained wedded" (1991: 356).

But Sturtevant was not blind to biological variability.[5] Sturtevant and Dobzhansky were interested in different evolutionary questions. Kohler is correct to claim that Sturtevant was committed to a traditional approach to evolutionary genetics that Dobzhansky was determined to leave behind. But is it also acceptable to assume that the two approaches can be placed on an equal footing so as to permit the judgment that one is intrinsically superior to the other and thus to conclude that Sturtevant's "typological thinking" and old-fashioned ways led him to miss out on evolutionary biology's future? This is suggested when, in reference to Sturtevant's approach, Kohler writes: "Its traditional aims and laborious but meagrely productive methods point up by contrast the novelty and remarkable productivity of the new mode of practice that Dobzhansky invented to compete with it" (1991: 363). The traditional methods certainly could not address very well the questions Dobzhansky was interested in. But the question remains whether they are adequate for the "historical problems" that interested Sturtevant. These problems and methods, after all, still find homes in fields of biology like molecular systematics. As Kohler does note, for Sturtevant "to construct phylogenies it was... essential to limit variability by using just a few standard types" (1991: 364). It might be more useful, therefore, instead to ask the pragmatic question: How do divergent theoretical interests lead scientists to conceive of biological variability in different ways?

Conclusion

We have argued that an understanding of the historical development of genetic mapping requires attention to continuities of the technical means by which experimental systems may be reproduced as well as to discontinuities of application of those means to distinct problems and projects. Stories and models of discontinuity, by themselves, leave processes of historical change unexplained (Griesemer 1996). We have also suggested that tracking the deflections of experimental systems through visual representations such as maps can provide valuable markers of changing theoretical interests, goals, commitments, and values. A pragmatic view of the ways in which Sturtevant's and Dobzhansky's theoretical preferences were manifested in such representations enriches historical assessment of their experimental practices, commitments, and productivity.

Acknowledgments

We are grateful to the organizers of the workshop from which this book sprang, Jean-Paul Gaudillière and Hans-Jörg Rheinberger, for inviting us to participate, to Jean-Paul in particular for inspiring the formulation of our project, and to the workshop participants for an exciting meeting. Lisa Gannett thanks Robert S. Cox, manuscript librarian at the American Philosophical Society Library, for assistance with correspondence in his care, and also the American Philosophical Society, Philadelphia, PA is acknowledged for the permission to use these correspondences.

Notes

1 Our story, it should be noted, concerns only the published maps. An equally compelling picture should also be painted of the "working maps" used to operate the experimental systems involved. Kohler (1994: 76) gestured at this other side of the mapping story in his comments about Bridges' four-sided "totem pole" working and valuation maps.

2 On the history of these linkage calculations and their complexities, see Wimsatt (1992).

3 We doubt very much that a mere technical limitation would have provoked sadness in Sturtevant. He was a supreme puzzle solver, as Provine (1991) points out, and would have received these results as a challenge to be overcome rather than a limitation to be accepted, as is evident in his solution of 1921.

4 The methods developed by Creighton and McClintock in maize, correlating chromosome morphology and genetic factor co-segregation in 1930 and 1931, are germane to the general history of genetic mapping, but not relevant to our story about the Drosophila system.

5 We are familiar with evidence of Sturtevant's attention to biological variability in his collaborative research with Dobzhansky into the geographical distribution of chromosomal variants and the "sex ratio" gene in natural populations of *pseudoobscura* during the mid-1930s. However, throughout his career, Sturtevant carried out work independently of Dobzhansky that was also attentive to biological variability. Sturtevant (1921c) presents evidence that mutational differences within species give rise to species-level genetic differences. Sturtevant (1937) suggests heterosis as a possible explanation for the "unexpectedly high" number of autosomal lethals in wild populations of *pseudoobscura.* An essay on selection in social insects argues that selection is operating interactively at three levels in ant species (Sturtevant 1938). A 1941 coauthored paper scolds Dobzhansky for interpreting chromosomal variations found in different members of the affinis group as interspecific differences given "the considerable variation in gene sequence within each species" (Sturtevant and Novitski 1941: 518).

Bibliography

Allen, G.E. (1978) *Thomas Hunt Morgan: The Man and His Science*, Princeton, NJ: Princeton University Press.

Anderson, W.W., Dobzhansky, T., Pavlovsky, O., Powell, J.R., and Yardley, D. (1975) "Three Decades of Genetic Change in *Drosophila pseudoobscura*," *Evolution*, 29: 24–36; reprinted in R.C. Lewontin, J.A. Moore, W.B. Provine, and B. Wallace (eds) (1981) *Dobzhansky's Genetics of Natural Populations, I–XLIII*, New York: Columbia University Press.

Dobzhansky, T. (1937) *Genetics and the Origin of Species*, New York: Columbia University Press.

—— (1939) "Mexican and Guatemalan Populations of *Drosophila pseudoobscura*," *Genetics*, 24: 391–412; reprinted in R.C. Lewontin, J.A. Moore, W.B. Provine, and B. Wallace (eds) (1981) *Dobzhansky's Genetics of Natural Populations, I–XLIII*, New York: Columbia University Press.

—— (1944) "Chromosomal Races in *Drosophila pseudoobscura* and *Drosophila persimilis*," in T. Dobzhansky and C. Epling *Contributions to the Genetics, Taxonomy, and Ecology of Drosophila pseudoobscura and its Relatives*, Washington, DC: Carnegie Institution of Washington.

—— (1948) "Altitudinal and Seasonal Changes Produced by Natural Selection in Certain Populations of *Drosophila pseudoobscura* and *Drosophila persimilis*," *Genetics*, 33: 158–76; reprinted in R.C. Lewontin, J.A. Moore, W.B. Provine, and B. Wallace (eds) (1981) *Dobzhansky's Genetics of Natural Populations, I–XLIII*, New York: Columbia University Press.

—— (1957) "Chromosomal Variability in Island and Continental Populations of *Drosophila willistoni* from Central America and the West Indies," *Evolution*, 11: 280–93; reprinted in

R.C. Lewontin, J.A. Moore, W.B. Provine, and B. Wallace (eds) (1981) *Dobzhansky's Genetics of Natural Populations, I–XLIII*, New York: Columbia University Press.

Dobzhansky, T. (1958) "The Genetic Changes in Populations of *Drosophila pseudoobscura* in the American Southwest," *Evolution*, 12: 385–401; reprinted in R.C. Lewontin, J.A. Moore, W.B. Provine, and B. Wallace (eds) (1981) *Dobzhansky's Genetics of Natural Populations, I–XLIII*, New York: Columbia University Press.

Dobzhansky, T. and Queal, M.L. (1938) "Chromosome Variation in Populations of *Drosophila pseudoobscura* Inhabiting Isolated Mountain Ranges," *Genetics*, 23: 239–51; reprinted in R.C. Lewontin, J.A. Moore, W.B. Provine, and B. Wallace (eds) (1981) *Dobzhansky's Genetics of Natural Populations, I–XLIII*, New York: Columbia University Press.

Dobzhansky, T. and Sturtevant, A.H. (1938) "Inversions in the Chromosomes of *Drosophila pseudoobscura*," *Genetics*, 23: 28–64.

Dobzhansky, T. and Epling, C. (1944) *Contributions to the Genetics, Taxonomy, and Ecology of Drosophila pseudoobscura and its Relatives*, Washington, DC: Carnegie Institution of Washington.

Dobzhansky, T., Anderson, W.W., and Pavlovsky, O. (1966) "Continuity and Change in Populations of *Drosophila pseudoobscura* in Western United States," *Evolution*, 20: 418–27; reprinted in R.C. Lewontin, J.A. Moore, W.B. Provine, and B. Wallace (eds) (1981) *Dobzhansky's Genetics of Natural Populations, I–XLIII*, New York: Columbia University Press.

Dobzhansky, T., Anderson, W.W., Pavlovsky, O., Spassky, B., and Wills, C.J. (1964) "A Progress Report on Genetic Changes in Populations of *Drosophila pseudoobscura* in the American Southwest," *Evolution* 18: 164–76; reprinted in R.C. Lewontin, J.A. Moore, W.B. Provine, and B. Wallace (eds) (1981) *Dobzhansky's Genetics of Natural Populations, I–XLIII*, New York: Columbia University Press.

Griesemer, J. R. (1996) "Periodization and Models in Historical Biology," in M.T. Ghiselin and G. Pinna (eds) *Memoirs of the California Academy of Sciences, No. 20: New Perspectives on the History of Life*, San Francisco: California Academy of Sciences.

Griesemer, J.R. and Wimsatt, W.C. (1989) "Picturing Weismannism: A Case Study of Conceptual Evolution," in M. Ruse (ed.) *What the Philosophy of Biology is: Essays for David Hull*, Dordrecht: Kluwer Academic Publishers.

Kohler, R. (1991) "Drosophila and Evolutionary Genetics: The Moral Economy of Scientific Practice," *History of Science*, 29: 335–75.

—— (1994) *Lords of the Fly: Drosophila Genetics and the Experimental Life*, Chicago: University of Chicago Press.

Koller, P.C. (1939) "Gene Arrangements in Populations of *Drosophila pseudoobscura* from Contiguous Localities," *Genetics*, 24: 22–33; reprinted in R.C. Lewontin, J.A. Moore, W.B. Provine, and B. Wallace (eds) (1981) *Dobzhansky's Genetics of Natural Populations, I–XLIII*, New York: Columbia University Press.

Lewis, E.B. (1961) *Genetics and Evolution: Selected Papers of A.H. Sturtevant*, San Francisco and London: W.H. Freeman.

—— (1995) "Remembering Sturtevant," *Genetics*, 141: 1227–30.

Lewontin, R.C., Moore, J.A., Provine, W.B., and Wallace, B. (eds) (1981) *Dobzhansky's Genetics of Natural Populations, I–XLIII*, New York: Columbia University Press.

Painter, T.S. (1933) "A New Method for the Study of Chromosome Rearrangements and Plotting of Chromosome Maps," *Science*, 78: 585–6.

—— (1934) "Salivary Chromosomes and the Attack on the Gene," *Journal of Heredity*, 25: 464–76.

Provine, W.B. (1981) "Origins of The Genetics of Natural Population Series," in R.C. Lewontin, J.A. Moore, W.B. Provine, and B. Wallace (eds) *Dobzhansky's Genetics of Natural Populations I–XLIII*, New York: Columbia University Press.

—— (1986) *Sewall Wright and Evolutionary Biology*, Chicago: University of Chicago Press.

—— (1991) "Alfred Henry Sturtevant and Crosses between *Drosophila melanogaster* and *Drosophila simulans*," *Genetics*, 129: 1–5.

Rheinberger, H.-J. (1997) *Towards a History of Epistemic Things: Synthesizing Proteins in the Test Tube*, Stanford: Stanford University Press.

Sturtevant, A.H. (1913) "The Linear Arrangement of Six Sex-Linked Factors in Drosophila, As Shown by Their Mode of Association," *Journal of Experimental Zoology*, 14: 43–59.

—— (1920) "Genetic Studies on *Drosophila simulans*: I. Introduction: Hybrids with *Drosophila melanogaster*," *Genetics*, 5: 488–500.

—— (1921a) "Genetic Studies on *Drosophila simulans*: II. Sex-linked Group of Genes," *Genetics*, 6: 43–64.

—— (1921b) "A Case of Rearrangement of Genes in Drosophila," *Proceedings of the National Academy of Sciences USA*, 7: 235–7.

—— (1921c) *The North American Species of Drosophila*, Washington, DC: Carnegie Institution of Washington.

—— (1937) "Autosomal Lethals in Wild Populations of *Drosophila pseudoobscura*," *Biological Bulletin*, 73: 542–551; reprinted in E.B. Lewis (ed.) (1961) *Genetics and Evolution: Selected Papers of A.H. Sturtevant*, San Francisco and London: W.H. Freeman.

—— (1938) "Essays on Evolution: II. On the Effects of Selection on Social Insects," *Quarterly Review of Biology*, 13: 74–6; reprinted in E.B. Lewis (ed.) (1961) *Genetics and Evolution: Selected Papers of A.H. Sturtevant*, San Francisco and London: W.H. Freeman.

Sturtevant, A.H. and Dobzhansky, T. (1936a) "Geographical Distribution and Cytology of 'Sex-Ratio' in *Drosophila pseudoobscura* and Related Species," *Genetics*, 21: 473–90.

—— (1936b) "Inversions in the Third Chromosome of Wild Races of *Drosophila pseudoobscura*, and Their Use in the Study of the History of the Species," *Proceedings of the National Academy of Sciences USA*, 22: 448–50.

—— (1937) "Observations on the Species Related to *Drosophila affinis*, with Descriptions of Seven New Forms," *American Naturalist*, 70: 574–84.

Sturtevant, A.H. and Plunkett, C.R. (1926) "Sequence of Corresponding Third-Chromosome Genes in *Drosophila melanogaster* and *D. simulans*," *Biological Bulletin*, 50: 56–60.

Sturtevant, A.H. and Novitski, E. (1941) "The Homologies of the Chromosome Elements in the Genus Drosophila," *Genetics*, 26: 517–41.

Wimsatt, W.C. (1992) "Golden Generalities and Co-opted Anomalies: Haldane vs. Muller and the Drosophila Group on the Theory and Practice of Linkage Mapping," in S. Sarkar (ed.) *The Founders of Evolutionary Genetics*, Dordrecht: Martinus-Nijhoff.

Part II

Mapping work, mapping collectives, mapping cultures

5 Mapping and seeing

Barbara McClintock and the linking of genetics and cytology in maize genetics, 1928–35

Lee B. Kass and Christophe Bonneuil

In April 1929, Rollins A. Emerson, head of the Plant Breeding Department at Cornell University, sent a summary of linkage data in maize to his colleagues (Emerson 1929). He had gathered maize geneticists in his hotel room in late 1928 at the AAAS winter science meetings in New York and formalized a cooperative group that he had informally initiated around 1920. In this first communication of what later became the "*Maize Genetics Cooperation News Letter*" he listed 10 linkage groups and gave a provisional genetic map for each of them. These maps were rather vague and the "rainbows" (Figure 5.1) indicated that much work needed to be done. All of the approximately 60 references he cited were based purely on the analysis of genetic crosses (Emerson 1929).

Three years later, in August 1932, Cornell welcomed the 6th International Congress of Genetics. Emerson summarized the state of the art in maize genetics (Emerson 1932). At that meeting he presented a much fuller map, including linkage groups assigned to chromosomes numbered from the largest to the smallest, and with no rainbows (Figure 5.2). His "Literature Cited" listed 16 articles, among them seven included cytological and cytogenetical research. A monograph in 1935, providing a revised and more complete and refined map and detailed linkage data, soon followed his summary (Figure 5.3).

During these years, maize genetics reached a major turning point. This chapter explores this shift and the way the cytogenetics work involving Barbara McClintock contributed to and transformed the genetic mapping of maize. Between 1928 and 1935, driven by the "Emerson School" at Cornell, maize genetics was in its golden age. The network of the students of Emerson and E.M. East constituted the nucleus of the maize genetics cooperative that was strengthened in 1928 and again in 1932. It was on maize, not on *Drosophila*, that a "Cooperative News Letter" was first initiated. By then, maize rivaled *Drosophila* as an experimental organism until the significance of the banded nature of the giant salivary chromosomes of *Drosophila*, was recognized (Painter 1933; Bridges 1935).[1] Parallel to Painter and Müller's cytogenetic work on *Drosophila*, McClintock's cooperative efforts fostered a strong connection between genetic mapping and cytogenetics using maize (identification of the ten chromosomes,[2] and a correlation with each of the ten known linkage groups between 1929 and 1933; cytogenetical proof of genetic crossing over in 1931; cytological determination of the physical location of

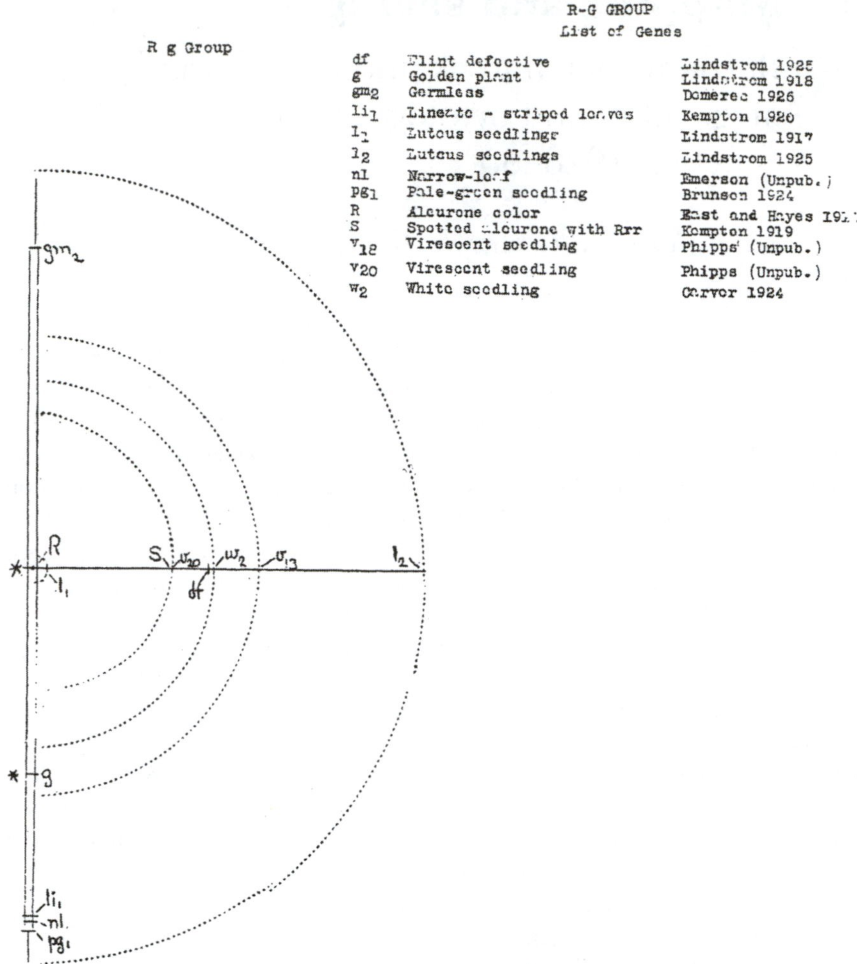

Figure 5.1 Rainbow map of the R–G linkage group in maize sent to "Student of Maize Genetics," April 12, 1929. Reproduced with permission from *Maize Genetics Cooperation News Letter*, No. 53: 117–30, 119–20.

genes within the chromosomes using reciprocal translocation, inversions or deficiencies, etc.; Rhoades 1984).

Emerson, maize, and genetics[3]

R.A. Emerson (1873–1947) received a BS degree in 1897, from the University of Nebraska's College of Agriculture. Emerson then worked for the USDA, Washington, DC until 1899, when he returned to his alma mater as Horticulturist

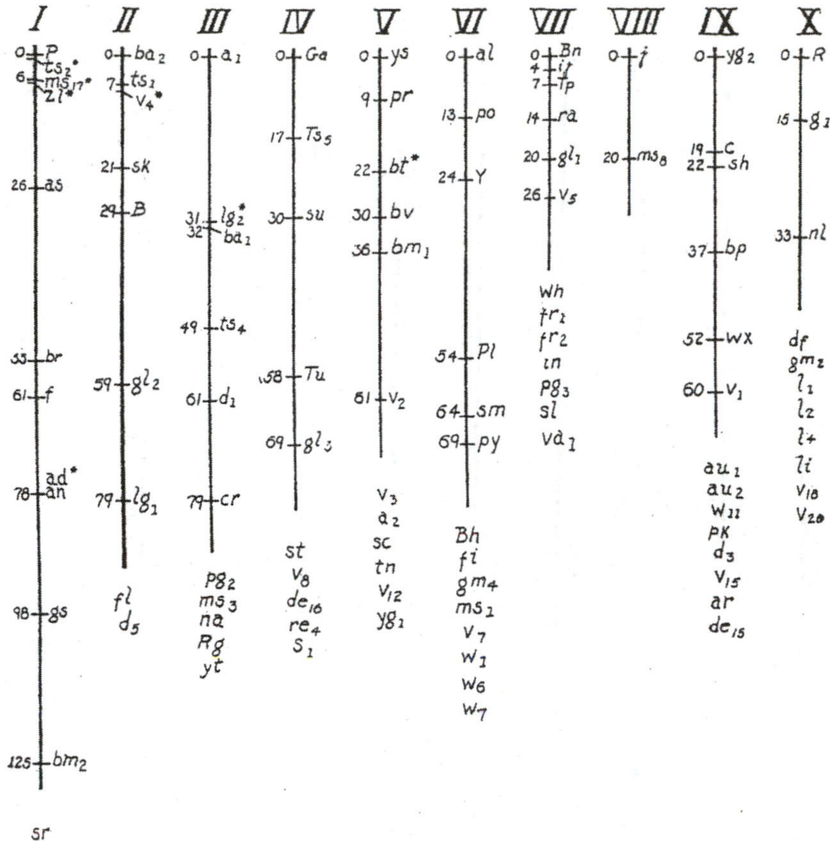

Figure 5.2 Maize linkage map and associated chromosomes published in December 1932. Reprinted with permission from Emerson, R.A. (1932) "The Present Status of Maize Genetics," *Proceedings of the Sixth International Congress of Genetics*, I: 141–52, 145, fig. 1. Plant Breeding Department Paper No. 190, Cornell University (paper presented in August published in December 1932).

in the Nebraska Agriculture Experiment Station and Assistant Professor of Horticulture. Taking his part in the agricultural science community's promotion of Mendelism in America, Emerson used beans and corn in his classes to demonstrate and validate Mendel's laws (Kimmelman 1987). During an experiment that was conducted to demonstrate a 3 : 1 ratio of starchy to sugary kernels he found aberrant ratios. Thus, the quest to determine the cause of his aberrant results led to his studies of maize genetics. In 1908, Emerson began a study of quantitative inheritance in maize. His experiments were designed to test whether or not these differences were due to numerous factors inherited in a strictly Mendelian manner. Three years later, Emerson took a year's leave of absence from Nebraska to

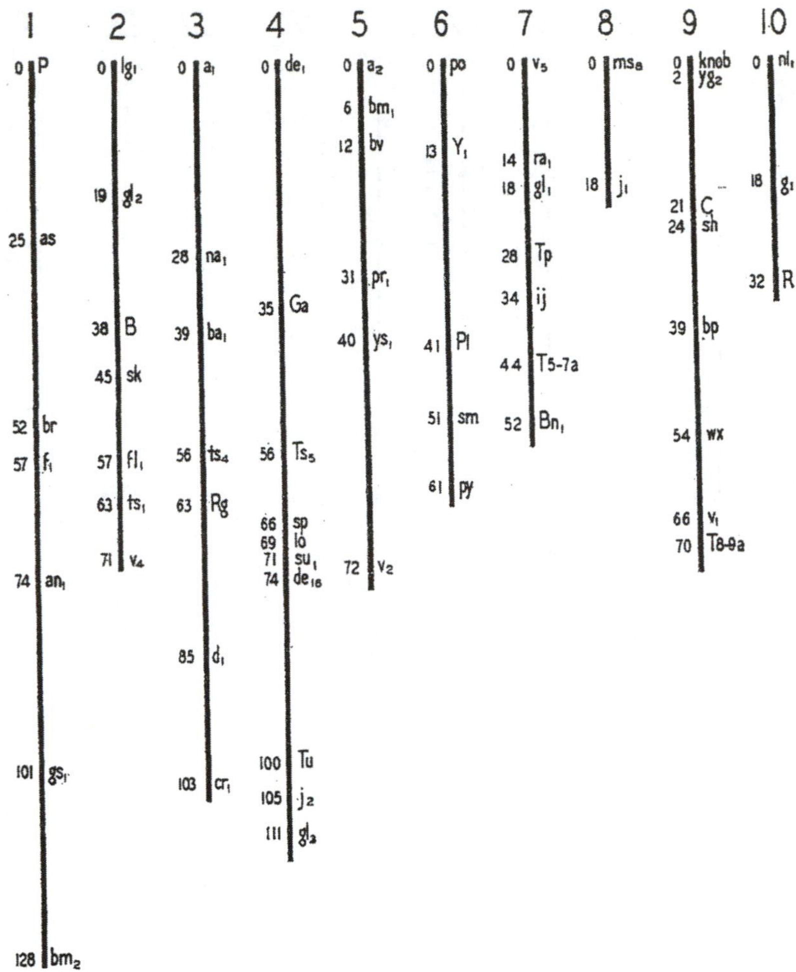

Figure 5.3 Maize linkage map and associated chromosomes completed in March 1935, published in June. Reprinted with permission from Emerson, R.A., Beadle, G.W., and Fraser, A.C. (1935) "Summary of Linkage Studies in Maize," *Cornell University Agricultural Experiment Station Memoir,* 180: 71. Plant Breeding Department Paper No. 212, Cornell University and Cornell University Agriculture Experiment Station.

pursue graduate studies at Harvard's Bussey Institution with the distinguished geneticist Edward M. East. Around this time (and independently of the studies of the Swedish geneticist Nilsson-Ehle), East (1910) and East and Hayes (1911) published papers that proposed multiple factor inheritance in corn. Emerson was awarded his DSc in 1913 and that same year Emerson and East published a collaborative paper titled "The Inheritance of Quantitative Characters in Maize." This paper applied and corroborated the multiple factor hypotheses and constituted a very important milestone in quantitative genetics, because for the first time the theoretical aspects were strongly supported by adequate data.

In 1914, Emerson was called to Cornell University to head the Department of Plant Breeding which he did until 1942. Two of Emerson's students at Nebraska, Ernest G. Anderson and Ernest W. Lindstrom, followed him to Cornell and continued to work on corn problems. On recommendations from distinguished plant-breeders and geneticists (i.e. East at Harvard, Etheridge at Missouri, and Jones at the Connecticut Agricultural Research station), students and established researchers from around the country and throughout the world soon joined Emerson's group and studied corn breeding and genetics at Cornell. C.B. Hutchison, a former Cornell graduate,[4] was appointed Professor of Plant Breeding in 1916 and taught the courses in genetics. By 1920, he had decided to discontinue his work on flax and devote the time he had for research to corn. He continued Emerson's unpublished study of C–Sh linkage and established that Sh was part of the C–Sh–Wx linkage group (Hutchison 1921, 1922). When A.C. Fraser succeeded Hutchison, he also turned (from wheat) to maize. In addition to Anderson and Lindstrom, several other students pursued graduate work with Emerson on corn genetics: Thomas Bregger, William H. Eyster, Milislav Demerec, Paul Kvakan, Helen Trajkovitch, George Sprague, Marcus Rhoades, George Beadle, Hsien W. Li, Swarm Singh, etc. (Table 5.1).[5] In 1934, among the 53 maize geneticists engaged in cooperative work on genetic mapping, it appears that not fewer than 30 were either Emerson's collaborators at Cornell, or had been graduate students there, or had done some post-doctoral work in his department. Of the 24 cooperators identified as "most actively engaged in genetic studies," 16 had been graduate students and two had been "post-doctorate fellows" at Cornell (Table 5.2).[6]

Emerson's physiological agenda as an alternative to mapping

Since Emerson's early work on multiple factor inheritance, his maize genetics' school contributed simultaneously to the progress of corn breeding and to general knowledge in genetics. In this respect, Emerson's program may be considered a corollary with Morgan's group and Emerson's students had close scientific associations with the *Drosophila* geneticists. Concepts, methods, standard nomenclatures and students (including E.G. Anderson, M. Demerec, G. Beadle, and M. Rhoades), who were trained in corn genetics and later also worked on *Drosophila*, circulated between the two communities. Nevertheless, Emerson had a different agenda from Sturtevant and Bridges' mapping enterprise (Kohler 1994). Until 1918, he still had not pursued a systematic study of linkage groups in corn (linkage studies were "stumbled into" in the progress of other work), and showed little

Table 5.1. Students of R.A. Emerson 1918–42, whose research involved corn, and the date they received their degree. Emerson was major professor for doctoral students (PhD) and master's students (MS) listed here

Name of student	
	Date of PhD
Ernest W. Lindstrom	1918
Ernest G. Anderson	1920
William H. Eyster	1920
Arthur M. Brunson	1923
Milislav Demerec	1923
Pavao Kvakan	1924
Thomas Bregger	1928
Ivan F. Phipps	1928
John B. Wentz	1928
George W. Beadle	1930
Hsien W. Li	1930
George F. Sprague	1930
Johannes D.J. Hofmeyr	1931
Max M. Hoover	1932
Harold S. Perry	1932
Marcus M. Rhoades	1932
Swarn Singh	1934
Derald G. Langham	1939
James E.Welch	1942
	Date of MS
Chao C. Feng	1923
Helen Z. Trajkovick	1923
George E. Ritchey	1927
Baburao S. Kadam	1928
Gabriel A. Lebedeff	1931
Carlos A. Krug	1932
Salomon Horovitz	1933
Sylvia M. Allen	1935[a]
Maurice L. Shapiro	1936

Source: Data used with permission from Dr R.P. Murphy's, *A History of the Department of Plant Breeding in the New York State College of Agriculture and Life Sciences at Cornell University*, appendices L and K, draft manuscript, May 22, 2002.

Note

a She acknowledged McClintock for suggesting problem.

interest for genetic mapping. He explained to D.F. Jones:

> This type of work does not interest me as much as working out some complex Mendelian Case for the reason that it is more or less mechanical & from the added fact that we cannot hope to do other than trail along behind

Table 5.2 Exhibit E, "List of Maize Geneticists," sent to the Rockefeller Foundation in support of a request for funds to further cooperation in maize genetics

List of Maize Geneticists

Anderson, Edgar, Bussey Inst., Harvard University, Cambridge, Mass.
o*Anderson, E. G., Institute of Technology, Pasadena, Calif.
o*Beadle, G. W., Institute of Technology, Pasadena, Calif.
*Brink, R. A., University of Wisconsin, Madison, Wisc.
o Brunson, A. M., Kansas State College, Manhattan, Kansas.
o*Burnham, C. R., Yale University, New Haven, Conn.
Collins, G. N., Bureau of Plant Industry, U.S.D.A., Washington, D.C.
Cooper, D. C., University of Wisconsin, Madison, Wisc.
o*Creighton, Miss H. B., Cornell University, Ithaca, N.Y.
o*Demerec, M., Carnegie Inst., Cold Spring Harbor, Long Island, N.Y.
o Dorsey, E., Cornell University, Ithaca, N.Y.
Down, E. E., Michigan State College, East Lansing, Mich.
o*Emerson, R. A., Cornell University, Ithaca, N.Y.
o*Eyster, W. H., Bucknell University, Lewisburg, Penn.
o*Fraser, A. C., Cornell University, Ithaca, N.Y.
Garber, R. J., University of West Virginia, Morgantown, W. Va.
Gurney, H. C., Waite Research Inst., Adelaide Univ., Adelaide, Aust.
*Hayes, H. K., University of Minnesota, Univ. Farm, St. Paul, Minn.
o Hill, Henry, Botany Dept., Cornell University, Ithaca, N.Y.
o Hofmeyr, J. D. J., P.O. Marabastad, Pietersburg, South Africa.
o Hoover, M. M., University of West Virginia, Morgantown, W. Va.
o*Horovitz, S., University of Buenos Aires, Buenos Aires, Argentina.
Hull, Fred, Agric. Exp. Station, Gainesville, Florida.
*Jenkins, M. T., Iowa State College, Ames, Iowa.
*Jones, D. F., Conn. Agric. Exp. Station, New Haven, Conn.
Kempton, J. H., Bureau of Plant Industry, U.S.D.A., Washington, D.C.
o Krug, Carlos A., Inst. Agronomica do Estado Campinas, Sao Paulo, Brazil.
Kuleshov, N. N., Inst. of Applied Botany, Herzen St. 44, Leningrad, Rus.
o Kvakan, Paul, Dobricevo Cuprija, Jugoslavia.
o Lebedeff, G. F., Carnegie Inst., Cold Spring Harbor, Long Island, N.Y.
o*Lindstrom, E. W., Iowa State College, Ames, Iowa.
o*McClintock, Miss Barbara, Institute of Technology, Pasadena, Calif.
Maines, E. B., Botany Dept., University of Michigan, Ann Arbor, Mich.
*Mangelsdorf, P. C., Texas Agric. Exp. Station, College Station, Texas.
Meyers, M. T., Farm Crops Dept., Ohio State University, Columbus, Ohio.
o Miles, L. Gordon, Brisbane, Queensland, Australia.
o*Perry, H. S., Botany Dept., Duke University, Durham, N. Caro.
o Phipps, Ivan, Waite Research Inst., Adelaide Univ., Adelaide, Aust.
o*Randolph, L. F., Cornell University, Ithaca, N.Y.
Reeves, R. G., Texas Agric. Exp. Station, College Station, Texas.
o*Rhoades, M. M., Cornell University, Ithaca, N.Y.
Richey, F. D., Bureau of Plant Industry, U.S.D.A., Washington, D.C.
o Sharp, L. W., Cornell University, Ithaca, N.Y.
o*Singh, S., Cornell University, Ithaca, N.Y.
*Singleton, W. R., Conn. Agric. Exp. Station, New Haven, Conn.
o*Sprague, G. F., Bureau of Plant Industry, U.S.D.A., Washington, D.C.
o*Stadler, L. J., University of Missouri, Columbia, Mo.
o Tavcar, A., Dept. of Plant-Breeding, Univ. of Zagreb, Zagreb, Jugoslavia.
Thomas, H. C., Dept. of Genetics, University Farm, St. Paul, Minn.
Taboada, E. R., Direccion Gral. de Agric., Sn. Jacinto, Mexico, D.F.
Weatherwax, Paul, University of Indiana, Bloomington, Indiana.
o*Wentz, J. B., Iowa State College, Ames, Iowa.
o Wiggans, R. G., Cornell University, Ithaca, N.Y.

Total = 53   * = 24
o = 31   o* = 18

Source: Reprinted with permission from the Rockefeller Archives Center, RF RG1.1 200D Box 136 f. 1684.

Notes
* = 24, names of researchers "most actively engaged in genetic studies with maize."
o = 31, persons who are at Cornell University or who have been at cornell either as graduate students or . . . post-doctorate fellows.
o* = 18. Total = 53.

> Morgan and his co-workers. I am hoping that all the men in this country who are working on related problems with corn may cooperate to such an extent that we can cover the field more quickly.[7]

Emerson saw greater scientific value in more theoretical questions such as multiple factor inheritance, and in the more chemical and physiological studies involving biochemical processes. As Barbara Kimmelman has shown, in the years 1917–25, Emerson developed and promoted research on the genetics and biochemistry of kernel pigment patterns and hoped that maize would be the right tool for such a job. He envisioned a physiological genetics that would connect the genetic aspects of heredity with physiological studies. Furthermore, these studies (useful for the country's agriculture) would interest American agricultural scientists, whose initial leading position in genetics were challenged by the shift to research in *Drosophila* genetics after 1910 (Kimmelman 1992).

The achievements of this physiological genetics agenda on maize remained meager. Emerson's former student, George Beadle, made decisive contributions to such a research program in the late 1930s, but not with maize as an experimental organism. By 1928, few significant general contributions to genetics were achieved with corn, and maize linkage studies and genetic mapping stood nearly a decade behind *Drosophila*. The diploid number of chromosomes in *Zea mays* ($2n = 20$) was in question when L.F. Randolph, Emerson's collaborator, commenced his cytological investigations in 1923 (and was still under investigation in 1928), and—contrary to *Drosophila* (Dobzhansky 1929a[8])—no linkage group had been assigned to any determined chromosome. The ten linkage groups in corn were not all clearly identified and the mapping work in each group was still very rough, as illustrated by the "rainbow maps" drawn by Beadle and Emerson in April 1929 (Emerson 1929).

Toward a cooperative enterprise to map maize

During the period 1918–20, Emerson had realized that he could not avoid investigating the linkage of maize, which was crucial both to breaching the gap with *Drosophila* workers and to providing a deeper basis for the breeding work on corn. Whereas *Drosophila* linkage mapping remained, from 1913 to 1928, the concern of a few laboratories, Emerson promoted the idea that maize genetic mapping should be a larger cooperative enterprise. To our view, four elements can account for this approach: (1) Emerson's cooperative and enthusiastic, yet trustworthy, personality; (2) his belief that collaborative work on the "more or less mechanical" job of genetic mapping would allow individuals to devote the best of their research time to more fundamental research projects; (3) his concern for building a network of former students so as to limit a brain drain to *Drosophila* genetics; (4) his striving to benefit from opportunities opened by massive USDA funding for corn research from 1920 onward.[9] When Frederick D. Richey took charge of corn breeding at the USDA, a regular collaboration was solidified between Emerson and the USDA.[10] This provided scientific background for validating the latter's corn breeding programs (Emerson acted as advisor, and trained many USDA people at Cornell, including Randolph who attended the advanced genetics course at Cornell in 1924), and lent some support to the former's projects and students (T. Bregger and several other of Emerson's students found jobs at the USDA; Randolph was appointed a USDA Agent in 1923 to do corn cytology at Cornell, etc.).

It seems that it was in 1920 that Emerson convened the first "cornfest" (later "cornfab") to draw together maize geneticists at an informal gathering during the AAAS meetings. From then on, such "cornfabs" seem to have taken place annually and informally, and Emerson circulated letters "to students of corn genetics."[11] The Cooperation was reinforced at the 1928 "cornfab" when the mapping of the ten linkage groups was divided among ten groups of researchers with the aim of publishing a general linkage monograph. Beadle acted as secretary and he and Emerson prepared a state of the art summary for each linkage group, with provisional maps (Emerson 1929). A meeting of Corn geneticists was convened during the 6th International Congress of Genetics at Ithaca in August 1932, which led to further development of the cooperation. The maize investigators elected a committee (Emerson, Brink, Mangelsdorf, Jones, and Stadler) to coordinate the work and seek funding support. The group's newsletter began to act as a stock exchange for tester strains. Cornell was chosen to host the repository for all genes and gene combinations (especially tester strains), with Marcus Rhoades as custodian.[12]

In 1934, 300 genetic stocks were grown at Cornell, which acted as the central clearinghouse.[13] The USDA supported this cooperative work. In 1933, Emerson submitted a grant proposal to the Committee of the Division of Biology and Agriculture of the National Research Council (NRC), to fund the maize cooperation at Cornell. The NRC rejected his application, and he subsequently submitted the proposal to Rockefeller Foundation officers, Warren Weaver and Frank B. Hanson. They funded his program beginning in March 1934, for a five-year annual grant of $1,000 a year for the Maize Cooperation.[14] A few months later Weaver accepted Emerson's proposal to extend the support with a Grant-in-Aid for McClintock.[15]

The USDA also supported the maize network. In the early 1930s, in addition to Randolph, two technical assistants were paid by the USDA to maintain the stock collection and assist in hand pollination and other such tasks.[16] In September 1934, the USDA Bureau of Plant Industry convened a conference of corn geneticists at Wooster (Ohio) in cooperation with The Rockefeller Foundation.[17]

The news circular that united the maize genetics group (later called the "Maize Genetics Cooperation") soon was not limited to offers and demands for strains but also disseminated unpublished results among the researchers. The rule was that any data appearing there could not be cited in publications without the direct consent of the contributor. So the News Letter became a vehicle for the exchange of non-published information, which accelerated the progress and the mapping work and allowed the diffusion of partial data not yet submitted or accepted in journals. In 1932, Emerson could proudly assert that no other group of researchers had yet so freely shared materials and unpublished results and praised this "unique, unselfishly cooperative spirit" (Emerson 1932: 142).[18] In his first call for cooperation between the laboratories doing *Drosophila* genetics, Milislav Demerec, a former Emerson student, stated in 1933:

> For several years now workers on genetics of maize have been receiving mimeographed circulars prepared in Professor Emerson's laboratory, containing information contributed by various investigators. This service proved to be so useful that steps are being taken to extend it and make it a permanent institution.[19]

Maize as a tool for genetics and cytogenetics[20]

By 1930, Maize and *Drosophila* were the two organisms whose genetic features were most thoroughly known to investigators. To Emerson's concern, in comparison with *Drosophila* and some other plants, corn had the disadvantage of having a long life cycle, which in temperate regions permits only one generation a year or two generations within greenhouse facilities (instead of two weeks for *Drosophila*!). Because corn is a self-compatible plant, corn ears (silks) had to be covered to prevent unknown self or cross-pollination. The relatively large haploid number of chromosomes ($n = 10$) also complicated the cytological and linkage studies compared with *Drosophila* ($n = 4$).

Nevertheless, corn also had many advantages as a tool for genetic research. It is easy to pollinate, many seeds result from a single pollination, and consequently up to 10,000 seeds can be collected from only "a single hour of work." Additional advantages are the wealth of variability in maize plants, providing much genetic material because of prevalent cross-fertilization. Many weak recessive mutations are perpetuated when in a heterozygous condition with their dominant normal alleles. Yet these are easily exposed by inbreeding, in contrast to naturally self-fertilized species. In addition the phenomenon of xenia and double fertilization favors genetic investigation on endosperm and aleurone [$3n$ tissues] characters, and maize lends itself readily to cytological examination because the chromosomes are much bigger than *Drosophila* chromosomes.[21] Maize haploid mitotic stage chromosomes are readily observed microscopically allowing their identification by size, form, and other morphological features (McClintock 1929d); and when they are long in the meiotic prophase stage, the distinction of signposts on the chromosomes (knobs, chromosomal alterations, etc.) can be observed with greater clarity (McClintock 1930). Moreover, there were a large number of maize genetics investigators, and more was known about its genetics than any other crop plant, due to the economic importance of maize in the United States. Since the late nineteenth century, when the Land Grant Colleges and experiment stations and the USDA started systematic corn breeding research, many mutants had been detected and studied (200 genes studied by 1932 and almost 400 by 1935), and by 1930 several linkage tester strains were available for "three-point-tests." The maize cooperation rapidly distributed these strains.

For these many reasons, Rhoades hardly exaggerated when he asserted that:

> In depth of knowledge of its genetic constitution and in its cytological resolution, maize remained unsurpassed as an experimental organism until the significance of the banded nature of the giant salivary chromosome of *Drosophila* was recognized.
>
> (Rhoades 1984: 24)

McClintock's work needs to be understood in the context of both of these opportunities and constraints. For instance, her fortuitous collaboration with Charles Burnham permitted her to describe cytologically a reciprocal translocation between chromosomes.[22] Yet, it is not by chance that she used chromosome 9 to establish the cytological proof of crossing over (Creighton and McClintock 1931; or to locate genes on the chromosome, McClintock 1931a): it combined ease of genetic study of three aleurone and endosperm genes C–Sh–Wx and facilitated cytological observations because of its easily detected knob.

Cytology meets corn genetics

Since Bridges' (1916) demonstration of non-disjunction, the chromosomal basis of heredity was largely accepted. He had shown by cytological investigation that offspring of the exceptional white eyed females of a mating of red-eyed males ($X^{W}y$) with white-eyed females ($X^{W}X^{W}$) were trisomics ($X^{W}X^{W}y$); an occasional egg being produced during oogenesis that contained two X-chromosomes (non-disjunction). Combining cytological observation with *genetic-cross* analysis, he pioneered work in what would later be called cytogenetics. However, the difficulty of observing *Drosophila* chromosomes prevented further rapid development. Rearrangements of chromosomal material were first detected in *Drosophila* by genetic methods: crossing over, deficiencies (Bridges 1917), duplications (Bridges 1919a,b), heterologous translocation (Bridges 1923a,b), inversion (Sturtevant 1926) but correlation with cytological events only came later (Dobzhansky 1929a; Sturtevant 1965).[23] Although *Drosophila's* small number of chromosomes ($n = 4$) was a favorable factor, it was not until 1929 (Dobzhansky 1929a,b[24]), that linkage groups' 3 and 2 were assigned respectively to the longest and second longest chromosomes.

Maize proved to be (until 1933) the right tool for the (cytogenetic) job. Although, linkage studies in maize were approximately ten years behind *Drosophila*, until 1928, Emerson soon had the satisfaction of seeing maize cytogenetics rival *Drosophila*. The (10) linkage groups were cytologically assigned to the (10) *Zea* chromosomes only a few years after similar studies began in *Drosophila*. The cytological proof of crossing over was demonstrated in corn and published by Harriet Creighton and Barbara McClintock only a few weeks before an equivalent study in *Drosophila* was reported by Curt Stern (1931). The union of cytology and genetics stimulated genetic mapping, and these accomplishments brought maize to the forefront of genetics research.

Cornell: a favorable place

For an understanding of how McClintock became the link between the geneticists and the cytologists, thus advancing the new field of cytogenetics at Cornell, one must look at the connection between the plant-breeders and the cytologists. Until about 1931, Plant Breeding was housed in the Forestry Building east of the main buildings of the College of Agriculture. Botany was in the Agronomy Building (Stone Hall), which was a wing to the west of the main building of the College of Agriculture. Emerson, head of the Plant Breeding Department, understood the value of cytology. He therefore encouraged Randolph's pursuit of corn chromosome numbers to correlate with the linkage groups that students of maize genetics were finding.[25] In addition, Emerson knew that a cooperative effort with a cytologist should prove valuable because of the work that was coming from the laboratories of Morgan and Blakeslee. Emerson's former students, E.G. Anderson and M. Demerec worked with both Morgan's and Blakeslee's and E.B. Babcock's groups and wrote to Emerson at Cornell about the exciting advances in those laboratories.[26]

Randolph had studied cytology with Lester W. Sharp in the Botany Department at Cornell and minored in Plant Breeding with Emerson. Emerson recommended a USDA appointment for Randolph at Cornell to investigate corn chromosome cytology. Cornell's Botany Department provided research space, laboratory equipment, and some funding for their project. The Plant Breeding Department provided field space for growing plants. When Randolph continued his intensive cytological investigations in 1924, the base number for chromosomes in many corn varieties was still in question. By spring of 1924, Randolph had applied John Belling's iron-aceto-carmine smear technique to clarify chromosome numbers reported in the literature (Belling 1921a,b, 1923; Longley 1924).[27] He realized the value of this technique for associating extra chromosome plants with genetic characters, and would soon share it with his new assistant Barbara McClintock.[28]

During McClintock's second and third years in graduate school (1924–26) she held an Assistantship in the Botany Department. From September 1924 through February 1926, she was a teaching assistant to Sharp and a research assistant to Randolph.[29] In February of 1925, McClintock began work for her PhD: Her interest was in the "B" or accessory chromosomes of corn—a project in which Randolph was much involved. However by the summer of 1925, they discovered, in A.C. Fraser's corn cultures, a plant that had three complete sets of chromosomes (a triploid).[30] They applied Belling's smear technique to study the chromosomes in the pollen-mother-cells of this plant and hypothesized the origin of polyploidy in maize (Randolph and McClintock 1926).[31]

But this collaboration did not last. McClintock was displeased that Randolph's name appeared first on their 1926 publication.[32] Additionally, their approach to experimental work was very different. Randolph was extremely careful, meticulous, and cautious. McClintock was notably bright and liked to explore and to modify new experimental techniques, which apparently caused discomfort for her employer. Upon finding the triploid maize plant, McClintock changed the focus of her dissertation project and decided to investigate the cytology and genetics of this unusual plant. Upon ending her service with Randolph, Cornell continued to employ McClintock in the Botany Department as a teaching and research assistant to Professor Sharp. McClintock taught Cytology labs with her Major Professor, who was at the time revising his Cytology text and hence had access to the latest references in the field. Sharp referred both Botany and Plant Breeding graduate students and Post Docs to McClintock for advice and consultation on their research. It was during this time, in 1926, that McClintock met both L.J. Stadler and George Beadle.[33]

When McClintock received her doctorate in June of 1927, Sharp recommended her for an Instructorship in Botany. This appointment gave her the opportunity to write and prepare her PhD thesis for publication and to continue to pursue her studies on the triploid corn plant and its offspring. As we shall see, these investigations led her to devise a technique for distinguishing the plant's ten individual chromosomes (1928–29) and to correlate linkage groups with their chromosomes.

In September of 1928, Marcus Rhoades, encouraged by E.G. Anderson and Sterling E. Emerson, came to Cornell from the University of Michigan to begin his doctoral work with R.A. Emerson. Rhoades became excited by McClintock's project to assign linkage groups to chromosomes. Their astonishing breakthroughs of 1928–29 led Emerson, possibly formerly closer to Randolph than to McClintock, to bring her "back in the fold" of the Plant Breeding Department (Keller 1983: 47–50).[34] In a letter to Stadler in January 1930, he wrote:

> graduate students as Beadle and Rhoades and also Dr. Burnham went to McClintock who was willing to spend any amount of time in helping them with the cytological aspects of their problems. These three men with McClintock's help have turned up more interesting and important things the past season [corn growing season 1929] than usually come to light in several years.[35]

McClintock's reputation as the cytology expert who could see what others could not see and who was willing to cooperate with geneticists soon extended beyond Cornell and was established in the maize genetics community. For this reason Burnham came to learn cytology with her. He hoped to corroborate Belling's translocation hypothesis, which he and Brink had proposed as the underlying mechanism in their semi-sterile corn stocks. This is also why Stadler sought her cooperation for his cytogenetic studies on his X-rayed strains.

By this time and until Botany moved out of Stone Hall, McClintock worked in a laboratory that Dr Sharp had established for graduate students and visiting researchers. There they undertook the preparation and observation of cytological specimens, from 1926, until the winter of 1930–31, when the Botany and Plant Breeding departments moved into the Plant Science Building. In this cramped space McClintock worked with graduate students that Sharp[36] referred to her: G.W. Beadle (September 1927 through late 1930), M.M. Rhoades (from September 1928–summer 1929, at Caltech 1929–30), Charles Burnham (an NRC Post Doctoral Fellow who had recently obtained his PhD with R.A. Brink at the University of Wisconsin, summer–fall 1929 and summer 1930), Harriet Creighton (from September 1929–fall 1930), Henry Hill (from 1929–fall 1930).[37] Faculty members in Cornell's Botany Department often gave the most promising research problems to ambitious young graduate students. McClintock did not hesitate to give the cytological proof of crossing over to Creighton and the trisomic tests for correlating linkage groups with chromosomes to Henry E. Hill.[38] McClintock was also very helpful to Sharp's minor students, Beadle and Rhoades, although they were members of the Plant Breeding Department. McClintock taught them to make their own cytological preparations and she was pleased that they learned so quickly—but not as quickly as she did[39]—to interpret them. The large but crammed room, afforded everyone access to each other's preparations and easily allowed them to discuss results. This atmosphere, combined with McClintock's communicative enthusiasm and the ingenuity of the young research community, created a very stimulating scientific atmosphere.[40]

Assigning linkage groups to cytologically identifiable chromosomes (1929–32)

Assigning each linkage group to cytologically identifiable chromosomes was on Emerson's mind when he and Randolph began collaborative studies supported by the USDA. Randolph's usual method of preparing root tip sections, and observing their division figures with the microscope, afforded limited identification of chromosome morphology. Randolph quickly adopted Belling's "aceto-carmine smear technique," but the methods for morphologically identifying the chromosomes had not yet been devised. In his cultures (strains) late prophase (diplotene and diakinesis stage) chromosomes were visible and countable, but each chromosome was not readily distinguishable. While working as Randolph's research assistant, in 1925, McClintock found a triploid corn plant in the Cornell stocks. They successfully applied Belling's smear technique to study the meiotic behavior of the chromosomes in this triploid plant, and they described the chromosomes in late meiotic prophase. Still, they could not identify each chromosome individually (Randolph and McClintock 1926; McClintock 1927; Randolph 1928). While examining offspring from this triploid plant McClintock found a trisomic plant ($2n + 1$), which she used to correlate with a particular linkage group (McClintock 1927, 1929a), yet she had not determined the identity of the extra chromosome. She believed, however that it would not be long before she would find a technique to do so (McClintock 1927). Persistent and innovative McClintock modified staining techniques to enhance coloration in root tip preparations by warming (short of boiling) the sections after staining (McClintock 1927, 1929b). But this was not enough. While experimenting with different types of preparations under various conditions, she discovered that late prophase or metaphase in the first microspore mitosis (male gametophyte) gave clearer chromosome observations than did root tip preparations. Sometime between summer and fall of 1928, McClintock thought she had recognized a few of the individual distinctive features of the 10 maize chromosomes and a year later she published the first ideogram for maize (Figure 5.4).[41]

In her June 1929 paper on maize chromosome morphology, she reveals her project and experimental strategy: "it is desirable to determine what linkage group is represented by the extra chromosome in the several 2n+1 individuals" (McClintock 1929d). As described earlier, McClintock had investigated triploid maize for her PhD dissertation, and she immediately sought to assign linkage groups to chromosomes using Belling's and Blakeslee's trisomic test. During meiosis in trisomic plants (sometimes resulting from the mating of triploids and diploids), some spores and therefore gametes receive one of the triplicate chromosomes and others receive two. Consequently, the genetic characters carried by this chromosome (and associated with this linkage group) appear in abnormal proportions (a "trisomic ratio") while other characters, simultaneously, appear in normal Mendelian ratios. It then becomes possible to associate a linkage group with a chromosome by cytologically observing spores with extra chromosomes in the late mitotic prophase in the microspore, if that extra chromosome is also present in triplicate in the corresponding strain. McClintock prepared several crosses during the summer of 1929, put a graduate student, Henry Hill, on this hot problem, and secured the help of Marcus Rhoades and George Beadle for the genetic part. They found that in a strain of maize with an extra chromosome, the smallest of the set [number 10]—by 1932, maize geneticists and cytologists had

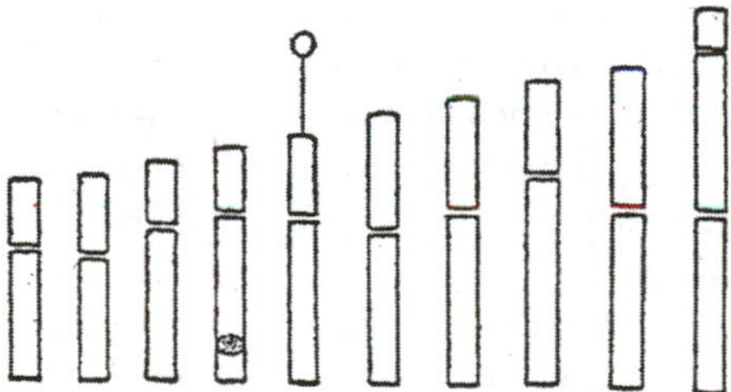

Figure 5.4 First identification of *Zea* chromosomes published by Barbara McClintock on June 14, 1929. Note that McClintock identified this haploid set of chromosomes during mitosis in the first division of the microspore (microgametogenesis). Reprinted with permission from McClintock, B. (1929d) "Chromosome morphology in *Zea mays*," *Science* 69: 629. Copyright 1929, American Association for the Advancement of Science.

decided to number the chromosomes from the largest to the smallest—was present in triplicate. At the same time they observed that an aleurone color, due to the gene R, showed trisomic ratios, contrary to characters in other linkage groups, which showed normal ("disomic") ratios. Therefore, by late 1929, they had identified the R–G linkage group with chromosome 10 (but simultaneously incorrectly identified the B–lg linkage group with chromosome 4, McClintock and Hill 1929[42]). By 1931, McClintock and Hill reported that between March 1930 and March 1931, five additional linkage groups had been assigned to chromosomes: P–br, B–lg, A–d1–cr, Y–P1, C–Sh–wx (chromosomes were not numbered in their paper).[43] In 1935, McClintock and Rhoades reported that by using trisomic methods six of the ten linkage groups had been associated with chromosomes: 2 [B–lg, initially incorrectly assigned to 4], 3[a1–rg], 5[pr–v2], 6 [Y–P1], 7[gl1–ra] and 10 [r–g]; and that other methods gave a definite check on previous trisomic determinations for linkage groups 1, 4 (su–Tu), and 9. Emerson *et al.*, (1935) reported that using trisomic ratios McClintock identified eight linkage groups with chromosomes: 2, 3, 5, 6, 7, 8(j), 9, 10. It is clear that by 1929, McClintock had first applied trisomic ratios and used mitotic chromosomes to correlate linkage groups with chromosomes and she was responsible for considerable progress in this area.

Before trisomic tests were completed for the remaining four linkage groups, other experimental strategies led to their correlation with chromosomes 1 (P–Br), 4 (su–Tu), 8 (j), and 9 (c–wx). One strategy used semisterile strains whose semisterility was due to a reciprocal translocation. While genetic studies could reveal the two linkage groups associated with a certain case of semisterility, cytological observation at meiotic prophase, showed cross-shaped, synaptic configurations involving all four chromosomes (resulting in a chromosome ring at diakinesis) and revealed thereby the identity of the chromosomes involved. McClintock first observed this interchange phenomenon in a translocation involving chromosomes 8 and 9 [T8–9] (chromosome numbers had not yet been assigned, see Figure 5.5). She first saw it in a *semisterile-2* stock that Burnham brought to Cornell, where he specifically came to learn cytology from McClintock in the summer of 1929. Once more, her attention to detail led to a cytological innovation. While collaborating with Burnham, McClintock had noted that the pachytene (mid-prophase) stage of the first meiotic division of the microsporocyte (pollen-mother-cell) showed long chromosome threads (with translocation or interchange chromosomes staining quite darkly), and afforded much finer resolution than preparations of root tip sections or microspore smears of first division mitosis to demonstrate where translocation breaks occurred. Following this breakthrough, the first use of an interchange to assign linkage groups to chromosomes was Burnham's and Brink's work on *semisterile-1*, which was shown, by late 1931, to be associated with linkage groups P–Br and B–lg and to involve the two largest chromosomes (1 and 2 respectively). Since the B–lg linkage group was assigned to chromosome 2, P–Br could be attributed to chromosome 1 (Rhoades and McClintock 1935).[44] In a similar way, a study of a strain carrying a translocation

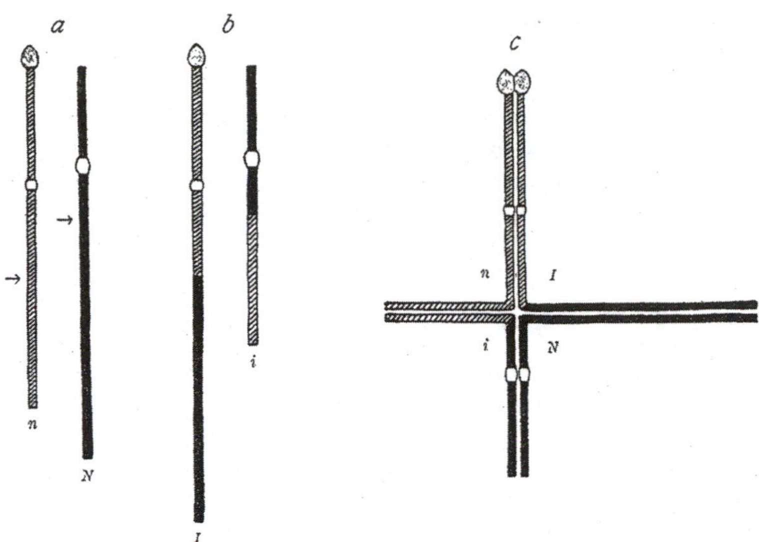

Figure 5.5 This illustration published in December 1930, demonstrates that chromosomes involved in a segmental interchange in *semisterile-2* are the second and third smallest chromosomes in maize [chromosomes 9 and 8]. McClintock used the pachytene stage (mid-prophase of meiosis) to identify this heterozygous translocation involving chromosomes 9 and 8 [T 8–9]. The chromosomes identified as *n* and *N* are chromosomes 9 and 8 respectively. Chromosomes identified by *I* and *i* are the interchange chromosomes. Reprinted with permission from McClintock, B. (1930) "A Cytological Demonstration of the Location of an Interchange between Two Non-Homologous Chromosomes of Zea mays," *Proceedings of the National Academy of Sciences*, 16 (12): 791–6, 793.

in chromosomes 8 and 4 [T8–4] led Anderson to assign linkage group su–Tu to Chromosome 4 (Emerson *et al.* 1935; Rhoades and McClintock 1935).

A third strategy utilized cytological and genetic studies of chromosome deficiencies. During a cytological study using Stadler's X-ray mutant line, which had lost the normal allele of the gene japonica (as shown by recessive backcross analysis), McClintock observed the loss (deletion) of a fragment in chromosome 8. Further cytogenetic study showed linkage between japonica and the cytologically identified "chromosome 8 deficiency" (McClintock 1931b).

Very quickly, results from trisomic tests, reciprocal translocations, and deficiencies, either independently or combined, corroborated each other (Emerson *et al.* 1935). At the Ithaca Congress in August 1932, Emerson could confidently present a genetic map with linkage groups correlated with numbered chromosomes. McClintock had accomplished most of the enterprise. Between 1929 and 1931, she associated a total of eight linkage groups with their chromosomes; six using trisomic methods (2, 3, 5, 6, 7, 10) between 1929 and 1931, one using deletions (8) in 1931, and she confirmed one using a combination of trisomic and reciprocal translocations involving chromosomes 8 and 9 in 1931 (McClintock and Hill 1929; Hill 1930; McClintock and Hill 1931). She also confirmed chromosome 10 linkage with a deficiency in the longer arm by a loss of R (McClintock 1931b). The remaining two chromosomes were associated with their linkage groups by Brink, Cooper, and Burnham, and by Anderson (1 and 4 respectively). The unpublished accounts by McClintock were later mostly confirmed in published accounts by Brink, Burnham, Anderson, and McClintock herself (Rhoades and McClintock 1935).

Cytogenetics helps genetic mapping

Cytogenetics did more than permit a correlation of chromosomes with linkage groups or provide cytological proof of genetic crossing over (the story of Creighton and McClintock's famous 1931 article has been told by E. Fox-Keller). It also accelerated and partly transformed the mapping work itself in the maize genetics cooperation group whose organization was strengthened by Emerson in late 1928 and again in 1932.

For mapping purposes, cytogeneticists tackled problems from two fronts and employed three main strategies: crossing over, chromosomal interchange, and deletions. The combined cytological and genetic study of crossing over allowed McClintock to position three genes between the exchange point and the terminal knob (deeper staining, a cytological character inherited in a simple Mendelian way) in chromosome 9. Thanks to the localization of a breakage point on the chromosome seen in synaptic configurations, the interchange also allowed qualitative positioning of genes relative to the breakage point (McClintock 1930, 1931a). The second strategy used mutual translocations. The first semisterile line was described in 1927, and in 1929 Brink and Burnham attributed the mechanism of semisterility to reciprocal translocation. By applying McClintock's cytological techniques their hypothesis was confirmed by Brink, Cooper, and Burnham between 1929 and 1931. McClintock's and Burnham's research stimulated interests in cytogenetics and soon geneticists actively searched for translocation mutants. By 1935, more than 50 such strains were produced (mostly by Burnham and by Anderson at Caltech[45]). Such lines were used to craft many tester lines that contained both usual (phenotypic) characters and a translocation. About one-third of the "three-point-tests" and "four-point-tests" whose results were reported in Emerson *et al.* (1935) linkage monograph involved a translocation. Such three-point-test combinations were extremely valuable, since they allowed confirmation of gene associations with specific chromosomes, and gave the order of genes and breakage points (Rhoades 1931).

The third major cytogenetic approach to mapping used deletions. In this way, and for the first time, McClintock placed a gene in a particular linkage group by other than purely genetic methods. The investigation was conducted at Missouri in the summer 1931; L.J. Stadler had observed that if a plant homozygous for a recessive gene or group of genes is crossed with X-rayed pollen from a plant homozygous for the dominant allele(s), a few of the progeny (F1) may show the recessive character instead of the dominant. Stadler suggested the problem to McClintock and furnished all the material in the growing state. She had previously studied plants cytologically (McClintock 1929c) and found among them 2*n*–1 individuals (loss of a chromosome), and now her cytological investigations at Missouri revealed individuals having translocations, inversions, and deficiencies, the latter having lost a small piece of a chromosome (McClintock 1931b). She correlated the recessive character (gene) with the piece of chromosome lost in these X-rayed mutants. In this way she showed that gene lg is very near the end of the short arm of chromosome 2, and that gene a1 was near the end of the long arm of chromosome 3 (McClintock 1931b).[46] In their use of X-ray deletions for mapping purposes, Stadler's and McClintock's corn investigations paralleled the experiments carried out at the same time by Muller and Painter using *Drosophila*. However, maize investigators were favored by better cytological methods, which furnished beautiful preparations for microscopic observations (until 1933 when more precise gene locations became possible using giant salivary chromosomes in *Drosophila*). Creighton (1934) used pachytene stage chromosomes to continue deletion-mapping studies and reported three deficiencies for *yg2* at or near the end of the short arm of chromosome 9. One deficiency (Df 9-1) covered about one-fourth of the arm including the conspicuous terminal knob. The absence of the knob demonstrated that the deficiency is really a terminal one.[47]

Conclusion: seeing and mapping

Early biographies of McClintock portrayed her at Cornell as a lone female genius not understood by traditional plant geneticists. This account may have been due to strong reliance on interviews and memories necessarily cloudy after 50 years, and often retrospectively biased by her later experiences on transposable ("controlling") elements (Keller 1983; Comfort 2001: 32–6). These stories told about the incomprehension met by McClintock's cytogenetics research program require reconsideration.

First, we showed that maize geneticists maintained strong relations with *Drosophila* geneticists during the 1920s. This connection was due primarily to Rollins Emerson, and to his students, who worked both with corn and *Drosophila*.[48] E.G. Anderson and M. Demerec studied with both Morgan's and Blakeslee's group and kept Emerson informed about the exciting work that was progressing in these laboratories. Rhoades had worked with Anderson before arriving at Cornell in 1928, and subsequently collaborated with him at Caltech during the 1929–30 academic year (Anderson and Rhoades 1930).[49] Consequently, Cornell maize geneticists were aware that the drosophilist's use of cytology had opened a fertile second front to tackle problems (Painter; Dobzhansky).

Second, we would argue that the association of cytology and genetics was important in several research programs in plant genetics in the 1920s so that McClintock did not arrive with a *tabula rasa*. John Belling and Albert F. Blakeslee, working on *Datura* at Cold Spring Harbor already had elegantly combined genetic-cross analysis and cytology. The use of trisomic strains and trisomic heredity to associate one specific chromosome (being present in three copies) with one specific linkage group was a strategy they used as early as 1923 (Belling and Blakeslee 1923). This work, decisive for McClintock's association of linkage groups with chromosomes, was known to Cornell's maize researchers since Randolph visited Belling in 1924 and applied his aceto-carmine smear technique.

Third, even if Emerson had favored Randolph's research project initially, and if there had been an early lack of understanding or acknowledgment of McClintock's work, this was reversed by her very productive summer of 1929. Emerson reported extensively on her cytogenetic achievements in his 1932 paper. It seems that after the relative failure of his physiological genetics program, in contrast with the Morgan group's achievements, Emerson was very pleased to see maize compete with *Drosophila* as a research organism for fundamental discoveries in the new field of cytogenetics.

Fourth and last, not only Beadle and Rhoades, but also Anderson, Stadler, Burnham, and Brink were geneticists who immediately grasped the significance of McClintock's work and consequently modified their research projects accordingly. Anderson and Burnham devoted their life's work to translocations in corn and trained their students in this field. Beadle left corn but brought McClintock to Stanford in 1944 to do cytology of *Neurospora*. Rhoades devoted his career to corn cytogenetics and trained many students in this area.

We end with a brief reflection on the ways in which McClintock's cytogenetical work transformed the mapping enterprise in the maize genetics group. Her cytological breakthroughs brought previously invisible objects and phenomena to light.[50] A new category of characters (knobs, chromomeres, centromeres, chromosome lengths, arm characterizations, chromosomal events like deficiencies, crossing over, or translocations) were brought into view under the microscope. These new cytological signposts were constructed in a way that made them legible to geneticists and comparable to the usual (phenotypic) characters they had worked with. These new characters were relevant because they showed a hereditary value and could be correlated with genetic findings (the "knob" of chromosome 9, which behaves like a Mendelian character, is a vivid example). Such cytological characters were new tools that improved linkage studies. They helped researchers to cope with the difficulty posed by crossing over in the establishment of linkage. As we saw, translocations also provided better distance data between genes as they resolved the problem of double cross-overs in three-point-tests.

New (cytological) objects and phenomena were therefore produced, which were genetically relevant. These boundary objects connected the practices of cytology and of genetic-cross analysis. The incorporation of cytological entities into the former genetic research tools transformed maize's form of life as an experimental organism. Maize was reconstructed as a cytogenetic tool for mapping. Dozens of new tester lines were constructed that integrated cytological landmarks, which were phenotypically expressed. Once this was done, it was not always necessary to use the microscope again for linkage studies.[51] By these methods many older tester strains were rendered out of date or useless: McClintock's early pioneering techniques and observations were routinely and repeatedly integrated, and partly blackboxed.

Cytogenetics may not have radically transformed the way the mapping work was divided and organized within the expanding Maize Genetics Cooperation. But, cytogenetic work fostered cooperative efforts and extended exchange practices, and provided the organization with a higher scientific status, which in this instance helped to secure two Rockefeller grants at Cornell during 1934–39.

Furthermore one may note that McClintock's early work in the context of the Maize Genetics Cooperation and the Emerson school have probably shaped her later work and her "feeling for the organism" (as Fox-Keller put it). Maize cytogenetics strongly developed as a new field of research in itself,[52] and McClintock's influence, in part or totally, may have diverted the attention of some scientists initially trained in maize genetics from mere mapping work (Beadle; Rhoades; Burnham; E.G. Anderson). In a collaborative article that synthesized the stunning advances of maize cytogenetics through 1935, Rhoades and McClintock (1935) mentioned several genes that affected chromosome behavior (asynaptic, polymitotic, sticky…), and proposed a hypothesis that would be at the heart of McClintock's subsequent work on transposons: "The effect of these genes suggest that not only development of the plant as a whole proceeds under the influence of genes but that the chromosomes themselves, which carry the genes, are under genic control." This view, departing from structural (mapping) toward a more physiological (regulation) approach, was indeed consistent with the particular culture Emerson had given to maize genetics, and the low scientific value that he had initially attributed to the mapping enterprise in itself.

Acknowledgments

LBK acknowledges funding from the National Science Foundation; NSF grants #SBR9511866, #SBR9710488, for support of archival research for this project; Faculty and Staff of the L.H. Bailey Hortorium, Department of Plant Biology, for providing logistical support during this study; special thanks to Rebecca Waldron for archival research assistance. We thank Professors R.P. Murphy and W.B. Provine, Drs Denise Costich, Richard Whalen, C. Husa, M.A. Gondolfo, Edward H. Coe, Paul Sisco, and the editors of this volume for reviewing drafts of this chapter and for helpful insights and discussions. We thank archivists, and friends and colleagues, who hosted us during our archival sojourns at the following institutions: Rare and Manuscript Collections, Karl A. Kroch Library, Cornell University, Ithaca, NY; US National Archives, College Park, MD; Rockefeller Archive Center, Sleepy Hollow, NY. We also thank Reference Librarians at Olin and Mann Libraries, Cornell University, Ithaca, NY; Dr W.B. Provine for unlimited access to the A.J. Cain/W.B. Provine library and reprint collection; Dr Margaret Smith for access to early volumes of The Maize Genetics Cooperation News Letter; and Dr Harriet Creighton for use of her personal copy of Emerson *et al.* (1935).

Notes

1 For a good history of the discovery of the salivary chromosomes and the attack on the gene see Painter (1934).
2 McClintock (1929d), the first published ideogram of Zea chromosomes; the chromosomes were identified in the "first division in the microspore" (Mitosis) not at pachytene stage of Meiosis I as mistakenly described by some text book authors.
3 Unless specifically noted, this section is based on Kimmelman (1992), and Morris (1969), an unabridged copy is in the Department of Plant Breeding Records, 21/28/889, Box 51, Rare and Manuscript Collections, Carl A. Kroch Library, Cornell University Library. See also Kimmelman (1987: 172–237), Rhoades (1949).
4 Hutchison had received his masters' degree from Cornell in 1913.
5 Murphy, Royse P., unpublished manuscript, *A History of the Department of Plant Breeding in the New York State College of Agriculture and Life Sciences at Cornell University*. Manuscript in preparation.
6 "Exhibit E" in file Materials supporting a request for funds to further cooperation in maize genetics, Rockefeller Archives Center (RAC), RF RG1.1 200D Box 136 f. 1684.
7 Emerson to Jones, November 8, 1918, Plant Breeding Records, 21/28/889, Box 4. File Jones, D.F., Rare and Manuscript Collections, Carl A. Kroch Library, Cornell University Library.
8 "The larger pair of the V-shaped chromosomes carries the third-chromosome linkage group of genes, the smaller pair carries the second-chromosome linkage group," p. 418.
9 On the last point see Fitzgerald (1990: 56–74).
10 See their exchanges in NARA 54–31 Box 43, NA-Emerson 1919–1935.
11 As he did in March 1923 to develop a standard notation for characters as adopted by *Drosophila* workers. Emerson to students of corn genetics (March 7, 1923), NARA 54–31 Box 43, *op. cit.*
12 "Materials supporting a request for funds to further cooperation in maize genetics studies," exhibit C, "Newsletter to maize geneticists," October 5, 1932, RAC, RF RG1.1 200D Box 136 f. 1679.
13 R.A. Emerson to F.B. Hanson, December 13, 1934, RAC, RF RG1.1 200D Box 136 f. 1679.
14 March 16, 1934, Appropriation of $5,000 for support of maize genetics clearing house at Cornell University directed by Professor R.A. Emerson, RAC, RF RG1.1 200D Box 136 f. 1679.
15 July 5, 1934, Grant-in-aid ($1,800) to provide the salary of Dr. Barbara McClintock, research assistant to Dr. R.A. Emerson, October 1, 1934– September 30, 1935; Renewal through September 30, 1936, RAC, RF RG1.1 200D Box 136 f. 1679.
16 McCall to Emerson (May 26, 1931), NARA 54-31 Box 43, *op. cit.*
17 Emerson to cooperators (March 28, 1934), NARA 54-31 Box 43, *op. cit.*
18 See also Kass (2001); Coe (2001).
19 Quoted in *Maize Genetics Cooperation News Letter* Vol. 4 M.M. Rhoades to Maize Geneticists, "Call for information," November 13, 1933, p. 2.
20 See Emerson (1932); Rhoades (1984).
21 This was an advantage until the discovery of the giant salivary chromosome in *Drosophila* by Painter in 1933.
22 See Coe (2001: 903). For an updated list of McClintock's publications see Kass (1999).
23 See Bridges (1919b): "Considerable cytological work was undertaken, but none of the slides were good enough technically to be able to demonstrate the deficiency *cytogenetically*" [our emphasis]. See also Bridges (1923a), cited by Dobzhansky (1929a: 408): "The phenomenon of 'translocation' was discovered by Bridges (1923a) (Anat. Record 24 S 426 1923). The *cytological evidence*, though not *entirely conclusive* ..." [our emphasis]. Note that years later Sturtevant (1965: 73) used the term heterologous (=non-homologous) translocation to describe Bridges' "translocation," which was not reciprocal.

24 Dobzhansky (1929b): "flies carrying a given translocation seem to be perfectly normal in their appearance, but when tested genetically, they show linkage of genes belonging to the third with genes belonging to the fourth linkage group."

25 L.F. Randolph to F.C. Richey, February 5, 1925: "A number of problems suggest themselves which seem to me to be of considerable importance . . . not only to learn about the behavior of these extra chromosomes, but also of characters [genes, factors] which may be associated with them. Also the origin of the extra chromosome is still open for definite solution." National Archives US, Box 121, Quisenberry, K.S. to Randolph, L.F., RG 54, records of the Bureau of Plant Industry, Soils & Agricultural Engineering. Correspondence 1917–35. File Randolph, L.F. 1922–1926.

26 For instance, see E.G. Anderson (then at Columbia University) to Emerson, December 21, 1918: "The drosophila work here is very interesting. Some notions have been changed very markedly during the last year or so. Among them deficiency. They now have several so called deficiencies, of which one at least shows a dominant effect in the wing . . . Then too reduplication is an interesting phenomenon. A piece of one chromosome gets detached from its proper position and gets hooked on somewhere else. That sounds fishy and I have to bolt a little to get some of the stuff down. But maybe they are right." Plant Breeding Records, 21/28/889 Box 1 File Anderson, Rare and Manuscript Collections, Carl A. Kroch Library, Cornell University Library. E. G. Anderson and Demerec often came back to visit and gave seminars at the Plant Breeding Department's Synapsis Club, a student/faculty organization that met weekly for social and intellectual get-togethers.

27 A.E. Longley (1924) and L.F. Randolph (1924) (unpublished) had studied a limited number of corn varieties and showed that the basic chromosome number in Zea "appeared" to be 10. See L.F. Randolph to F.D. Richey, May 21, 1924, August 14, 1924, July 1 1924, all letters in National Archives US, Box 121, Quisenberry to Randolph, *op. cit.*

28 L.F. Randolph to F.D. Richey, February 5, 1925: "The examination of pollen-mother-cells will begin soon," National Archives US, Box 121, Quisenberry to Randolph, *op. cit.*

29 L.F. Randolph to F.D. Richey, May 21, 1924, National Archives US, Box 121, Quisenberry to Randolph, *op. cit.*

30 L.F. Randolph to F.D. Richey, August 4, 1925, National Archives US, Box 121, Quisenberry to Randolph, *op. cit.*

31 McClintock's culture card, no 56 [=F1270, F is Fraser's culture number], McClintock MS Col 79, Series V, Box 68, APS. See also Provine, W. B. and P. Sisco, Interview with Barbara McClintock 1980, Rare and Manuscript Collections, Carl A. Kroch Library, Cornell University Library [interview restricted until 1998—see Kass and Provine (1998 and1999)]. Note that Navaschin's (1925) cytogenetical studies in *Crepis*, published a few months previously, had similar implications for understanding the origin of polyploidy and was of "extreme interests for genetics," because progeny of polyploid individuals "should permit a quick solution of the question as to the locations of different groups of genes . . . in the haploid set." An annotated copy in Sharp's reprint collection is now in the possession of W.B. Provine; the quoted statements are underlined in red pencil on Sharp's copy. Both Randolph and McClintock had free access to Sharp's reprints.

32 R.A. Emerson to L.J. Stadler January 14, 1930: McClintock "was quite displeased that her name appeared second on their 1926 publication when she had done most of the work . . . ," Plant Breeding Records 21/28/889, Box 18, File L.J. Stadler, Rare and Manuscript Collections, Carl A. Kroch Library, Cornell University Library. Shortly thereafter, the head of the Botany Department informed Randolph that it was not possible to furnish him an assistant for the coming year, L.F. Randolph to F.D. Richey, March 9, 1926, National Archives US, Box 121, Quisenberry to Randolph, *op. cit.*

33 Beadle was a student of Emerson's and had come to Cornell in 1926 from the University of Nebraska. He was at first in the Agronomy Department with a minor in Plant Breeding but he soon transferred to Emerson's department in 1927. Stadler came to Cornell as a National Research Council Fellow with Emerson, after spending the first part of the year with East at the Bussey Institution. Plant Breeding Department files, Beadle, G.W., Stadler, L.J. in Plant Breeding Department Archives. We thank R.P. Murphy for bringing these files to our attention.
34 See also Provine and Sisco interview with B. McClintock 1980, *op. cit.*
35 Emerson to Stadler, January 14, 1930, Plant Breeding Records 21/28/889, Box 18, File L.J. Stadler, Rare and Manuscript Collections, Carl A. Kroch Library, Cornell University Library.
36 Many plant-breeding graduate students minored in cytology with Sharp.
37 Beadle, Burnham, and Rhoades, who were members of the Plant Breeding department, had a table and a microscope in the Botany lab for cytological observations. (Provine and Sisco 1980 interview with Barbara McClintock, *op. cit*; Creighton 1992: 16; Harriet Creighton pers. com. 1996; Kass interview August 17, 1996).
38 Unlike Plant Breeding Department faculty, who, as Rhoades reported, would initially assign routine problems to students, "When a new student appeared, he would usually assign him some routine problem. . . . if the student were good, he would soon find a more interesting and exciting problem for his doctoral dissertation, while if the student were mediocre, it didn't matter what kind of a problem he had," (Rhoades 1949: 316).
39 Beadle recalled in 1980, that McClintock looked at his material and interpreted it before him (W.B. Provine pers. com., 1993) and in 1982, Burnham had similar recollections about his own cytological investigations (Paul Sisco pers com., 2002).
40 Creighton recalled the "excitement of seeing what someone else had found . . . open exchange of observations and interpretations," (Creighton 1992: 16).
41 McClintock's culture cards no.'s MC 121, 8/8/[1928]; McC 137 [summer 1928]; McC 138, 8/3/[1928]. On these cards she numbered three chromosomes counting from the smallest. McClintock MS Col 79, Series V, Box 68, APS. Rhoades (1984: 22) recalled that the maize chromosomes were not yet identified when he arrived at Cornell in the fall of 1928.
42 Their results were presented at the December/January 1929/30 winter meetings (AAAS in Iowa). They presented data for two linkage groups; the smallest chromosome carries the r–g linkage group and the fourth largest carries the b–lg linkage group. See McClintock (1933) for her correction of B–lg linkage group from chromosome 4 to chromosome 2.
43 See McClintock and Hill (1931) appendix, added after they submitted their paper in March of 1930, in which they explain that five additional linkage groups had been correlated with the chromosomes.
44 Burnham (1930) assumed that Pbr was associated with the largest chromosome; see Emerson (1932: 149) discussing reciprocal translocations, "By this means Burnham (1930) had shown that genes of the P–br linkage group (group I) are borne by chromosome 1." Note: Cooper and Brink (1931) reported that chromosomes in *semisterile-1* are not easily identified at the open spireme [Pachytene] stage; see also Brink and Cooper (1931), here they used diakinesis, anaphase I and metaphase 1 (not pachytene) chromosomes to confirm their association.
45 See Anderson's impressive stocks in *Maize Genetics Coop. News Letter* vol. 5, January 25, 1934, p. 11–12.
46 See also McClintock (1932).
47 For a good review of chromosomal aberrations in maize through 1934, see Anderson (1936), whose review was submitted in 1934.
48 See also Murphy, (unpublished ms.), *op. cit.*
49 "Paper from the Department of Botany of the University of Michigan No. 273."
50 For an interpretation of McClintock's visual style see Keirns (1999). On strategies of representations, see Rheinberger (1995).

51 For instance, once routine, three-point-tests with translocations did not require cytological observation.

52 See the impressive list of breakthroughs listed by Rhoades (1984) and Rhoades and McClintock (1935); see also Anderson (1936); Burnham (1992).

References

Anderson, E.G. (1936) "Induced Chromosomal Alterations in Maize," in B.M. Duggar (ed.) *Biological Effects of Radiation*, New York: McGraw-Hill Book Co. Inc.

Anderson, E.G. and Rhoades, M.M. (1930) [Published 1931] "The Distribution of Interference in the X-Chromosome of *Drosophila*," *Papers of the Michigan Academy of Sciences, Arts and Letters*, 13: 227–39.

Belling, J. (1921a) "The Behavior of Homologous Chromosomes in a Triploid *Canna*," *Proceedings of the National Academy of Sciences*, 7: 197–201.

—— (1921b) "On Counting Chromosomes in Pollen-Mother-Cells," *American Naturalist*, 55: 573–4.

—— (1923) "Microscopical Methods Used in Examining Chromosomes in Iron-Acetocarmine," *American Naturalist*, 57: 92–6.

Belling, J. and Blakeslee, A.F. (1923) "Trisomic Inheritance in the Poinsettia Mutant of *Datura*," *The American Naturalist*, 57: 481–95.

Bridges, C.B. (1916) "Non-Disjunction as Proof of the Chromosome Theory of Heredity," *Genetics*, 1: 1–52 and 107–63.

—— (1917) "Deficiency," *Genetics*, 2: 445–65.

—— (1919a) "Duplication," *Anatomical Record*, 15: 357–8.

—— (1919b) "Vermilion deficiency," *The Journal of General Physiology*, 9: 645–56.

—— (1923a) "The Translocation of a Section of Chromosome II upon Chromosome III in *Drosophila*," *Anatomical Record*, 24: 426–7.

—— (1923b) "Aberrations in Chromosomal Materials," *Eugenics, Genetics and the Family*, I: 76–81.

—— (1935) "Salivary Chromosome Maps," *Journal of Heredity*, 26: 60–4.

Brink, R.A. and Burnham, C. (1929) "The Inheritance of Semi-Sterility in Maize," *American Naturalist*, 63: 301–16.

Brink, R.A. and Cooper, D.C. (1931) "The Association of *semisterile-1* in Maize with Two Linkage Groups," *Genetics*, 16: 595–628.

Burnham, C.R. (1930) "Genetical and Cytological Studies of Semisterility and Related Phenomena in Maize," *Proceedings of the National Academy of Sciences*, 16: 269–77.

Burnham, C.R. (1992) "Barbara McClintock: Reminiscences," in N. Fedoroff and D. Botstein (eds) *The Dynamic Genome: Barbara McClintock's Ideas in the Century of Genetics*, Plainview: Cold Spring Harbor Laboratory Press.

Coe, E.H. Jr (2001) "The Origins of Maize Genetics," *Nature Reviews Genetics*, 2: 898–905. Available at <http://www.nature.com/reviews/genetics> (accessed November 2001).

Comfort, N. (2001) *The Tangled Field*, Cambridge: Harvard University Press.

Cooper, D.C. and Brink, R.A. (1931) "Cytological Evidence for Segmental Interchange between Non-Homologous Chromosomes in Maize," *Proceedings of the National Academy of Sciences*, 17: 334–8.

Creighton, H.B. (1934) "Three Cases of Deficiency in Chromosome 9 of *Zea mays*," *Proceedings of the National Academy of Sciences*, 20: 111–15.

—— (1992) "Recollections of Barbara McClintock's Cornell Years," in N. Fedoroff and D. Botstein (eds) *The Dynamic Genome: Barbara McClintock's Ideas in the Century of Genetics*, Plainview: Cold Spring Harbor Laboratory Press.

Creighton, H.B. and McClintock, B. (1931) "A Correlation of Cytological and Genetical Crossing-over in *Zea mays*," *Proceedings of the National Academy of Sciences*, 17: 492–7.

Dobzhansky, Th. (1929a) "Genetical and Cytological Proof of Translocations Involving the Third and Fourth Chromosomes of *Drosophila malanogaster*," *Biologisches Zentralblatt*, 49: 408–19.

—— (1929b) "A Homozygous Translocation in *Drosophila melanogaster*," *Proceedings of the National Academy of Sciences*, 15: 633–8.

East, E.M. (1910) "A Mendelian Interpretation of Variation that is Apparently Continuous," *American Naturalist*, 44: 65–82.

East, E.M. and Hayes, H.K. (1911) "Inheritance in Maize," *The Connecticut Agricultural Station Bulletin*, 167, New Haven Connecticut.

Emerson, R.A. (1929) "To Students of Maize Genetics," April 12, 1929; reprinted in *Maize Genetics Cooperation News Letter*, 53: 117–30.

—— (1932) "The Present Status of Maize Genetics," *Proceedings of the Sixth International Congress of Genetics*, I: 141–52 [paper presented in August, published in December 1932].

Emerson, R.A. and East, E.M. (1913) "The Inheritance of Quantitative Characters in Maize," *Nebraska Agricultural Experiment Station Research Bulletin*, no. 2.

Emerson, R.A., Beadle, G.W., and Fraser, A.C. (1935) "Summary of Linkage Studies in Maize," *Cornell University Agricultural Experiment Station Memoir*, 180: 1–83.

Fitzgerald, D. (1990) *The Business of Breeding: Hybrid Corn in Illinois, 1890–1940*, Ithaca: Cornell University Press.

Hill, H.E. (1930) *A Cytological and Genetical Study of Certain Trisomic Types in Zea mays L.*, PhD thesis, Cornell University.

Hutchison, C.B. (1921) "Heritable Characters of Maize. VII. Shrunken Endosperm," *Journal of Heredity*, 12: 76–83.

—— (1922) "The Linkage of Certain Aleurone and Endosperm Factors in Maize and their Relation to Other Linkage Groups," *Cornell University Agricultural Experiment Station Memoir*, 60: 1421–73.

Kass, L.B. (1999) "Current List of Barbara McClintock's Publications,"*Maize Genetics Cooperation Newsletter*, 73: 42–8. Available at <http://www.agron.missouri.edu/mnl/73/110kass.html> (accessed January 1999).

—— (2001) "Ethics in Science," *Plant Science Bulletin*, 47: 42–8. Available at <http://www.botany.org/bsa/psb/2001/psb47–2.html#ETHICS IN SCIENCE: PREPARING STUDENTS FOR THEIR> (accessed January 2003).

Kass, L.B and Provine, W.B. (1998 and 1999) "Formerly Restricted Interview with Barbara McClintock, now Available at Cornell University Archives," *Maize Genetics Cooperation Newsletter*, 73: 4. Available at <http://www.agron.missouri.edu/mnl/73/11kass.html> (accessed August 1998).

Keller, E.F. (1983) *A feeling for the Organism: The Life and Work of Barbara McClintock*, San Francisco: W.H. Freeman and Co.

Keirns, C. (1999) "Seeing Patterns: Models, Visual Evidence and Pictorial Communications in the Work of Barbara McClintock," *Journal of the History of Biology*, 32: 163–96.

Kimmelman, B. (1987) *A Progressive Era Discipline: Genetics at American Agricultural Colleges and Experiment Stations 1900–1920*, PhD thesis, University of Pennsylvania.

—— (1992) "Organism and Interests in Scientific Research: R.A. Emerson's Claims for the Unique Contributions of Agricultural Genetics," in A.E. Clark and J.H. Fujimura (eds) *The Right Tools for the Job: At Work in the Twentieth-Century Life Sciences*. Princeton: Princeton University Press.

Kohler, R.E. (1994) *Lords of the Fly. Drosophila Genetics and the Experimental Life*, Chicago: University of Chicago Press.

Longley, A.E. (1924) "Chromosomes in Maize and Maize Relatives," *Journal of Agricultural Research*, 28: 673–81.

McClintock, B. (1927) *A Cytological and Genetical Study of Triploid Maize*, PhD thesis, Cornell University.

—— (1929a) "A Cytological and Genetical Study of Triploid Maize," *Genetics*, 14: 180–222.

—— (1929b) "A Method for Making Aceto-Carmin Smears Permanent," *Stain Technology*, 4: 53–6.

—— (1929c) "A 2*N*–1 Chromosomal Chimera in Maize," *Journal of Heredity*, 20: 218.

—— (1929d) "Chromosome Morphology in *Zea mays*," *Science*, 69: 629.

—— (1930) "A Cytological Demonstration of the Location of an Interchange between Two Non-Homologous Chromosomes of *Zea mays*," *Proceedings of the National Academy of Sciences*, 16: 791–6.

—— (1931a) "The Order of the Genes C, Sh, and Wx in *Zea mays* with Reference to a Cytologically Known Point in the Chromosome," *Proceedings of the National Academy of Sciences*, 17: 485–91.

—— (1931b) "Cytological Observations of Deficiencies Involving Known Genes, Translocations and an Inversion in *Zea mays*," *Missouri Agricultural Experiment Station Research Bulletin*, 163: 1–30.

—— (1932) "A Correlation of Ring-Shaped Chromosomes with Variegation in *Zea mays*," *Proceedings of the National Academy of Sciences*, 18: 677–81.

—— (1933) "The Association of Non-Homologous Parts of Chromosomes in the Mid-prophase of Meiosis in *Zea mays*," *Zeitschrift fur Zellforschung und microskopische Anatomie*, 19: 191–237.

McClintock, B. and Hill, H.E. (1929) "The Cytological Identification of the Chromosomes Associated with the 'R-Golden' and 'B-Liquleless' Linkage Groups in *Zea mays*," *Anatomical Record*, 44: 291.

—— and —— (1931) "The Cytological Identification of the Chromosome Associated with the R–G Linkage Group in *Zea mays*," *Genetics*, 16: 175–90.

Morris, R. (1969) "Rollins Adams Emerson (1873–1947): Horticulturist, Pioneer in Plant Genetics, Administrator, Inspiring Advisor," *Proceedings of the Nebraska Academy of Sciences*, 79: 37.

Navaschin, M. (1925) "Polyploid Mutations in Crepis: Triploid and Pentaploid Mutants of *Crepis capillaris*," *Genetics*, 10: 583–92.

Painter, T.S. (1933) "New Method for the Study of Chromosome Rearrangements and the Plotting of Chromosome Maps," *Science*, 78: 585–6.

—— (1934) "Salivary Chromosomes and the Attack on the Gene," *Journal of Heredity*, 25: 465–76.

Randolph, L.F. (1928) "Chromosome Numbers in *Zea mays* L.," *Cornell University Agricultural Experiment Station Memoir*, 117: 1–44.

Randolph, L.F. and McClintock, B. (1926) "Polyploidy in *Zea mays* L.," *American Naturalist*, 60: 99–102.

Rheinberger, H.-J. (1995) "From Microsomes to Ribosomes: 'Strategies' of 'Representation,'" *Journal of the History of Biology*, 28: 49–89.

Rhoades, M.M. (1931) "Linkage Values in an Interchange Complex in Zea," *Proceedings of the National Academy of Sciences*, 17: 694–8.

——(1949) "Biographical Memoir of Rollins Adams Emerson 1873–1947," *National Academy of Sciences of the United States of America Biographical Memoirs*, 25: 313–23.

Rhoades, M.M. (1984) "The Early Years of Maize Genetics," *Annual Review of Genetics*, 18: 1–29; reprinted with slight modifications in *Dynamic Genome* (1992) Plainview: Cold Spring Harbor Press.

Rhoades, M.M. and McClintock, B. (1935) "The Cytogenetics of Maize," *Botanical Review*, 1: 292–325.

Stern C. (1931) "Zytologisch-genetische Untersuchungen als Beweise für die Morgansche Theorie des Faktorenaustauschs," *Biologisches Zentralblatt*, 51: 547–87.

Sturtevant, A.H. (1926) "A Crossover Reducer in *Drosophila melanogaster* due to Inversion of a Section of the Third Chromosome," *Biologisches Zentralblatt*, 46: 697–702.

—— (1965) *A History of Genetics*, New York: Harper and Row Pub.

6 The ABO blood groups

Mapping the history and geography of genes in *Homo sapiens*

Lisa Gannett and James R. Griesemer

Introduction

The ABO blood groups, and other blood group systems as they were discovered, provided an empirical foundation for human genetics research during the first half of the twentieth century. However, the legacy of the ABO blood group research is a matter of some debate, a debate that has emerged recently as a result of controversy surrounding the Human Genome Diversity Project (HGDP). HGDP proponents such as L. Luca Cavalli-Sforza and Mark Stoneking tend to regard the ABO blood group research as foundational to the discipline of anthropological genetics and the study of human genome diversity. Critics of the HGDP such as Jonathan Marks tend to view the ABO blood group work as marginal, in several ways: as scientifically suspect, as negative in its influence, as outdated, and even as racist. The controversy surrounding the HGDP heightens disciplinary tensions that preceded it, between geneticists, physical–biological anthropologists, and social–cultural anthropologists. Yet, the debate raises a number of methodological and conceptual issues concerning the investigation of human genome diversity, issues too important to allow these disciplinary maneuverings to obscure. The methodological and conceptual issues we focus on here concern classification: relations between a priori and a posteriori groupings in classification, intersections and tensions between social–political and biological–anthropological categories of classification, the privileging of genetic over traditional anthropological traits in classification, and "racial" classification.

Our approach is to examine these important methodological and conceptual issues within a theoretical framework that makes use of cartographic representations and situates these representations within the history of mapping more generally. Attention to approaches taken by several researchers in mapping ABO blood group distributions permits appreciation of the interplay between objectivity and judgment that is involved in the construction of maps as representations of reality (Galison 1998), the construction of different notions of objectivity at different periods in the history of Western science (Daston and Galison 1992), and the circulation of reference that occurs in the construction of objects of knowledge (Latour 1999). Maps, as historical products of scientific activity, become useful tools in the hands of analysts of science as indicators of changing practices and theoretical interests (Griesemer and Wimsatt 1989). In a companion chapter in this volume, "Classical Genetics and the Geography of Genes," we make use of gene and chromosomal linkage maps and geographic distribution maps as such indicators. These maps indicate how representational strategies in the Drosophila experimental system were exploited to maintain continuities of practice through the movement from laboratory to field to answer novel sets of questions *and* how deflections of the experimental system in given research contexts reflect particular theoretical and practical interests. How genes or chromosomes are ordered in space and time, whether or not they become bounded in populations, and the extent to which genetic continuities or discontinuities are epistemically or historigraphically privileged depend on pragmatic features arising within specific contexts of investigation.

According to Pauline Mazumdar, "The blood-grouping laboratory was the fly-room of the human species" (1996: 620). In this chapter, it is the ABO blood group maps that are of interest to us.

Karl Landsteiner discovered the ABO blood groups in 1900. This discovery explained why blood could not always be successfully transfused from one person to another: a person's red blood cells sometimes become clumped together, or agglutinated, when mixed with another person's serum. Landsteiner called the agglutination factors *A* and *B* (Lawler and Lawler 1957). The inheritance of the *A* and *B* antigens had yet to be worked out. Based on their studies of dogs and then human families, Emil von Dungern and Ludwik Hirszfeld proposed, in 1910, that factors *A* and *B* are inherited as dominant alleles segregating at two independent loci. Felix Bernstein challenged this account in 1924, arguing that the data did not support a presence–absence theory of inheritance at two independent loci. Bernstein went on the following year to advance the theory that ABO inheritance involves a single multi-allelic locus, identifying three alleles, and calling these *A*, *B*, and *R*. Most researchers in the field had accepted Bernstein's account by 1928 (Mazumdar 1996).[1] In 1931, inspired by the chromosome mapping in Drosophila that had been carried out by the Morgan lab, Bernstein developed a mathematical technique for the study of genetic linkage using blood groups and this provided the opportunity for geneticists to begin to map the human genome (Mazumdar 1996: 631).

However, whereas in Drosophila, genetic linkage mapping preceded the geographical mapping of chromosomal variants in populations, the study of geographical variation in human blood group frequencies had commenced over a decade earlier, during the First World War. Ludwik and Hanna Hirszfeld took advantage of the circumstances of the war that led to their presence in the Aegean Sea port of Salonika (now Thessaloniki, Greece) as army physicians. The Hirszfelds recognized the anthropological value of the agglutination properties of blood: "It seemed . . . that it would be of interest to make use of hitherto unknown and anatomically invisible relationships between different races" (1919b: 36). With access to soldiers and refugees from different parts of the world, the Hirszfelds were able to compare blood groups in diverse human groups without the extensive international travel that would otherwise have been necessary.

They published their findings in 1919, in two articles: in *L'Anthropologie*, "Essai d'Application des Méthodes Sérologiques au Problème des Races," and, in *Lancet*, "Serological Differences Between the Blood of Different Races: The Results of Researches on the Macedonian Front." It is the Hirszfelds' research that is portrayed today as marking the inception of a new discipline, anthropological genetics, by proponents of the HGDP like Cavalli-Sforza and Stoneking. By 1961, ABO data for over seven million people living in areas stretching across the globe had been published (Mourant 1961: 1).

The human genome diversity project: contesting disciplinary boundaries and the historical legacy of ABO blood group research

The use of the ABO blood groups to map the history and geography of genes in *Homo sapiens* throughout much of the twentieth century is considered by some scientists to provide methodological and theoretical foundations for contemporary human genome diversity research. The serological research carried out by Ludwik and Hanna Hirszfeld during the First World War is portrayed as marking the inception of a new discipline.

According to human population geneticist L. Luca Cavalli-Sforza, "This early work with ABO gave birth to anthropological genetics" (2000: 15). In a recent article in *Nature* that introduces that issue's presentation of single nucleotide polymorphism (SNP) data, anthropological geneticist Mark Stoneking similarly represents the Hirszfelds' work as a "seminal study," the first attempt to study genetic variation in human populations (2001: 821). Stoneking commends the Hirszfelds' research for its scientific rigor: "This work was notable for its broad coverage of the world's populations, large sample sizes and scrupulous attention to anthropological details" (2001: 821). He believes that the significance of the Hirszfelds' contributions has finally been recognized by the scientific community because of increased appreciation of the importance of human genome diversity: "Happily, times have changed, [and] diversity is all the rage" (2001: 821).

Cavalli-Sforza traces a path of continuous linear progress in the investigation of human evolution since these beginnings—from the use of biological reagents to determine blood group differences in the first decades of the twentieth century, to the mid-century introduction of electrophoresis to discern protein differences, to, finally, during these past couple of decades, the availability of restriction enzymes and PCR to identify DNA differences. He sees the latest developments as building upon but in no way replacing earlier research: "The future of the analysis of genetic variation is clearly in the study of DNA, but results accumulated with the old techniques based on proteins have not lost their value.... Results with DNA have complemented but never contradicted the protein data" (2000: 18). Cavalli-Sforza's own career path follows this same trajectory. After gaining his MD in the 1940s, he studied population genetics, immunology, and blood group techniques at Milan's serum institute. While at Cambridge on a research post-doc from 1948–50, he worked with R.A. Fisher who was using the blood groups to study human evolution (Cavalli-Sforza and Cavalli-Sforza 1995: 106). During the early 1960s, while at Pavia University, Cavalli-Sforza and Anthony Edwards launched a comprehensive study of human evolution. They developed quantitative methods that calculated genetic distances based on blood group differences between populations in order to establish a phylogenetic tree. An evolutionary tree they constructed in 1962 was based on five blood group systems in fifteen populations, with three populations taken from each continent (Cavalli-Sforza *et al.* 1994: 31–2; Cavalli-Sforza and Cavalli-Sforza 1995: 111–3). Cavalli-Sforza's current research expands the project he began in the 1960s, with a great deal more data available. A 1984 evolutionary tree was constructed on the basis of 110 genes in forty-two "native" populations from around the world (Cavalli-Sforza and Cavalli-Sforza 1995: 119). His vision for the HGDP calls for the immortalization of cell lines from up to 500 "aboriginal" populations worldwide, many of which are at risk of disappearing. He estimates that comparing approximately 100 gene loci for each cell line will allow researchers to address a variety of questions about the history of human evolution and patterns of human genome diversity (Bowcock and Cavalli-Sforza 1991; Cavalli-Sforza *et al.* 1991).

This representation of the historical legacy of ABO blood group research, which sees the contributions of the Hirszfelds and their successors as providing methodological and theoretical foundations to contemporary human genome diversity research and physical–biological anthropology, is, however, contested. Prominent among the critics is biological anthropologist Jonathan Marks (1996, 2000). Marks is dismissive of the significance of the blood group research, and genetics more generally, for developments in his discipline. While he agrees with Cavalli-Sforza and Stoneking that there is historical continuity leading from the blood group research to contemporary approaches to the study of human genome diversity and human evolutionary history, Marks does not characterize this legacy in positive terms. The ABO blood group research is viewed by Marks, not as foundational, but as marginal to contemporary research efforts in a number of ways: outdated, scientifically suspect, negative in its impact on anthropology, and even racist. This contrasts with Stoneking's commendation of the scientific rigor of the Hirszfelds' efforts and regret for the delay of scientists in recognizing the importance of these efforts. Marks claims that, already in the 1920s, anthropologists were skeptical of the ABO blood group research because of the unlikely groupings that resulted. Marks contends that "racial serology" managed to "reinvent" its hold on physical anthropology from the 1920s to the 1940s only by making illegitimate use of blood group data to "confirm" racial divisions that, in actuality, were "imposed" on the data. By 1945, according to Marks, the ruse was up, with serological methods cast, deservedly, to the margins of the discipline of physical anthropology. The HGDP, Marks writes, "seems to fit snugly with the mold established earlier in the century by racial serology—high technology wedded to folk concepts about human biological diversity and conceptually antiquated approaches to the study of the peoples of the world" (1996: 360–1).

This distance between hagiographies presented by Cavalli-Sforza and Stoneking, on the one hand, and Marks, on the other hand, is unsurprising. The debate over the historical legacy of ABO blood group research has been shaped by controversies surrounding the HGDP. Proponents like Cavalli-Sforza and Stoneking tend to portray the history of ABO blood group research and its contributions to the contemporary study of human evolution in a favorable light. An opponent like Marks' interpretation of the historical record is couched in terms of disciplinary differences, whereby ignorant and narrowminded geneticist outsiders repeatedly challenge the authority of experienced and broad-thinking anthropologists. Marks believes that the successful use of genetic techniques and DNA data requires anthropological knowledge, and it is at their peril that geneticists try to supersede anthropologists. He draws an analogy between the failure of "racial serology" and the difficulties that the HGDP, as conceived by molecular geneticists, has faced in gaining support.

Of course, the debate over the historical legacy of ABO blood group research, as it has emerged within the context of controversies concerning the HGDP, is embedded in longstanding disciplinary conflicts over the study of human biological and cultural diversity and the history of human evolution. Jennifer E. Reardon's recent doctoral dissertation, *Race to the Finish: Identity and Governance in an Age of Genetics*, details ways in which these conflicts structured negotiations over the HGDP by a number of stakeholder groups, including population geneticists, physical–biological anthropologists, social–cultural anthropologists, and indigenous peoples. Physical–biological anthropologists questioned the qualifications of geneticist organizers of the HGDP to study human, rather than zoological, populations and criticized their focus on genetic, instead of phenotypic, differences. When HGDP organizers responded by inviting anthropologists to participate, the hand extended did not unequivocally welcome fellow experts in place of assistants who could facilitate access to populations of interest. These difficulties were compounded by HGDP organizers' surprising lack of awareness of other sources of conflict: politically charged disciplinary disputes between physical–biological and social–cultural anthropologists, the growth in political activism among indigenous groups, and the history of racism and colonialism. Reardon argues that the HGDP could not proceed without the "co-production" of accommodating natural and social orders (for example, workable categories of "race" and "expertise"),[2] and this explains its failure.

Although disciplinary conflicts between geneticists, physical–biological anthropologists, and social–cultural anthropologists, heightened by recent controversies concerning the HGDP, play a significant role in shaping understandings of the historical legacy of the ABO blood group research, it would be unfortunate were these maneuverings to obscure the importance of the methodological and conceptual questions raised. Rhetoric that fosters discipline formation in the relative short term by minimizing continuities and exaggerating discontinuities with neighboring disciplines may, in the long term, impoverish the methodological and conceptual foundations of all of these disciplines by failing to interrogate, in an intellectually honest and fruitful manner, those interesting questions that are prone to arise, sometimes unexpectedly, in border regions. In the case of the HGDP, the politics of representation associated with discipline formation is embedded in, and incorporates the meanings of, wider social discourses surrounding the history of racism and colonialism. Consequently, historiographic choices, and the continuities or discontinuities they privilege or downplay, receive moral signification. Diane B. Paul's (1994a,b, 1995) work on eugenics, human genetics, and the Human Genome Project beautifully illustrates similar developments in a related area and how contesting politics of representation can result in important questions being overlooked. In assessing the implications of the history of eugenics for contemporary human genetics, supporters of the project emphasize discontinuities while critics of the project emphasize continuities. The result is not only the selective misrepresentation of historical developments, but that questions we ought to take seriously, like what it is people fear about eugenics, become overlooked.

The debate between HGDP proponents and opponents over the historical legacy of ABO blood group research raises a number of methodological and conceptual issues. These issues concern the classification of human groups: relations between a priori and a posteriori classifications, intersections and tensions between social–political and biological–anthropological categories of classification, the privileging of genetic over traditional anthropological traits in classification, and the "racial" classification of groups. In the following sections, we examine these issues within the context of the debate over the historical legacy of the ABO blood group research.

Mapping the history and geography of genes in *Homo sapiens*

In a companion chapter (Gannett and Griesemer, Chapter 4), we argue that the historiography of discontinuity used to interpret the history of classical genetic mapping neglected important continuities of mapping practice that were deflected, but maintained, as fly researchers shifted their attention and operations from lab to field in order to address questions of the genetics of natural populations. Specifically, we trace a continuous historical chain of representational forms in linkage and geographical maps as Theodosius Dobzhansky, in collaboration with A.H. Sturtevant, adapted laboratory one-species linkage mapping practices to work on the geographical distribution of genes and chromosomes in natural populations.

Here, we take for granted the deflected continuities of mapping practice between lab and field to address a different historiographic problem about continuities of genetic mapping. An additional continuity of Dobzhansky's and other geneticists' mapping practices in the early twentieth century concerns the common use of mapping techniques by fly and human researchers, and recognition of these efforts as directed to similar ends. For instance, observations about the distribution of human genes appeared in Dobzhansky's publications, very often immediately following his observations about distributions of fly genes, with both represented through the technology of geographical distribution genetic mapping.

Human variation and its classification began to receive a great deal of attention in the nineteenth century, long before the genetic mapping carried out by Dobzhansky in flies and the ABO researchers in humans. Notoriously, "racial" classifications based on the physical characteristics of humans were subject not only to observations of the appearance of variation and difference, but also to judgments of categorical difference and to ethnic, cultural, and national biases that served as a priori classifications guiding sampling protocols for research on biological traits. As geneticists and physical anthropologists turned their attention to genetic mapping in humans, classification practices of population geneticists came into direct contact with classification practices of anthropologists. Classifying humans genetically, by mapping geographical distributions of serological traits—blood groups—seemed to afford mappers an opportunity to improve on the objectivity of human "racial" classifications based on physical characteristics because, they reasoned, distributions of blood group genes could not be affected by the mating choices and preferences of humans carrying the genes, nor would the measurement of human differences be affected by the racial judgments and biases of investigators (Davis 1935).

In this section, we examine methodological and conceptual questions associated with classification practices within a theoretical framework that makes use of cartographic representations, in particular, the geographical maps of ABO blood group distributions favored by researchers like Ludwik and Hanna Hirszfeld, Laurence Snyder, J.B.S. Haldane, and William C. Boyd, and spanning a period from 1919 to 1950. We attempt to situate these cartographic representations within the history and epistemology of mapping more generally.

Our historiographic project concerns the relation between classification judgments and scientific objectivity in the emerging epistemology of human blood group mapping. Peter Galison and Lorraine Daston have argued for a periodization of the historical development of notions of objectivity from the eighteenth to the twentieth century which opposes, as alternative stances between which investigators faced a fundamental epistemic choice, the judgment of the trained, twentieth-century scientific expert to the objectivity of the dispassionate, nineteenth-century mechanical recorder or the inspired discovery of the eighteenth-century genius (Daston 1992; Daston and Galison 1992; Galison 1998).

Galison and Daston argue that the eighteenth-century conception of being "true to nature" depended on a notion of artistic interpretation in the representation of nature's essences discovered through acts of genius. Artistic judgment was needed to extract truth from the distractions of accidental variation, for example, in the visual representation of the essential healthy body or organ from observations on individually varying, anachronistic, even diseased subjects (Daston 1992). Thus, accuracy in representation of objective, essential truths about nature was a product of judgment that transcended the brute facts presented to the observer.

By the late nineteenth century, Daston and Galison argue, a new vision of *mechanical* objectivity emerged, in which the potentially biasing judgments of an artist-representer who is not a professional scientist had to be removed from the path from data to visual representation of nature (Daston and Galison 1992). In his place would go a machine—a device lacking any capacity for judgment or bias—that would register and render visual the objective truth about nature, variation and all. Thus, objectivity in representations of nature was to be a product of machine discipline and the "self-abnegation" of the investigator, who would avoid the temptation to interpret and depict unseen essences as products of observation.

Galison (1998) extends this periodization of objectivity, arguing that somewhere between the 1920s and 1950s, judgment again gained ascendancy against (mechanical) objectivity in the stance of scientific atlas- and visual image-makers, though in a new form—that of the trained, self-confident scientific expert and judge rather than that of an inspired artistic and temperamental genius. Galison links his periodization to the professionalization and institutionalization of science. The profession of scientist emerged in the nineteenth century and mechanical objectivity can be seen as the stance of the dis-interested professional, with specialized equipment and training, against that of the biased, judgmental, interested artist-amateur. In the twentieth century, as science became bureaucratized and rationalized with an elaborate division of scientific labor, the mechanically-objective equipment operator became a technician—a low-paid, theoretically unmotivated, and therefore (it was assumed) unbiased helper, often a woman. The scientist, in contrast, became an expert trained in the exercise of scientific judgment.

This historiographic model, based on an opposition of judgment to objectivity and their conceptual transformation with the emergence of expertise, depends on a vision of the relation between representation and reality as a large and fundamental gap to be bridged. The "old settlement" of this relation by the linguistic turn toward correspondence between ontologically distinct categories of world and words ill fits the complexities of scientific practice in general and the historically and socially situated negotiations of scientific objectivity in particular (Latour 1999). We argue that Galison's periodization would be better served if the twentieth century is viewed in terms of an emerging conception of objectivity *with* judgment rather than against it.[3] The conceptual and material displacements in each of the many small steps it takes to extract representations through scientific work require a form of abstraction that supports a new image of objectivity. However, as we show in the case of human blood group mapping, there does remain a tension between the older mechanical view and the emergent vision of expertise in the attempt to discharge subjectivities of judgment in expert scientific practice. Thus, we endorse Galison's periodization of the changing rhetoric of epistemic virtue, but suggest that the history of scientific practice puts different music to the libretto. As judgment becomes essential to the circulation of reference between representations and reality, it becomes inextricable from scientific work.

The image of subjectivity

Bruno Latour's provocative account of the circulation of reference, which aims to solve sociologically the ontologist's problem of the relation between abstract wordly representations and concrete worldly nature, involves a chain of small abstractions (1999: ch. 2). At each step in the scientific process, he argues, matter extracted from a scene of investigation is converted into form for the purposes of the next step's extraction. Since each step represents only a small displacement from the context of the investigative scene, reference can "circulate." Representations of soil scientists in Paris can successfully refer to dirt in Brazil because the chain of connections, so carefully produced and maintained by back-breaking scientific work, can be successfully traced and retraced. Thus, the seemingly large, unbridgeable ontological gap between words and the world is made of a series of small, bridgeable ones. Understanding abstraction becomes an empirically manageable problem in the sociology of science.

We wish to analyze these small abstractions further to understand the way in which objectivity depends on the circulation of reference and, for our study of human blood group mapping, how objectivity can be understood as the "image" of subjectivity. Objectivity and subjectivity are reflections *along* the line of circulating reference created by scientific work, just as wordly abstractions and worldly concretions are reflections *across* the ontologists' "line of being" (Jubien 1997). In our study, the a priori subjective judgments of national, ethnic, and racial categories are used to initiate the scientific process of building a chain of circulating reference leading to a posteriori classification schemes. But in order to sustain the claim of objectivity for the resultant scientific classifications, it seems that the subjective a priori assumptions that bridged the gap between abstractions (hypotheses and a priori categories) and concrete research subjects to initiate research must be discharged. However, because they are linked to the a posteriori classifications through the reference chain, subjective judgments are ineliminable if science is to achieve objectivity.

Each of Latour's small abstractions is composed of a small extraction and a small judgment (see Figure 6.1). The abstraction is not a Platonic one as Latour suggests, as though matter itself could jump ontological categories into form. Rather, the abstraction is Aristotelian: a subtraction in thought of some of the properties of concrete matter, facilitated by the extraction of a material sample from its context.[4] A lump of dirt is extracted from a hole in Brazil. Thus, the dirt's qualities and structure can be contemplated in abstraction from its relations to the surrounding environment. The lump is trimmed to a neat cube—extracted from its irregular surfaces—so as to fit a cubicle in the pedocomparator, thus preparing the extracted lump for comparison with other, similarly prepared lumps. And so on, until the chain of references leads to a series of numbers in a published data table and a specimen cabinet.[5] Each step provokes a small jump, a small gap between one material object and another. The gaps allow the extracted matter to be moved away from the sampling point, but they open up new problems of judgment—what to do next with the extracted sample, where to take it, where should it go?—but always making a trail that can be retraced. Hence, reference can circulate back down the trail established by a sequence of small judgments, and it is this possibility of referential backtracking that secures objectivity, that is, a return to the subject as object.[6] The gaps are not the unbridgeable ones of

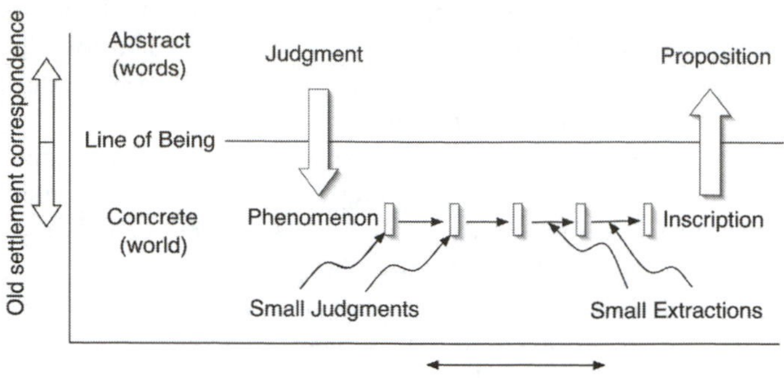

Figure 6.1 Correspondence and circulation models of reference, objectivity and abstraction. Vertical axis shows the "old settlement" correspondence model, where judgment and representation cross the "line of being" between ontological realms of abstract and concrete. Horizontal axis shows the "new settlement" circulation of reference model, where judgment and extraction leading to inscriptions keep reference and objectivity below the line of being, that is, in the realm of the concrete. Symbols are identified in the figure. See text for further explanation of the models.

words and world, but the eminently bridgeable ones of matter extracted and displaced from matter.

These small, bridgeable gaps are generated by means of the small judgments that also take place at each gap-forming extraction by choosing one path rather than another. Thus, judgments follow a logic of why-questions: why this path rather than another? The choice to chain the extractions in one direction, rather than another, implies a contrast class of options or roads not taken at each gap. Should we save the dirt or only record its color? Do we store the pedocomparator in a cabinet or only a photograph? As such, chains of judgments are amenable to social worlds commitment models of scientific work (Gerson 1998). Small judgments not only are necessary for extraction to occur, they are essential for reference to circulate—they put reference into circulation. Thus, objectivity in the twentieth-century form of expert judgment lies in the traceability from inscription back to the source, which is therefore the image of subjectivity, the forward-moving "push" toward objectivity.

In the human blood group mapping work described in the following section, we follow the objectifying moves that are produced by small judgments and small abstractions, and investigate the epistemology of cartographic objectivity.

A priori and a posteriori classifications of human groups

L. Luca Cavalli-Sforza's interpretation of the historical legacy of the blood group research credits the Hirszfelds for their demonstration of differences in ABO blood group frequencies among ethnic groups and recognizes one of their successors, William C. Boyd, for his use of three blood group systems (ABO, RH, MN) to differentiate populations on the five continents from one another (2000: 14–6). In other words, Cavalli-Sforza believes that the blood group researchers were able to discover existing genetic differences among ethnic and/or racial groups. Jonathan Marks, in contrast, is dubious about the validity of classifications based on blood group differences. He claims that serologists like Boyd, simply used blood group data to validate the existence of groups they had assumed from the outset, and not as an empirical basis for classification. Here, Marks finds continuity between the blood group researchers and contemporary geneticists associated with the HGDP. He contends that among the "conceptually antiquated approaches to the study of the peoples of the world" today's population geneticists share with their "racial serologist" predecessors is a reliance on a priori "racial" divisions (1996: 360–1): "population geneticists still commonly assign individual genotypes a priori into races, and ask their computers about the genetic relationships among the races they have constructed" (1996: 358).

This point of disagreement between Cavalli-Sforza and Marks raises important questions about the nature of a priori and a posteriori classifications of human groups and the relations between them. What is the status of the a priori groupings assumed by researchers? Must these a priori groups be validated by empirical data? Do the data alone determine a posteriori classification schemes or are unexamined a priori assumptions involved? The nature of biological variability in *H. sapiens* constrains the answers that are available to these questions. Researchers cannot forego a priori classification altogether or, on the basis of empirical evidence, reconstitute these a priori groups entirely. Methods of a posteriori classification inevitably impose discontinuities upon continuities. This is because historical and geographical patterns of genetic variability among human groups are overwhelmingly quantitative, not qualitative. Both closely and distantly related groups share most of their alleles in common and differ only in the frequencies with which these are found. And, at any given time slice, the geographical sampling of genes reveals that the vast majority of alleles are found throughout the world, though at varying frequencies in different places. In their mid-twentieth century efforts to integrate anthropology into the modern evolutionary synthesis through its incorporation of the methods and concepts of population genetics and the replacement of "typological thinking" by "population thinking," biologists like Theodosius Dobzhansky and Ernst Mayr emphasized the prevalence of genetic continuities over discontinuities across the distribution of *H. sapiens*.

The prevalence of genetic continuities over discontinuities was not news to serologists, however. When the ABO blood groups were discovered at the beginning of the twentieth century, researchers thought they might be able to identify qualitative serological differences among "races" that would be analogous to those blood characters that definitively sort individual organisms into distinct species. But, in 1919, the Hirszfelds found that blood group differences vary quantitatively rather than qualitatively among the "races" with A and B "present in all races examined" (1919b: 37), though "in different proportions in different races" (1919b: 41). It is unlikely that the Hirszfelds' failure to discover qualitative ABO blood group differences among national (presumed, as we discuss later, to be "racial") groups, and the resulting inability to rely on these differences to sort individuals into "racial" groups, would have been surprising. Because of inheritance studies of the ABO blood groups, and the use of blood group differences to sort donor and recipient individuals for transfusion services, it was well established by this time that individuals belonging to the same ethnic group, and even the same family, can have different blood types. The significant empirical finding would have been the variation in relative proportions of the blood types exhibited by different national groups. Further attempts to isolate blood group differences other than ABO that could serve as "racial" characters proved unsuccessful. Close to a decade later, serologists like Landsteiner and Levine had accepted "the idea that the serological make-up of races is determined by varying combinations of a number of characteristics" (1928: 130).

Given that genetic differences among human groups involve "varying combinations of a number of characteristics," the "typological" sorting of people into "racial" groups, based on specific alleles or genotypes each person possesses, is unavailable as a technique that can be used for a posteriori classification. Groups, not individuals, are the basic units of classification: a constellation of ABO blood group or allelic *frequencies* is a description of a group, not an individual, and the pattern with which these frequencies vary from one place to another sorts groups, not individuals, into "races." It is impossible to forego a priori classification altogether; some method of a priori grouping is required to establish a basis for calculating frequencies. Thus, judgment is required in a priori classification. Thrown into the mix of a priori classifications is quite a range of categories: political, linguistic, geographical, religious, national, racial, and ethnic. The methods of a priori classification used by several ABO blood group researchers like the Hirszfelds, Snyder, and Boyd reveal the nature of the categories used and the relations of their classification schemes to the empirical data. We need to consider whether the data—for example, differences in blood group allele or genotype frequencies—can be used to validate or reconstitute these groups, or whether the data simply classify, on the basis of a biological criterion, groups that may be of dubious biological significance. In addition, because alleles are rarely wholly present in one group and/or absent in another, a posteriori classification methods cannot be entirely objective but must involve judgment about where to draw lines of statistical distinction. We need also to consider, then, what a priori assumptions are implicated in the imposition of discontinuity upon continuity in a posteriori classification and in the illusions of continuity in map representations of frequency data that seem to discharge the a priori assumptions.

A sampling from anthropological genetics research—as the field is identified by Cavalli-Sforza—over its early decades reveals a transition in views on a priori classification. The Hirszfelds, pioneers of the field, simply assumed that the prevailing ways in which people were categorized in the social milieu were both biologically and anthropologically meaningful. In their a priori groupings, the Hirszfelds used the term "race" or "people" to refer to the group membership of the soldiers and refugees they tested. They understood such "racial" designations to be based on nationality or "national type." The "races" or "nationalities" identified by the Hirszfelds, in examining "500–1000 persons of each race" (1919b: 37), were: "English," "French," "Italians," "Germans," "Austrians," "Serbs," "Greeks," "Bulgarians," "Arabs," "Turks," "Russians," "Jews," "Malagasies," "Negroes (Senegal)," "Annamese," and "Indians." At least to our ears, the Hirszfelds' "nationalities" are not strictly political groups. Some of the designations like "English" and "German" carry the sense of "ethno-nation" that is prevalent in Europe. Others are more evidently what might be considered to be "ethnic" categories, for example, "Jewish" and "Arab." Religion becomes a determinant of national identity in the use of "Mohammedean Macedonians" to represent "Turks." When they questioned this designation because the "Mohammedean Macedonians" "must certainly contain a large admixture of Slav blood" (1919b: 37), the Hirszfelds seem to be assuming an ethnic category of "Slav" that is broader than "Serb," "Bulgarian," or "Russian." And the representation of the Senegalese as "Negroes" appears to import the racial categories of the nineteenth century. The Hirszfelds' demonstration that these "national types" differed in their frequencies of *A* and *B* was, in the late 1910s, a novel discovery. The Hirszfelds did not use the blood group data to reconstitute these groups in an a posteriori classification, though they did, in a sense, appeal to the data as validation for the a priori groups, in remarking that "the distribution of *A* and *B* corresponds with surprising accuracy to geographical situation" (1919b: 41).

During subsequent decades, we find increased attention to the biological and anthropological validity of a priori groupings. Snyder, during the 1920s, was skeptical about the Hirszfelds' assumption that the ways in which people are classified in the social milieu are necessarily meaningful from the perspective of biology or anthropology. He believed that, while some prevailing modes of classification will be biologically or anthropologically significant, others are merely social or political. Snyder exhibited a greater wariness than the Hirszfelds in employing the term "race" to describe these categories. He referred to the groups he sampled as "nationalities" or "peoples" and insisted that these "nationalities" or "political groups" were not the units of "racial classification." "[T]he German nationality," he wrote, "is not a racial unit" (1926: 236). The "real races" that are the objects of anthropological research were those that have been identified by "a true 'racial' study of blood groups" (1926: 235). Snyder considered his serological research on indigenous peoples of the Americas to come close to this standard.[7] Presumably, then, "real races" cannot be identified on an a priori basis, but require a posteriori sanction. Nevertheless, a priori groups identified by Snyder such as "American Indians," "Senegalese," "Turks," "Spanish Jews," and "French" remained intact in his table of blood allele correlation (1926: 248, figure 4). So, while Snyder was skeptical about the Hirszfelds' assumption that prevailing modes of classification were biologically and anthropologically meaningful, and though he hoped that blood group data would pick out "real races," these data were not used to reconstitute the a priori groupings, which therefore remained the units of "racial" classification.

By the 1940s and 1950s, the evolutionary synthesis had influenced human geneticists like Boyd. Boyd's fundamental units of "racial" classification were populations presumed to be random mating and in genetic equilibrium (Boyd 1953: 496); his a priori classification used the terms "population" or "ethnic group" instead of "race," "nationality," or "people." Boyd's tables of blood group frequencies included the geographical location where sampling took place, as well as "ethnic" or "tribal" identities. Whereas an earlier tabulation of blood group frequencies made only occasional reference to the geographical location where sampling took place (Snyder 1926),[8] this was standard practice by the time Boyd published his *Genetics and the Races of Man* in 1950. Sample a priori designations found in Boyd's charts detailing ABO frequencies include "American Indians (Kwakiutl), British Columbia," "Basques, San Sebastián," "Irish (Dublin)," and "Chinese (Peking)" (1950: 223–5). While Boyd's a posteriori racial classification was to be established on the basis of differences in blood group frequencies among these groups, it can be seen that there was a mélange of identities involved in his a priori designations—racial, ethnic, national, and geographical. These designations were supposed to be justifiable on biological, and therefore, at least potentially, empirically ascertainable grounds. Individuals belong to the same biological population because of the increased likelihood that they will find a mate within the group. For Boyd, then, there were biological and anthropological criteria that justify a priori groupings: breeding populations are the basic units of "racial" classification. However, it is rare for these initial groupings to be arrived at empirically; more often, they are simply assumed, and therefore remain a priori designations that have been influenced by already-existing, but often highly contested, social and political categories. In the section that follows, we consider the intersection of social–political and biological–anthropological categories of classification.

Blood group data—similarities and differences in frequencies of alleles among these designated groups—are the basis for a posteriori (or "racial") classification. These data achieve objective status through a chain of extractions carried out in the scientific work of: (1) identifying subjects from a priori classified populations; (2) sampling their blood; (3) determining blood type from hemeagglutination tests; (4) aggregating data into population frequencies; and (5) locating frequencies on geographical maps or in quasi-geographical tables (Figure 6.2).

Objectivity is achieved, notwithstanding questions surrounding the scientific status of the a priori groups themselves, because of the abstraction of results (represented in maps and tables) from the particular, local, material, social, and cultural circumstances to which the scientists were led by their judgment in the use of a priori classifications of potential research subjects. However, it does not follow from scientific success in such objectifying movements that the subjectivities of judgment are dispatched. The notion of abstraction must first be resolved. Under the "Platonic" large gap notion of abstraction as the identification of a nonconcrete entity, subjective judgments are discharged when the formal relation between abstract (proposition, model) and concrete (inscription, phenomenon) is discovered. Subjectivity is mere means to that formal end. Under the

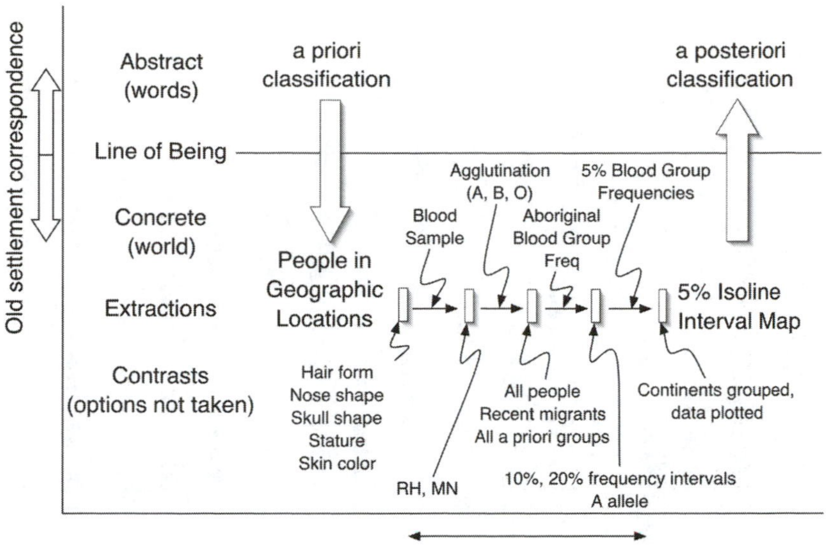

Figure 6.2 Blood group mapping and a posteriori classification following Latour's circulation model. Illustration of the research process of constructing objective representations of geographic frequencies of human blood groups according to Latour's circulation model. Compare to Figure 6.1.

"Aristotelian" small gap notion of abstraction as the extraction in thought of a concrete entity from some of its properties, subjective judgments are integral, not only to the production of objectivity, but to its maintenance. The extracted data, results, and even representations alone do not determine a posteriori classifications; a priori assumptions remain involved. Indeed, what is depicted in map and table representations of population blood group frequencies could be said to be objectified judgments. Given that historical and geographical patterns of genetic variability between human groups are overwhelmingly quantitative, not qualitative, a posteriori (or "racial") divisions inevitably impose discontinuity, represented by vertical jumps across the "line of being," on continuity, represented by the horizontal chains of extractions and judgments (see Figure 6.2). There is interplay between objectivity and judgment, and cartographic representations are indicative of tradeoffs that are made.

Although the Hirszfelds remarked on the geographical pattern of variability in the blood group frequencies of national groups, the articles in *L'Anthropologie* and *The Lancet* contain no geographical maps. The data are presented in a bar graph that orders the "national types" according to the relative frequency of *B* and a measure, invented by the Hirszfelds, called the "biochemical race-index" that represents the ratio of *A* to *B*. The bar graph exhibits general geographical

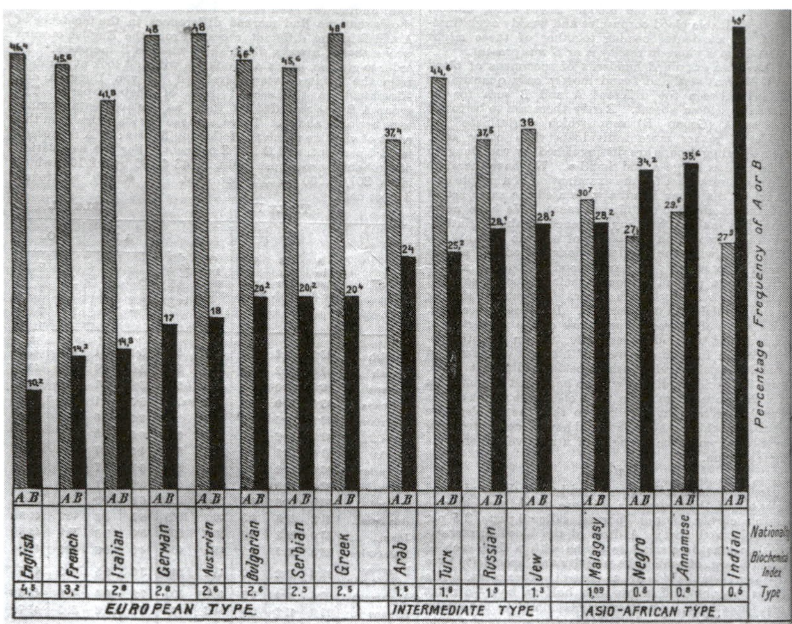

Figure 6.3 Hirszfeld and Hirszfeld 1919 bar graph representation of A and B human blood type frequencies according to "national type." See text for explanation. Reprinted with permission from Elsevier (*The Lancet*, 1919, 2: 675–9).

trends: the frequency of *A* is most pronounced in Europe and diminishes in southward and eastward directions and the frequency of *B* is most pronounced in India and diminishes in northward and westward directions. The empirical data were not used by the Hirszfelds to reconstitute the a priori "national types" but to characterize, compare, and then combine them into higher-order groups. On the basis of the "biochemical race-index," the "national types" were also grouped into three higher-order, remotely geographical, "types": "the European type," "the intermediate type," and the "Asio-African type" (Figure 6.3). These "types," in turn, were treated as cohesive units with characteristic blood group frequencies; reference was made, for example, to "the European A frequency" (1919b: 39). But the discontinuities of these "types" were imposed; although the relative frequencies of *A* and *B* blood types distribute along a geographical gradient in moving from one national group to another, the pattern is one of continuity.

The Hirszfelds' bar graph representation reveals the interplay of objectivity and judgment. *A* and *B* frequencies and the "biochemical race-index" that combines them are presented as objective, numerical quantities. The "national types" are ostensibly ordered along the horizontal index by "biochemical race-index," but there are accompanying judgments with respect to relative order, spacing, and the higher-order division into "European," "Intermediate," and "Asio-African types." While the order imposed by the percentage frequency of *B* and "biochemical race-index" generally coincide, the percentage frequency of *B* wins out where the indices are equal and, in the one case, the "Arab" and "Turk" groups, where these measures differ. Ordering by percentage frequency of *A* instead would have altered the representation significantly, for example, by moving "Turks" from the "intermediate type" to the "European type" and "Italians" in the opposite direction, and placing "Greeks" into proximity with the "French" and "Serbians" alongside the "English." While the bar graph representation permits a visualization of the gradual variation moving from one "national type" to another, it also reveals that the boundaries of the three "types" impose discontinuity upon a continuous, roughly geographical, distribution pattern of percentage frequencies of *A* and *B* agglutination reactions. Clearly, there was a judgment to forego proportional spacing in the graph of the "national types" relative to one another in a way that corresponds to the quantitative differences among them. Increased and equal graph spacing is used to separate the three "types"—"European," "Intermediate," and "Asio-African"—from one another. Within the "Asio-African type," the "Indian" group is offset more from the African groups than these are from each other. Thus, the space separating "Bulgarians" ("European type") and "Arabs" ("Intermediate type") is greater than the space separating the "English" and the "French" (both "European type") though the differences in "biochemical race-index" and percentage frequency of *B* are less (index difference of 1.0 versus 1.3 and percentage frequency difference of 3.6 versus 4.0). The overall effect is that between-group differences are exaggerated and within-group differences are minimized in the Hirszfelds' study.

Despite Snyder's later insistence that the "nationalities" or "political groups" sampled by blood group researchers were not units of "racial classification" and that "real races" must be identified a posteriori on the basis of empirical evidence, it was the higher-order classification of the "nationalities" or "political groups" that the evidence bore on and not the constitution of these groups themselves. In his a posteriori classification, Snyder drew a distinction between "races" and "types." He stipulated that when groups exhibiting similar blood group allele frequencies are classified as belonging to the same "type," it should not be assumed that they belong to the same "race." Two groups classified as belonging to the same "type" may have arrived at their similar allelic frequencies in different ways, for example, by mixture rather than descent. In other words, contemporary genetic composition alone determines "type," whereas ancestry, in addition, determines "race."

Snyder recognized the arbitrariness of the boundaries he drew. In his correlation table grouping "peoples" "more or less" into "natural groups," he noted that it is, of course, arbitrary to use *five-percent* intervals of allelic frequencies to distinguish groups. The boundaries of these "natural groups" may just as well have been drawn at two-percent or ten-percent intervals (Figure 6.4). Snyder also stated explicitly that his combination of these "natural groups" into seven "types" ("European," "Intermediate," "Hunan," "Indomanchurian," "Africo-Malaysian," "Pacific-American," and "Australian") was done "for convenience." These "convenient" boundaries were not wholly arbitrary, however; certain a priori assumptions can be observed to lead to preferences for some boundaries over others. For example, although on the correlation table, "Danes" are as similar to "Australians" as they

q \ p	0 – 5	6 – 10	11 – 15	16 – 20	21 – 25	26 – 30	31 – 35
0 – 5	AMERICAN INDIANS	AMERICAN INDIANS			AUSTRALIANS		
6 – 10		FILIPINOS		ICELANDERS	DANES	AMERICANS ENGLISH FRENCH ITALIANS MALTANS GERMANS GERMAN JEWS AUSTRIANS DUTCH SERBS GREEKS	NORWEGIANS SWEDES
11–15			SO. AFRICANS	AMER. NEGROES MADEGASCANS MELANESIANS	ARABS TURKS RUSSIANS SPANISH JEWS CZECHS	ROUMANIANS BULGARIANS POLISH JEWS	ARMENIANS
16–20			SENEGALESE SUMATRANS	ANNAMESE JAVANESE SUMATRAN CHINESE	SO CHINESE	SO. CHINESE NO. JAPANESE HUNGARIANS POLES	MID. JAPANESE SO. JAPANESE ROUMANIAN JEWS
21–25				NO KOREANS	MID. KOREANS		SO. KOREANS UKRANIANS
26–30			NATIVES OF INDIA GYPSIES	NO. CHINESE MANCHUS		AINUS	

Figure 6.4 Correlation table grouping "peoples" into "natural groups," using five-percent allelic frequency intervals in the columns and rows to distinguish groups. Reprinted from Snyder L.H. "Human Blood Groups: Their Inheritance and Racial Significance," *American Journal of Physical Anthropology*, © 1926, by permission of Wiley-Liss Inc., a subsidiary of John Wiley & Sons Inc.

are to (white) "Americans" or "Germans," they are included in the "European" and not the "Australian" type. And discrete boundaries for the "types," indicated by definite bounding lines, are also incorporated on the geographical distribution maps that appear at this time (Figure 6.5). These judgments, therefore, combine with more objective features of the maps such as the locations where sampling took place and the frequencies of the a priori groups themselves.

Boyd's mapping approach, a quarter century after Snyder, reveals a similar interplay between objectivity and judgment. Boyd's a posteriori "racial" classification, one he claimed to base on gene frequencies, includes a "hypothetical Early European group" "[r]epresented today by their modern descendants, the Basques," a "European (Caucasoid) group," an "African (Negroid) group," an "Asiatic (Mongoloid) group," an "American Indian group," and an "Australoid group" (1950: 268). Classification was based on the MN blood groups, Rh factor, PTC tasting, and the "secreting gene," in addition to ABO (1950: 268–9). On the

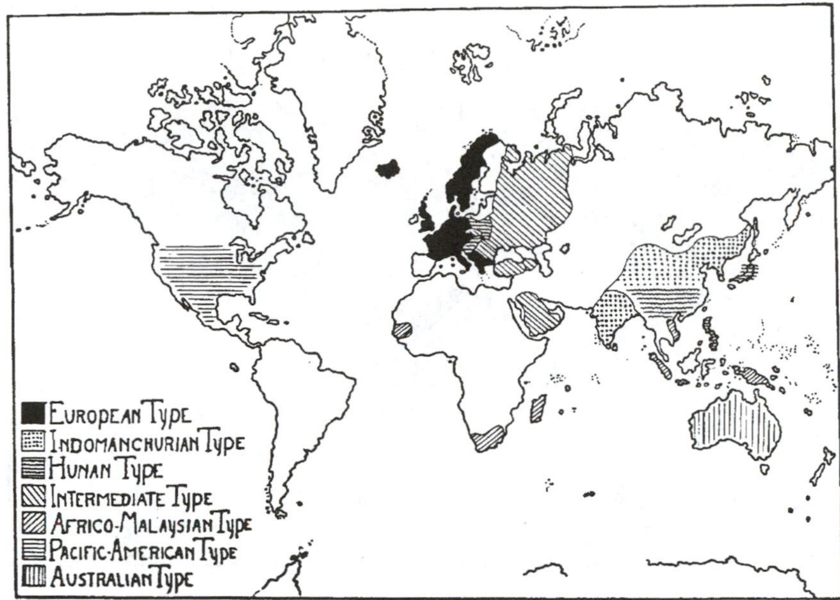

Figure 6.5 World-wide distribution of seven human "types" with discrete boundaries and definite bounding lines (Snyder 1926, figure 6.1).

accompanying geographical map, the six "racial" groups are represented as discrete homogeneous types, their boundaries (apart from the Basque) coinciding with continental divisions (Figure 6.6). Boyd appreciated the geographical pattern of variability in gene frequencies: "It is encouraging that this classification corresponds well, on the whole, with the facts of geography" (1953: 506).

However, the map's touted demonstration of the "correspondence" of Boyd's "racial" classification with "the facts of geography" belies the interplay of objectivity and judgment involved in its construction. Boyd, like Snyder, made explicit mention of several of these judgments. He recognized that the discrete boundaries between a posteriori "racial" groups were imposed: "The method of gene frequencies is completely objective (subject to the qualification that our decision as to what boundary between frequencies is to separate two races remains always a man-made and arbitrary decision)" (1950: 273). He justified the inclusion of only indigenous peoples by appealing to the theoretical preferences of researchers:

> Since we are not most interested in recent historical migrations, we have tried to avoid the confusing effect of recording data on recent migrants, and for America, the Pacific Islands, and Australia, we have plotted information only on the aborigines, omitting the results for the modern inhabitants, whose blood group frequencies, of course, are characteristic of their origins.
>
> (Boyd 1950: 226–7)

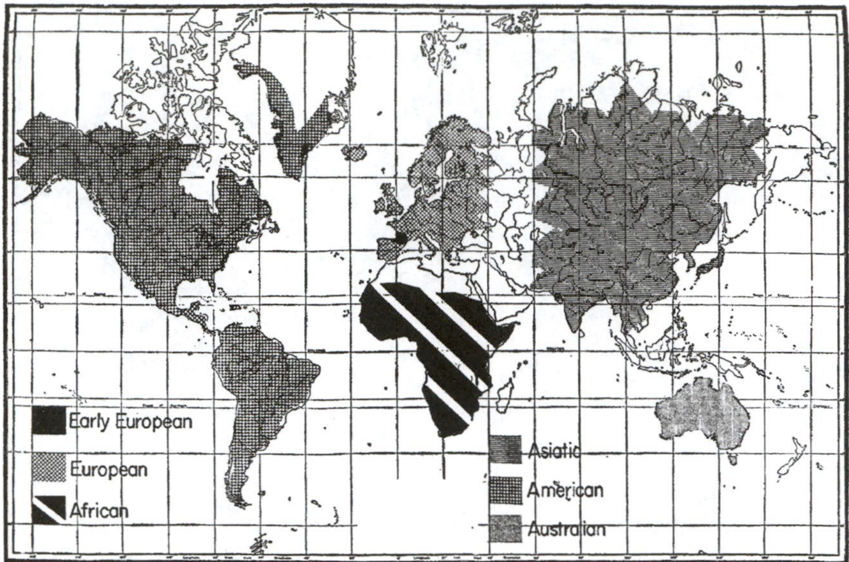

Figure 6.6 World distribution of six genetically defined "races" (Boyd 1950, figure 37). The figure purports to show a correspondence between a posteriori race classfication and geographic distribution.

Additional judgments, though, are obscured. There are no "objective" *frequencies* of blood group alleles at all, without categories of a priori group classification. Recall that Boyd's a priori classification attempted to identify populations that are random mating and in genetic equilibrium, groups he referred to as "tribes" or "ethnic groups." These populations would presumably be the units of a posteriori "racial" classification, placed into higher-order types on the basis of blood group allele frequencies. Although Boyd justified his use of an additional a priori category of classification—a distinction between "aborigines" and "nonaborigenes" (or "original inhabitants" and "modern inhabitants")—in terms of researchers' lack of interest in recent migrations, this lack of interest itself calls for explanation. There is also judgment involved in deciding *which* contemporary populations to count as indigenous to a geographical location—Boyd believed in a single origin for *H. sapiens*, but not that all regions of the world were settled only once, each by a single group. The fixing of population to place is accompanied by an additional a priori category of classification that yields an a posteriori "racial" classification that is based on the comparison of blood group frequencies among continental groups, *not* the local populations that are supposed to be the units of classification. Justification is provided by the potential for continental borders to serve as barriers to migration and gene exchange. But judgment is involved in privileging these over other potential barriers and thereby ignoring the possibility of intra-continental frequency gradients more pronounced than inter-continental frequency gradients.

That humans differ quantitatively, not qualitatively, in the distribution of blood types among groups means not only that a priori classification is necessary, since it is groups not individuals that are the units of a posteriori classification, but that there is significant room for blood group researchers to diverge in their a posteriori approaches to classification. That judgment plays this role leaves the blood group researchers vulnerable to charges of lack of objectivity by HGDP proponents like Marks. It is important not to overlook that researchers like Snyder and Boyd explicitly recognized at least some of the "convenient" or "arbitrary" aspects of their classification schemes. It is also important to realize that this dichotomy between arbitrary/subjective and objective is misleading, and risks the too rapid dismissal of some interesting questions. The play of judgment is unlikely to be entirely arbitrary; theoretical preferences and commitments, practical concerns, or social values may well be implicated. And, crucially, as we argue in this chapter, such judgments may well be *necessary* for scientific objectivity. If we are to reach an adequate understanding of the historical legacy of the ABO blood group research and its implications for contemporary studies of human genome diversity, it is beneficial to explore reasons why particular choices are made, rather than others. In subsequent sections, we consider judgments and choices implicated in disputes that have arisen in a posteriori classification regarding the relative weight to assign serological data over traditional anthropological traits and whether "racial" classifications based on differences in blood group frequencies are unwarranted impositions of invented discontinuity on actual continuity.

Intersections of social–political and biological–anthropological categories of classification

As we saw in the last section, the Hirszfelds treated the "races," "peoples," and "national types" they sampled as biologically and anthropologically meaningful, despite the political foundations of these groups. Snyder recognized the Hirszfelds' assumption to be problematic and argued that "nationalities" and "political groups" are not the appropriate units of "racial" classification, but he proposed no genuine solution. For Boyd, influenced by the evolutionary synthesis, breeding populations were the basic units of "racial" classification. Although such populations can be identified by ostensibly biological and anthropological criteria, social and political categories are frequently imported: groups referred to by Boyd include the "Irish" and the "Basque." Contemporary population geneticists like Cavalli-Sforza consider the substitution of social–political group boundaries for biological–anthropological group boundaries to be expedient in many cases. This facilitates resampling and averts problems with statistical significance that arise in applying Hardy-Weinberg to small populations (Cavalli-Sforza *et al.* 1994: 20–1). Biological–anthropological entities—Mendelian populations or demes—are assumed to exist independently of the social–political units that substitute for them, even if they are not always easy to delineate or retrieve. However, Latour's (1999) concept of circulating reference suggests that social–political categories may not be theoretically expendable. In this section, by exploring the relationships between the groups delineated by the Hirszfelds and the political boundaries and social categories of their time, we consider ways in which social–political and biological–anthropological categories of classification intersect.[9]

The social–political origins of the a priori classification used by the Hirszfelds can be understood, in part, due to the context provided by the First World War. Most of the "national types" identified by the Hirszfelds correspond to the nation-states at war: Britain, France, Italy, Serbia, Russia, and eventually Greece, on the side of the allied powers, and Germany, Austria, Bulgaria, and Turkey, on the side of the central powers. The allied forces occupied Salonika throughout the war. British and French naval forces landed at Salonika in October 1915, just over a year after the war began, and too late to save Serbia from the attack launched by Germany, Austria, and Bulgaria the preceding month. With the assistance of local Greeks, British and French soldiers fortified the city of Salonika, building an "entrenched camp" during the first four months of 1916 (Price 1918). By the summer of 1916, the Anglo-French forces in Salonika had been joined by Russian and Italian troops, as well as Serbian forces reconstituted after their retreat across Albania and evacuation to Allied-occupied Corfu. Greece was neutral when the British and French landed at Salonika in the fall of 1915, but eventually entered the war on the side of the Allies in 1917. The Hirszfelds drew blood from soldiers who found themselves in Salonika, both members of the allied forces and, in the case of captured POWs, members of the central power forces. The uniforms worn by these soldiers provide the evident basis for the Hirszfelds' classification into "national types."

This classification is less straightforward than it may appear at the outset, however. British forces included English, Welsh, Irish, and Scottish battalions, and therefore these categories were also available to the Hirszfelds. It is possible that the soldiers were collectively designated as "English," because the other categories would not be as meaningful to the Polish Hirszfelds, as they would be to Britons. And not all soldiers belonging to the British and French forces were classified as "English" or "French": colonial subjects of Britain and France, originating from India (a colony of Britain) or the Malagasy Republic (Madagascar), Annam (Vietnam), or Senegal (colonies of France), were grouped according to the boundaries of these colonial possessions. The Senegalese were the only "national type" that was also described in terms of the traditional racial categories of the nineteenth century, in this case, as "Negroes." This is no doubt because European eyes saw "race," not just "nationality," when it came to sub-Saharan Africans. In this respect, the Hirszfelds' classification is not so different from the characterization of the composition of the Allied forces present in Salonika by official war correspondent, G. Ward Price, of the *Daily Mail*:

> SALONICA is a very museum of the Allies. Of the principal Allied Armies in the field only representatives of the Americans and Portuguese are lacking, and there used to be rumours that even they were coming. In the Balkans there is none of the isolation that keeps the armies of different nationalities apart in France. All of us rub shoulders at our common base of Salonica. The Annamite and the Serbian sit side by side in the tram without either

> finding the juxtaposition odd. A brigade of blond Russians may be relieved by a brigade of black Senegalese. Italian, Frenchman, Englishman and Greek will share a table in a restaurant, and it is very satisfactory to find that in spite of his customary ignorance of any language but his own,—in which respect he is no worse than the average Frenchman, however,—the Englishman seems as generally popular all round as any of the Allies.
>
> (Price 1918, in Chapter IX, The Coming of the Russians and the Italians)

Not all individuals from whom blood was taken as representatives of the "national types" mentioned thus far were uniformed soldiers. Some of the designations, such as "Jews," also fall outside of the "national type" categories as constituted by the at-war nations. To understand the origins of these designations, the history of the region of Salonika also needs to be considered.

Salonika was a pluralistic and cosmopolitan port city, part of the Ottoman Empire from the fifteenth century until Turkey's defeat in the Balkan wars of 1912–13. Greece occupied Salonika in the war and formally took it over in 1913, despite Austria's preference that it become an international city and Bulgaria's own claims upon it. Surrounding Macedonia was divided between Greece, Serbia, and Bulgaria.[10] Thus, at least for residents of the Salonika region, "Greek" had become only very recently a national identity when the Hirszfelds were taking blood samples at the end of the 1910s. Ottoman administrative units, *millets*, were based on religious affiliation. The 1900 census has Salonika's 173,000 residents divided among some 80,000 Jews, 60,000 Muslims, and 30,000 Christians. Muslims answered to the Ottoman caliph (who was also the sultan); non-Muslims had their own patriarchs in Constantinople. These religious identities intersected with a range of linguistic, ethnic, and national identities. Ladino-speaking Sephardic Jews vastly outnumbered Azkhenazi Jews. There were Greek- and Slavic-speaking Orthodox Christians who answered to the Greek patriarch and Bulgarian-speaking Orthodox Christians who had by this time gained their own patriarch. The Armenian patriarch oversaw the affairs of Armenian Christians whose church had always been independent of the Roman and Byzantine churches. There were also Gypsies, and when Serbia, Greece, and Bulgaria became independent states in the nineteenth century, and sought to extend their boundaries to include their Macedonian compatriots, Serbian, Greek, and Bulgarian became available as national identities.[11] The decade leading up to the Balkan wars (1912–13) was a time of much repression in the region during the rule of Abdul Hamid who played these groups and the European powers off one another, and due to the failure of the "Young Turks" upon seizing power in 1908 to unify these groups under a secular Turkish national identity. Hence, the "national types" that comprised the Hirszfelds' a priori classification were quite contested identities. Local "Mohammedean Macedonians" were used to represent "Turks," but this substitutes a religious identity for nationality and ethnicity. Similarly, refugees from Monastir, whom the Hirszfelds used as representatives of a Jewish "national type," shared a common religious identity but had varied ancestral roots.

Thus, the a priori classification used by the Hirszfelds reflects the composition and structure of WWI military forces, regional and global geo-political struggles, and local history. H.R. Wilkinson's book *Maps and Politics: A Review of the Ethnographic Cartography of Macedonia* looks at how maps have been used as political devices in the region of Macedonia, put forward to substantiate the claims of rival powers. Any assignments of individuals to one "national" category or another will necessarily privilege some set of competing interests over others. Yet, "national type" and the particular array of nationalities used in their study were not assumed by the Hirszfelds to be at all problematic as an a priori categorization for anthropological research.

The access the Hirszfelds had to soldiers and refugees from different parts of the world because of the war provided them with an unusual opportunity, but even they used the results of studies that had been previously carried out for a portion of their data. Subsequent efforts by blood group researchers to map the global distribution of the ABO alleles relied to a far greater degree on data from multiple sources. Researchers like Snyder and Boyd were responsible for some of the data included in their comprehensive studies; these were data obtained from the analysis of blood samples they themselves collected, or blood samples sent to them by anthropologists in the field or physicians in the clinic. Other data were taken from the published or unpublished results of researchers working in genetics, physiology, medicine, and anthropology. Extensive data, especially for large cities in industrialized countries, became available to researchers through the cooperation of agencies involved in transfusion services and paternity testing. Hence, the data that are presented in comprehensive global surveys of blood group distributions have been gleaned from a vast number of sources and a wide array of research studies. These studies have been informed by a diversity of aims and interests, both practical and theoretical. This raises questions about methodology: how people are sampled, how samples are transported, stored, and analyzed, and how classifications travel between lab and field. Do the group classifications found in published tables and maps of ABO frequencies refer to *real* human groups?

Latour criticizes philosophers for attempting to solve the problem of reference while ignoring the details of scientific practice. Latour's concept of circulating reference calls attention to the careful and painstaking work scientists perform that establishes and maintains concrete ties to and in the world, in their travels to the field and back to the lab and desk. Adopting an empirical approach to the problem of reference, Latour travels to the Amazon basin with a botanist, a geographer, and two soil scientists. The goal of the scientific study is to collect data on the characteristics of the soil in a region where the savanna borders the forest (a "natural" not "man-made" boundary, Latour points out) in order to address the question whether the forest is receding and the savanna advancing, or vice versa. Latour follows the "movement of abstraction" that proceeds from the Amazonian landscape to its diagrammatic representation in the publication that ensues, in a series of intermediary steps that "pack the world into words" (1999: 24). Each of these steps involves the extraction of matter to be used subsequently as a form in the representation of a new phenomenon, or referent. The bagged soil sample is marked with the number of the hole and the depth at which it was taken. The field notebook records, for each sample, the location's coordinates, the number of the hole, the time and depth at which it was taken, and qualitative data like color and texture. Soil samples are sorted by depth and compared by being placed into location-coded cardboard cubes arranged in a coordinate system within a transportable wooden frame. Soil color is attributed a numerical value according to a common standard. These quantities and relations are represented in charts, diagrams, equations, maps, or sketches. Latour points out that at no point along this chain of reference is an opening created that resembles the traditional "gap in representation" that must be bridged by "correspondence." Discontinuity is introduced: the diagram does not resemble the tray of samples, the notebook etchings do not resemble the landscape. But continuity is always maintained; in each successive phenomenon, there is a "trace" of the former. This means that the chain of reference is reversible. "Traceability" in the "downstream" direction permits the circulation of truth-value in scientific discourse and connects the scientific text, and its internal referents like charts and diagrams, to the world through each intermediary step.

Latour emphasizes that the circulation of reference that is responsible for the construction of objects of scientific knowledge, and the ability to make truth claims about these objects, would not be possible without preexisting formal structures: "Yes, scientists master the world, but only if the world comes to them in the form of two-dimensional, superposable, combinable inscriptions" (1999: 29). At no point do investigators engage in the "observation of raw data," as traditional empiricists assume. The Amazonian field site is a "minimalist" laboratory: the botanist tags trees to establish a system of Cartesian coordinates for her plot of land, the soil scientist marks his holes by using a compass for angles and the unraveling spooled thread of a "topofil" for distances, a numbering system is devised for the soil samples, the protocol for notebook records is agreed upon, the "pedocomparator" furnishes a two-dimensional coordinate system that can be transposed to a paper diagram, soil scientists join cartographers and painters in adopting the Munsell code of colors as a common standard, and so on. And knowledge of this small part of the world is possible only if the investigators can locate the site and make their way there. For this, they need the help of additional inscriptions, an atlas map of Amazonia juxtaposed with aerial photographs—inscriptions—Latour notes, that would not exist without the disciplines of trigonometry, cartography, and geography, the labor of draftspeople, engravers, and printers, and technologies like plane radar and orbiting satellites. They also need access to funding sources and institutional support. This entire network is required for the circulation of reference. If the network breaks down, reference disappears.

Just like the atlas map and aerial photographs that permit this research team to travel to the Amazonian location that interests them, political maps are far more useful than geographical maps in facilitating field work in biological and anthropological studies of most human populations. Planes and trains travel to countries and cities, not river valleys and mountaintops. Because human population geneticists and biological anthropologists rely on multiple sources for genetic data and may be involved in collaborations with cultural anthropologists, linguists, medical researchers, and others, social and political boundaries may provide the best common denominator. The group consent model for population-based biological and anthropological research also relies on establishing contact with leaders of social or political units (Reardon 2002: ch. 5). There are many reasons why researchers find it expedient to substitute social–political categories of classification for biological–anthropological ones. At the same time, they consider these to be practical concerns; from a theoretical point of view, they do not doubt the independent existence of biological–anthropological entities (Mendelian populations or demes), and they seek to eliminate the social and political "contaminants" of "objective" knowledge. However, Latour's concept of circulating reference suggests that these assumptions may be false. If reference is lost once the network that supports its circulation breaks down, any social–political categories imported by a priori classifications cannot simply be abandoned.

Recall Latour's remark that the researchers he was accompanying were interested in a boundary between savanna and forest that was "natural," not "man-made." Biological–anthropological categories of classification similarly aim to represent "natural" discontinuities. Presumably, adopting a naturalistic approach to the study of human genome diversity would avoid making a priori assumptions about population or, for the Hirszfelds, "racial" boundaries, permitting such boundaries to be revealed instead by existing genetic discontinuities. This approach might take blood samples from a specified number of individuals found at, or within a specified distance from, intersecting points of a geographical grid where the coordinates of the grid have been established by a map that includes natural landmarks such as oceans, rivers, or mountain ranges. This would conceivably establish a chain of reference, connecting sampling location, the individual sampled, the labeled blood sample transported from field to lab, the coded vial of blood stored in the lab refrigerator, the written record of the blood group based on agglutination tests, and, finally, the data point on a chart or map. The avoidance of social–political categories of classification would also protect objectivity, understood in the traditional sense.

There are problems with the above scenario, however. As we have already discussed, blood group or allelic *frequencies* describe groups, not individuals, and it is these values that are tabled and mapped as the bases for a posteriori classification. To retrace the chain of reference for a particular data point on a geographical map is to end up with the *collection* of individuals from whom blood was drawn *and* at the location where blood was drawn. Of course, specific individuals do not interest the population geneticist or biological anthropologist; just as the numbered bag of soil is understood to be representative of soil found at a given location, so the sampled individuals are taken to be representative of a larger group that resides at the location. Continuity in reference over time is also assumed for both the soil and the group; an increase in clay content of the soil or a decrease in frequency of a particular allele is likely to be of theoretical interest. The chain of reference will be broken if researchers return to the field location at a later date and do not encounter individuals belonging to the *same* group that had been sampled. While, for the soil scientist, geographical location may suffice to fix reference, it cannot satisfy the population geneticist or biological anthropologist. This is reflected in the limitations of an ostensibly naturalistic geographical grid strategy for sampling human genome diversity.

As plans for the HGDP unfolded, a debate arose concerning whether a geographical grid or population-based approach should be used for sampling (Roberts 1991). Even proponents of the grid approach like Allan Wilson did not rely simply on geographical location to fix reference. They called for only "indigenous" peoples to be sampled at each point in the grid. This is a strategy that permits reference to circulate by maintaining a connection between people and place. But, at the same time, it demands the creation of boundaries, both spatial and temporal. What are the boundaries of a person's territory to which she is indigenous? How many of a person's ancestors must have lived in that territory, and for what duration of time, for him to be indigenous? The natural landmarks of geographical maps that serve as grid coordinates cannot provide the basis for a priori classification. Natural landmarks serve as boundaries for people only if these people represent them as boundaries, that is, imbue them with social–cultural meanings and transmit these meanings across generations. And if people represent these as *group* boundaries, social organization into groups must already exist. Thus, social–political categories of a priori classification are not simply a matter of practical expedience for biologists and anthropologists. The naturalistic approach is unrealistic because it prohibits the circulation of reference. If we expect evolutionary narratives and explanations to say something about the world, social–political categories of a priori classification are not even theoretically expendable.

Privileging blood groups over traditional anthropological traits in classification

Particularly significant to Cavalli-Sforza, in his consideration of the historical legacy of ABO blood group research, is the pioneering by the Hirszfelds of a new approach to the study of human variation through "the introduction of genetic markers, which are strictly inherited and basically immune to the problem of rapid changes induced by the environment" (Cavalli-Sforza *et al.* 1994: 18). The use of biological reagents to determine blood group differences continued to be used over the next few decades, until the mid-century introduction of electrophoresis to discern protein differences, and, finally, in recent years, the availability of restriction enzymes and PCR to identify DNA differences. In contrast, Marks (1996) regards the serological research initiated by the Hirszfelds as an early attempt by non-anthropologists to supersede physical anthropologists by treating their own data, for example blood group frequencies, as more important in the classification of human groups than traditional anthropological characters like skin color and stature. Marks contends that the "racial serologists" improperly substituted data on blood groups for data on a range of characteristics, including those traditionally used by physical anthropologists. According to Marks, physical anthropologists had "effectively" integrated genetics into their discipline by the 1960s, analyzing blood samples they collected in the field. But blood group data never trumped other data. Today's focus on DNA data continues this usurping trend.

Given the interplay between objectivity and judgment, it is worth examining the justifications blood group researchers like the Hirszfelds, Snyder, Haldane, and Boyd provided for abandoning the anthropometric data traditionally used by physical anthropologists for "racial" classification and the study of human evolution. The blood groups are not evidently useful traits for classification. Since the Hirszfelds' time, it has been recognized that blood group allele frequencies vary quantitatively, not qualitatively, which means that the blood groups cannot provide "racial" characters, or markers, that sort individual humans into discrete groups. Also, since the Hirszfelds' time, it has been recognized that serological characteristics appear to vary independently of the characteristics that anthropologists had traditionally used for classification (Davis 1935).

The Hirszfelds noted that the blood groups appeared to be inherited as independent traits in conformity with Mendel's law (though mistaken in their belief that A and B are inherited as dominant alleles segregating at two loci), to stay constant in individuals over time even in the presence of conditions affecting the blood like anemia, malaria, and typhoid, and to remain intact when passed from parents to offspring. They also noted that environmental factors like climate, diet, and disease could not have affected the differences in blood group frequencies because these were shared by members of all of the "national types" represented in Salonika during the war (aside from the vegetarianism of the Indians). It was thus the hereditary nature of the blood groups that recommended them to the Hirszfelds. Their decision to privilege serological over traditional anthropological traits in classification therefore did not deviate from, but concurred with, anthropologists' views that "racial" characters should be inherited traits and, by implication, that "races" should be hereditary groups.

Snyder took a similar tack: "In the human race the blood groups occur as fixed bio-chemical conditions, subject to the laws of heredity. As such they provide a method of studying racial origins and relationships" (1926: 233). Snyder presented a couple of additional reasons for adopting a serological approach to "studies of racial relationships": the blood groups appeared to be unaffected by constitutional factors like age or sex and environmental factors like climate, living conditions, or x-rays, and, apart from the unresolved question of linkage to disease traits, "it is difficult to conceive of any effect of selection on the proportions of the groups" (1926: 251). For Snyder, then, the constancy of the blood groups over time promised access to knowledge of genealogical origins and relations; "races" became not just hereditary, but genealogical, groups. However, in his 1929 book, likely in response to serology's critics, Snyder emphasized that serology is not to be taken as authoritative: "the blood groups are simply additional anthropological characters which must take their place along with other longer-known criteria in the study of racial relationships" (1929: 117). This served as no more than a disclaimer, though; Snyder proceeded to use only blood groups for "racial" classification and even to invent four "laws of serological race-classification" based on the correlation of proximity of genealogical relationships to similarities in blood group frequencies.

Haldane (1931) defended outright the superiority of "racial" classification on the basis of blood group frequencies. In contrast to traits traditionally used by anthropologists, ABO differences appeared to be monogenic, genetically determined, unsusceptible to environmental modification, and selectively neutral. Haldane believed that traditional anthropological traits like skin color are often adaptive and consequently of limited value for the study of evolutionary history. One reason is convergent evolution: adaptive traits may arise independently in different populations exposed to similar environments—for example, dark skin color across tropical regions in response to sunlight—and thus confuse questions of origins. In contrast, Haldane asserted, "we may take the proportions of the blood group genes in any population as indicating racial origin rather than effects of climate or other environmental influences" (1931[1933]: 67). A second reason is that adaptive traits may increase in frequency relatively quickly in populations, whereas selectively neutral traits, unless the population size is small, will stay fairly constant in frequency. As a result, Haldane concluded, adaptive and neutral traits can serve different purposes for "racial" classification:

> We may perhaps compare the information given by different characters on the structure of a population with that given by different rocks on the structure of a country. The more highly adaptive characters, such as pigmentation, give most information on the immediate past (for example, the racial origins of the peoples of the United States), just as the recent and Pleistocene deposits tell of recent glaciation, vulcanism, and so on. The blood-groups on the other hand give information of a more fundamental character on racial structure, just as do the palaeozoic rocks on geological structure. The contradiction between the two sources of information is thus only apparent.
>
> (Haldane 1940: 477)

Haldane, along with the Hirszfelds and Snyder, by privileging the blood groups as inherited traits, constructed a hereditary "race" concept and "races" as hereditary groups. For Haldane, like Snyder, "race" was about origins and genealogical relations, not adaptive similarities; "races" were genealogical groups or clades, not ecotypes. In Haldane's case, the deepest origins and most distant genealogical ties were "fundamental"; the blood groups were preferred not just because they provide the most reliable passport to our human evolutionary past but because they are supposed to be the longest persisting record of that past.

On the one hand, the blood group researchers privileged serological over traditional anthropological traits because they shared a desire for objectivity: the hereditary transmission of ABO was believed known and environmental influences on the development of the blood group phenotypes were believed controlled or irrelevant. On the other hand, judgments were involved, judgments which at the same time served to construct a concept of "race" and "racial" groups themselves. Such judgments are not arbitrary; they reflect the researchers' shared theoretical interests in historical questions concerning origins, migrations, and genealogical relations rather than causal questions directed to mechanisms of evolutionary change like selection and drift. These judgments, and the theoretical preferences and commitments that direct them, are implicated at each link of the chain of reference that connects blood samples in the field to published tables and maps of blood group frequencies. Although this "movement of abstraction" obscures such subjectivities as judgment, it may be possible to recover them by attending closely to the mapping representations.

Besides the bar graph and geographical distribution map representations found in papers by the Hirszfelds and Snyder, blood group researchers made use of geographical frequency maps to address historical evolutionary questions about origins, migrations, and genealogical relations. In a 1931 article, "Prehistory in the Light of Genetics," Haldane published a geographical frequency map for the *B* allele that made use of isolines to connect equivalent values for allelic frequencies (using five-percent intervals) at different geographical sites. Assumptions built into a diffusion model allow the isolines to represent a third dimension on the map, that of time. The model assumes that a given allele originated at the geographical location where its present frequency is greatest. The allele is assumed to have "diffused" outwardly from its site of origin in all directions—witness the curvature of the isolines that connect points of equal frequency on the map (Figure 6.7). The movement of people is assumed to account for the "diffusion" of alleles. Historical migrations are assumed to have extended as far in distance from the site of origin as the particular allele is found. Multiple sites of origin for an allele are entertained as a possibility if centers of high frequency accompanied by a radiating pattern of diminishing frequencies occur in different regions of the globe. Additional assumptions permit the further temporalization of events. If a gene mutates a number of times, and it is possible to ascertain which alleles are ancestral to others, the relative timing of different historical migrations might be surmised. Haldane assumed that the most geographically widespread alleles are the oldest.

On the basis of the map of *B* allele frequencies, and discussion of the geographical distribution of *A* allele frequencies, Haldane concluded: "The general result of blood group studies... is to point to a migration in all directions from Central Asia into a more primitive population" (1931[1933]: 71). Haldane held that the *B* allele arose in Central Asia with migration outward during prehistoric times extending as far as Western Europe but not reaching the Americas or Australia. The more widespread *A* allele he believed arose either far earlier than the *B* allele or in several locations. Since the *O(R)* allele was found to be most prevalent across the globe, Haldane considered it to be the ancestral state and characteristic of the most "primitive" humans. This ruled out a historical migration outward from the center of the *O(R)* allele's highest frequency in North America.

In a 1935 article, "Human Blood Groups and Anthropology," Leland C. Wyman and Boyd presented geographical frequency distribution maps using isolines for

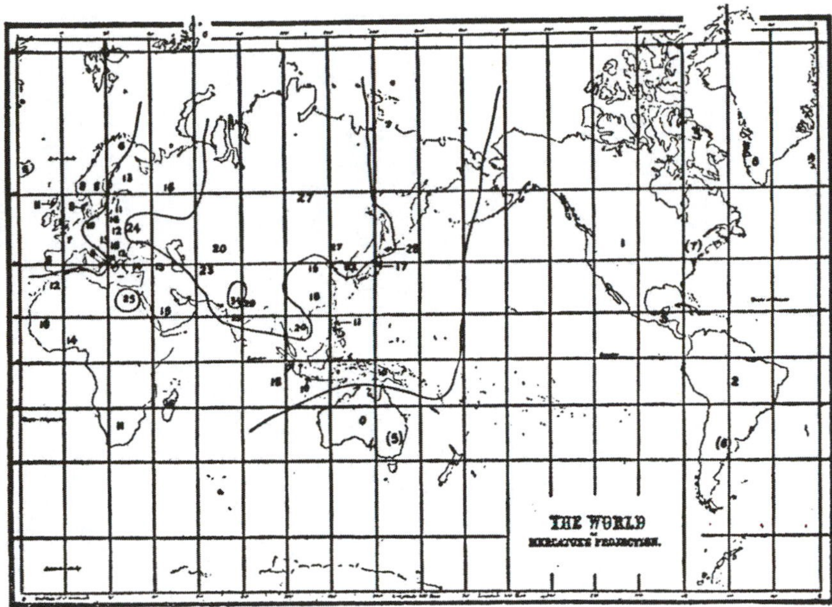

Figure 6.7 Geographical frequency map for the blood-group *B* allele in human populations using isolines to connect equivalent allelic frequency values (five-percent intervals) at different geographical sites. Both values and isolines are plotted (Haldane 1931, figure 1). Reprinted by permission of HarperCollins Publishers Inc.

the *A* and *B* genes (*p* and *q* alleles). The map for *B* was based on Haldane's 1931 map and additional data (Figure 6.8). One notable difference is that where Haldane's map superimposes isolines on raw frequency data at five-percent intervals, Wyman and Boyd's map includes only the isolines themselves, a judgment that maximizes the map's appearance of continuity in frequencies. Wyman and Boyd noted that their map seemed to support Haldane's hypothesis: "If the map for the gene *B* (*q*) is examined, it will be seen that the high center in Asia near the Punjab, and the way the contour lines surround it, are strongly suggestive of the origin of this factor in the region of northern India, and its subsequent spread into other parts of the world, including Europe" (1935: 186). However, Wyman and Boyd did not accept this hypothesis. They contended that blood group differences reflected a pattern of dispersal that was older than "the differentiation of the present races" (1935: 192). They believed that there had been inadequate time for multiple independent mutations of *A* and *B* to have arisen and spread following inhabitation of the New World, unless the blood groups are affected by selection which appeared unlikely. In addition, the *B* gene had been discovered in indigenous South Americans, its frequency higher than could be accounted for by recent mixture with Europeans and without additional genetic evidence of

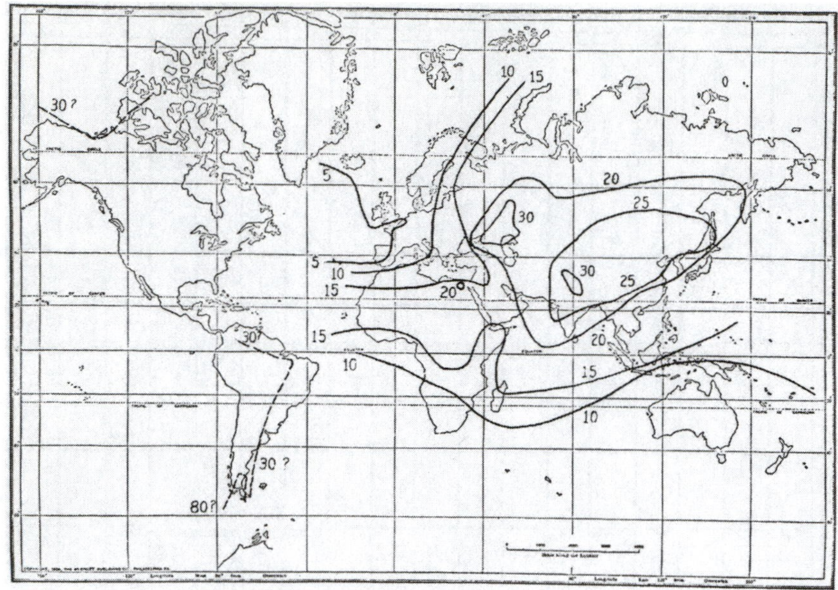

Figure 6.8 Distribution of frequencies of the gene for *B*(*q*) in percent, based on Haldane's 1931 map (cf. Figure 6.7). Isolines but not data are plotted in support of the view that blood group differences reflected a pattern of dispersal older than the differentiation of the present races (Wyman and Boyd 1935, figure 2). See text for discussion.

genealogical proximity to central Asians. Wyman and Boyd leaned toward the hypothesis that we inherited the ABO blood groups from our nonhuman primate ancestors.

The "isogene" geographical frequency maps (as Boyd [1950] referred to them) accompanied by diffusion model assumptions, then, are suggestive of common ancestral origins and the directions in which historical migrations occurred, as well as, perhaps, their relative timing. This is similar to Sturtevant and Dobzhansky's use of geographical distribution maps of chromosomal inversions to construct phylogenetic maps in *Drosophila pseudoobscura* and hypothesize about historical migrations (Gannett and Griesemer, Chapter 4). There is an important difference, though. The Drosophila phylogenies were of individual chromosomes. Ancestral–descendant relations between chromosomal types were established according to the number of inversions that separate them: under the assumption of parsimony, the fewer the number of inversions, the more closely related the chromosomes are judged to be. This assumes material continuity between chromosomes. But as we have already emphasized, gene frequencies are properties of groups, not individuals (whether organisms, chromosomes, or genes). Although isoline maps represent frequencies of single blood group alleles, the relevant ancestral–descendant relations hold between groups of people. The use of isolines (and isopleths where intervening spaces are filled in) effaces the discontinuities of assumed group boundaries. By replacing discontinuities with continuities, this step in the "movement of abstraction" attempts to discharge the subjectivities associated with the application of a priori categories of group classification that is required for the objectification of quantitative differences in blood group allele frequencies.

To this point, we have interpreted the maps in terms of a fairly straightforward Latourian story of small judgments and small extractions generating a reference chain and objectivity secured by the possibility of backtracking to the source. The steps needed to produce geographic maps, particularly the isoline maps we have been discussing, require further cartographic consideration.

Thematic mapping represents the geographic occurrence and variation of one or a few phenomena. This cartographic form matured in the mid-nineteenth century as a result of advances in cartographic technique such as lithography and the use of tones, shading, and color, of advances in world-wide base map production (as, for example in Berhaus' 1848 atlas and Johnson's English language reprint), and with increased interest in and development of statistical data (Robinson 1982).

The epistemology of thematic mapping work—the discovery of geographical structure through mapping phenomena—we argue, is caught between the imagery of nineteenth-century mechanical objectivity and twentieth-century scientific expertise. On the one hand, maps epitomize a form of mechanical, if humanly constructed, objectivity. The rhetoric of mapping places humans outside the epistemic loop since maps are supposed to express isomorphisms between representation and geographic reality. Thus, thematic mapping, which involves plotting data on maps, is a quintessential "objectifying move" in the mechanical sense that data are extracted from the geographic setting and plotted in a mechanical way according to a mathematical coordinate system that avoids human bias, judgment, and interpretation. Thus, any discovered patterns are "there" to be discovered. On the other hand, the discovery of geographic pattern requires some classification system, else the pattern is a mere report of uninterpreted data. This "perennial cartographic problem" (Robinson 1982: 139) is reflected in the tension between mechanical objectivity and expert judgment in the mapping of human blood group frequencies. "The method of gene frequencies is completely objective," Boyd (1950: 273) wrote, in the cartographic sense that frequency data correctly plotted on accurate base maps cannot lie. However, the method is dependent on initiating and continuing scientific judgments of an appropriate classificatory scheme if geographical patterns in the data are to be discovered. Without an a priori classification of either data groups or geographic units, there can be no pattern "in" the data.

The maps do not plot actual blood type data, but rather, blood group frequencies. Frequencies are population properties which thus do not occur at points on geographic maps, but rather cover geographic regions. The numbers indicating frequencies are instances of "map generalization." Awareness of the man-made and arbitrary decision to assign a mapped point to cover a geographic area is carried throughout the debate about anthropological genetics as evidenced, for example, by this statement of Cavalli-Sforza's: "Gene frequencies are not geographic features like altitude or compass direction, which can be measured precisely at any point on the earth's surface; rather, they are properties of a population that occupies an area of finite extent" (2000: 26). Moreover, because geographic patterns might not be discernible even if the frequencies are plotted, isolines are often drawn to connect equal blood group frequencies. Similar to topographic lines of equal elevation, albeit not applying literally to geographic points as do elevations, blood group frequency isolines seem to indicate geographically continuous frequency distributions. However, the isolines represent deliberate falsehoods in two respects.[12] First, the lines very rarely connect all the equal frequencies on the world base map and sometimes they connect areas that cannot represent equal frequencies. Continents and other widely separated geographic areas having equal frequency points are typically not connected by isolines and, just as clearly, frequencies of blood groups across continents could not be so connected since blood group frequencies in the oceans (and across other remote geographical features) are zero. Second, there is the arbitrary and man-made decision to choose a frequency interval between isolines to plot data on geographic maps, with the implication that the interpolated values between isolines represent valid inferences of blood group frequency. Both of these idealizations reflect the view that frequency data must be continuous, but the lines are no mere interpolations: they give the impression of data where none exists.

Once it is recognized that the ABO system has always existed in *H. sapiens*, leaving room neither for material overlap of ancestral and descendant genes nor for hypothesized mutation events or "pure races" of A, B, and O individuals, historical narratives about origins and migrations become problematic. Left are similarities in relative ABO frequencies as the basis for inferring the proximity of genealogical ties between populations separated in space. The continuity of these populations over time is assumed, just like the continuity of chromosomes over time is assumed when numbers of inversions are used in *D. pseudoobscura* as a measure of genealogical proximity. It is also assumed that selection is not operating, as geographical location would then matter. Latour's concept of circulating reference is again helpful. We have seen that attempts to discard social–political categories of a priori classification interrupt the "traceability" of the chain of reference and consequently interfere with the circulation of reference. Historical questions concerning origins, migrations, and genealogical relations make further demands on fixing reference. Reliance on an a priori category of classification like indigenous–nonindigenous to fix people to place becomes unavailable to the researcher whose interests lie with these historical questions. Migrations occur between geographical locations and genealogical ties connect people living in different places. For the circulation of reference to be maintained, researchers need to fix group identity across space and time. This need is reflected in Boyd's (1950) presentation of a series of four maps that postulates a hypothetical history of human migration that could account for contemporary distributions of blood allele frequencies. The series begins with an original population in Asia that possesses a characteristic distribution of blood allele frequencies and then traces the dispersal of descendant populations of this group to all continents of the world (Figure 6.9). In contrast to "isogene" maps, these geographical frequency maps are more strongly suggestive of the existence of underlying groups since the relative frequencies of all alleles are included.

In his critique of the HGDP, Marks takes contemporary human population geneticists to task for sharing with "racial serologists" a reliance on simplistic migration hypotheses: "the major historical processes invoked to explain contemporary patterns of diversity are essentially the same as the most quickly discredited ideas of early serologists: mass invasions of pure and qualitatively distinct primordial races imposing their gene pools upon others" (1996: 359). The Hirszfelds did indeed subscribe to the a priori assumption that groups once existed that were "pure" or genetically homogeneous—an *A* "race" and a *B* "race." The story of human evolution became a narrative of originally "pure" races blending through migration to become the "mixed" groups—the "national types" and the continental "types"—of our time. Without doubt, the Hirszfelds were mistaken in this assumption, but historical explanations of blood group frequencies in terms of migration and mixture were common among the serologists, and such evolutionary narratives continue to be employed today. But more important than this continuity itself are a number of issues implicated in it.

Vestiges of long-disproved assumptions of "pure and qualitatively distinct primordial races imposing their gene pools" persist because of the need to fix group identity across space and time if circulating reference is to be maintained when historical questions concerning origins, migrations, and genealogical relations are addressed. We cannot speak of group origins or unique common ancestors without well-delineated "primordial" groups locatable in space and time. We cannot speak of dates and routes of group migrations without assuming the constancy and integrity of these groups over space and time. We cannot speak of genealogical relationships other than between "qualitatively distinct" groups for which there are sorting criteria for inclusion and exclusion. We cannot speak of the admixture of groups without some modified sense of "purity" in terms of the relative homogeneity and heterogeneity of "qualitatively distinct" "gene pools" with characteristic compositions. The bounding of genes—and the people who possess and pass on these genes—across space and time is a necessary a priori assumption for all such narratives or explanations. Strict endogamy will, of course, do the trick, if it can be established that there exists a socially discernible group such that mates are chosen only within the group and group members can trace *all* of their ancestral roots back to that group, or to a well-delineated ancestral group.

Hence, we find in Haldane's interpretation of the Hirszfelds' results, an attempt to establish the legitimacy of a priori assumptions that are required if blood group frequencies are to be informative about "racial" origins and relationships. Haldane noted the anthropological value of the human blood groups as nonselective traits that made it possible to "determine the proportions of *pure*

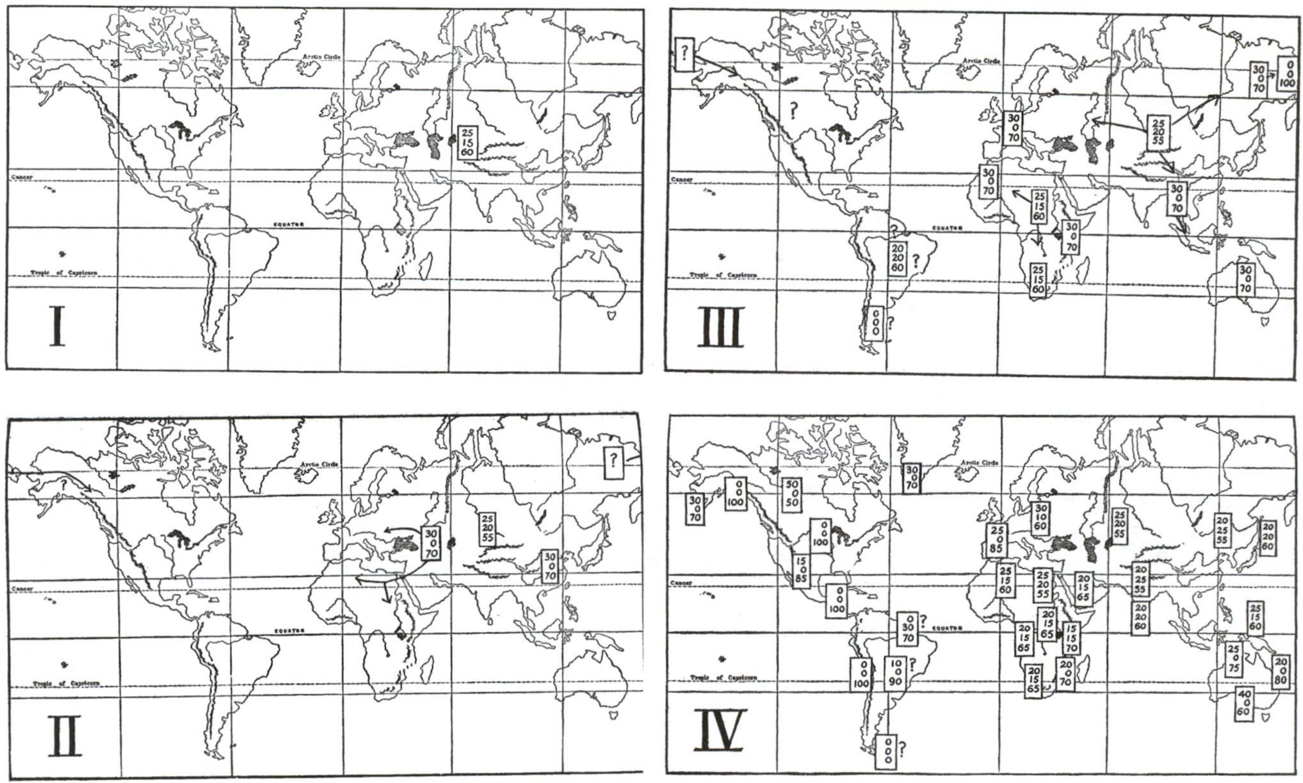

Figure 6.9 Series of four geographical maps postulating a hypothetical history of human migration to account for contemporary distributions of blood allele frequencies. The series traces four stages of historical dispersal, beginning (I) with an original population in Asia and tracing the dispersal of descendant populations (II–IV) to all continents of the world. Note that relative frequencies of all alleles (A, B, and O) are included (boxed columns of numbers) rather than just a single allele, Boyd 1950 (figures 46a–d).

races which have gone to make a mixed people from its present composition" (1931[1933]: 64; italics added). He also referred to the endogamy of Salonika's various groups and the ability to draw conclusions about the "racial" origins of these people as a result:

> The proportions [of genes A, B, and R] are constant in a given race, and are not affected by changed environment in the course of a few centuries. Thus at Salonika there have been endogamous Greek, Turkish, and Jewish communities since the late fifteenth century. The Greek proportions are typically Balkan. The Jews are much the same as Arabs. The Turks are decidedly Asiatic. . . .
>
> Clearly, then, we may take the proportions of the blood group genes in any population as indicating racial origin rather than effects of climate or other environmental influences.
>
> (1931[1933]: 67)

This mention of "purity" seems uncharacteristic of a scientist Elazar Barkan describes as one of a small group of British biologists who contributed to the fight against scientific racism prior to the Second World War by demonstrating the incompatibility of Mendelian principles with notions of "racial purity" and the construction of "racial" typologies (1992: 162). Haldane appealed to "purity" in a relative sense. Because according to Hardy-Weinberg, genetic equilibrium is reached in one generation of random mating, it is possible to determine the relative proportions two or more parental populations have contributed to a "mixed" or "heterogeneous" population. The parental populations are regarded as relatively unmixed or homogeneous and in possession of characteristic constellations of allelic frequencies treated as genetic identities that remain constant across space and time.

We see this today in HGDP plans to sample "isolated" and "primitive" populations, and the urgency attached to carrying this out before these groups disappear. Just as geneticists in the USA have used African-Americans and Asian-Americans as proxies for African and Asian populations that are difficult to access because of spatial distance, the peoples targeted by the HGDP are to be proxies—regarded as "remnants"—for temporally distant populations living centuries and millenia ago. Historical narratives about migrations and mixtures cannot be told without these proxies, and which groups become proxies will depend on researchers' interests—and assumptions about *which* groups' origins matter, a choice that is deeply embedded in social and cultural milieus. This is illustrated in Nurit Kirsh's (2003) "Population Genetics in Israel in the 1950s: The Unconscious Internalization of Ideology." Kirsh points out ways in which post-WWII population genetics research in Israel was shaped by the Zionist narrative. This narrative about the return of Jews to an ancient homeland from which they had long ago been dispersed assumes the maintenance of biological as well as religious identity across space and time. Kirsh presents evidence that Israeli geneticists were influenced, perhaps unconsciously, by Zionism. More so than their non-Israeli counterparts, they tended to stress genetic similarities and minimize genetic differences among Jews across space and time. When attention to genetic differences could not be avoided, explanations were preferred that did not make reference to intermarriage and gene influx from non-Jewish populations. Israeli Arabs, and therefore their genealogical ties to Israeli Jews, were virtually ignored in the studies.

Marks' criticism of population geneticist proponents of the HGDP for sharing "racial serologists'" reliance on simplistic migration hypotheses implicates an additional question, that is, whether alternate hypotheses, besides migration and "racial" mixture, were seriously entertained by the blood group researchers.

Recall the Hirszfelds' bar graph representation of frequencies of *A* and *B* in "national types" and their a posteriori grouping of these into three higher-order "types": "the European type," "the intermediate type," and the "Asio-African type" (Figure 6.3). The phenomena of interest to the Hirszfelds were "marked differences in the incidence of *A* and *B* in the different races" (1919b: 38) and "that the distribution of *A* and *B* corresponds with surprising accuracy to geographical situation" (1919b: 41). The Hirszfelds considered two possible explanations of the geographical distribution of blood group differences they observed, one causal and one historical. They rejected as "improbable" a role for natural selection due to climatic differences, pointing, for example, to similar proportions of *B* in people from Russia and from Madagascar. Instead, they favored a hypothesis that "two different biochemical races... arose in different places" and have since mixed (1919b: 42). Suggesting a "possible double origin of the human race," the Hirszfelds placed the "cradle of one part of humanity" in India where the frequency of *B* is highest and the "cradle" of the other part in "North or Central Europe" where the frequency of *A* is highest (1919b: 42).

The Hirszfelds' approach mirrors that of Latour's soil scientists who, from a sample of Amazonian soil, followed a "movement of abstraction" that generated factual support for a hypothesis about whether the savanna or the forest is advancing. The Hirszfelds' efforts began with blood samples of individuals grouped by nationality, proceeded through intermediary steps such as agglutination tests and statistical analysis, and culminated in a journal article where evidence depicted in words, tables, and a bar graph representation was marshaled in support of a hypothesis about human evolution. The Hirszfelds' hypothesis that *H. sapiens* originated separately in two places and subsequently spread across the globe through migration and "racial" mixture can aspire to explain the world in so far as the chain of reference is reversible. "Traceability" connects words to the world, beginning with the scientific text and its internal referents like charts and diagrams, proceeding through intermediary steps of statistical analysis and agglutination testing, and ending up with actual blood samples and people sampled.

"Packing the world into words" enables scientific theories to find, or fail to find, empirical support. The process of objectification that accompanies abstraction in the movement from blood samples to texts and purports to discharge the subjectivities of a priori and a posteriori classification makes this portrayal of the evidential weighting of competing hypotheses possible. However, the Hirszfelds' hypothesis can claim to provide a superior explanatory account of the blood group frequency data only if its competitors—a causal hypothesis about natural selection due to climactic differences or a historical claim of a single origin for the species—are genuine contenders. Genuine contenders share the same referent, or, rather, chain of reference. At each and every link along the chain of reference that connects words back to world, the abstract judgments that made material extraction possible must be shared. It is both abstract and material ties between world and word that make the circulation of reference, and the evidential weighting of competing hypotheses, possible.

As we have seen in this section, choices that privilege certain traits over others in a posteriori classification contribute to a process that constructs both "race" concepts and "racial" groups. The privileging of traits other than the blood groups may have resulted in quite different "race" concepts and different "racial" groups. This raises the question whether any particular system of "racial" classification can be authoritative, and on what basis. The next section looks specifically at "racial" classification.

"Racial" classification

Marks argues that the "real units of human diversity" are the "small biopackages" called populations, not "races" (1995: 116, 274). Races do not exist, because populations cannot be classified into higher-order types due to the fact that genetic differences between them are quantitative, not qualitative. Species genome diversity, Marks writes, is "geographically patterned": it is generally the case that "people are similar to those nearby and different from those far away" (2000: 9). Given that gene frequencies change gradually and continuously across neighboring populations, Marks rejects the typological division of humans into a small number of discrete "races" (corresponding, e.g., to the longstanding division of "Caucasoid," "Negroid," and "Mongoloid," or some related rendition).

Marks criticizes the "racial serologists" for failing to appreciate the clinal pattern of ABO blood group distribution. He believes that this was due to their a priori expectations of finding differences between groups they considered to be "races":

> Today we use ABO as a paradigmatic demonstration of the absence of discrete racial groupings among the aboriginal populations of the world. Populations differ from one another in a quantitative, gradualistic manner.... Curiously, though, that clinal pattern was not immediately put forth as inherent in these data by the earliest exponents of blood-group data for physical anthropology. What they presented as results, rather, was what folk wisdom and contemporary anthropology had led them to expect to find: qualitatively different major groupings of people, or races.
>
> (Marks 1996: 346)

These invented "racial" divisions are described by Marks as the imposition of discontinuities on an underlying reality of blood group frequencies continuously distributed across the species. The result was the biological reification of fictive "races" illegitimately assumed to exist from the outset. It is along these lines that Marks and Rachel Silverman (2000) characterize Boyd's "racial" classification as circular. Recall Boyd's a priori and a posteriori classifications discussed earlier—the a priori classification of breeding populations and an a posteriori "racial" classification consisting of six groups ("hypothetical Early European," "European (Caucasoid)," "African (Negroid)," "Asiatic (Mongoloid)," "American Indian," and "Australoid" (Figure 6.6)). Whereas Cavalli-Sforza credits Boyd for his use of three blood groups (ABO, RH, MN) to differentiate populations on the five continents from one another (2000: 16), Silverman argues that Boyd used blood group data simply to validate his a priori assumption that continental borders constitute "racial" divisions: "In essence, Boyd's races were based on large continental divisions on which he *imposed* gene-frequency differences. He first marked out racial delineations, and then made the blood group frequencies fit within these divisions" (2000: 14; italics in original).

Marks recounts a history of ambivalent relationships between blood group researchers and their anthropologist contemporaries. Anthropologists greeted the Hirszfelds' work with skepticism, according to Marks, because "racial" classification based on ABO differences failed to coincide with anthropological classifications of the time. From the 1920s to the 1940s, "racial serology" managed to "reinvent" its hold on anthropology, because the circularity of "racial" classifications based on blood group differences meant they corresponded more closely with anthropologists' expectations. Marks argues that anthropologists of Boyd's own time criticized this circularity, and by 1945, this contributed to "racial serology's" marginal status with respect to physical anthropology. Ultimately, Boyd's "racial" classification was undermined by the very blood group data on which it was supposed to be based. According to Marks, Frank Livingstone's 1963 argument for the nonexistence of human races given the clinal distribution of genetic variation among human groups demonstrated that Boyd's approach was "fundamentally archaic" (1996: 354). Marks characterizes Boyd's "racial serology" as "intellectually tangential to the main lines of thought in physical anthropology" during the 1960s. These years were a period when physical anthropologists were making increasing use of genetics to study the micro-evolution and demography of populations, and coming to recognize the "major qualitative divisions of the human species…as illusory" (1996: 357).

When considered from perspectives that recognize the interplay of objectivity and judgment and requirements for maintaining the circulation of reference, Marks' and Silverman's criticisms of Boyd and other blood group researchers raise some interesting questions. What is to be concluded when serological "racial" classifications fail to coincide with "racial" classifications based on other traits? One possibility is that there are no mind-independent "races," for otherwise, these objects would be picked out by numerous traits. Another possibility is that "race" concepts and "racial" groups themselves are constructed *by* the privileging of certain traits over others—different choices, different "race" concepts, different "racial" groups. What about the circularity of Boyd's approach to "racial" classification that Marks and Silverman point out? If attempts to discharge subjectivities associated with a priori assumptions—for instance, social–political categories of classification—compromise the circulation of reference, might it be the case that a posteriori classifications will inevitably be circular? Given that the blood group researchers were not ignorant of the fact that the populations they were classifying differed quantitatively not qualitatively in gene frequencies, how did they attempt to justify their imposition of "racial" divisions?

The Hirszfelds noted the difference in classifications produced by the blood groups and by "anthropological characteristics":

> We see thus that A and B are present in different proportions in different races. The serological formula for a particular race is in no way affected by the anthropological characteristics. The Indians, who are looked on as anthropologically nearest to Europeans, show the greatest difference from them in the blood properties. The Russians and the Jews, who differ so much from each other in anatomical characteristics, mode of life, occupation, and temperament, have exactly the same proportion of A and B.
>
> (Hirszfeld and Hirszfeld 1919b: 41)

The Hirszfelds did not speculate on reasons for this difference. They were confident, however, that common ancestry explained the geographical distribution of the blood groups. The Hirszfelds' successors were more pressed to account for differences between their classifications and those of their anthropologist peers. Although Snyder remarked that "in general the blood group data conform remarkably well to the known anthropological facts" (1925: 407), he addressed the "comparative value" of the blood groups and "racial characters" used by anthropologists. Snyder believed that the blood groups were potentially superior for investigating the "problem of the origin and relationships of races" (1925: 407). As particulate characters, they would remain intact across successive generations after "race crossing," providing an accurate record of the past, of even "a little crossing" (1925: 407). In contrast, "blending" characters like those traditionally used by anthropologists would be submerged. But Snyder saw no reason why suitable traits would not be useful alongside the blood groups: "It must not be thought…that because the groups are hidden in the blood, they possess some mysterious power of providing a basis for racial classification" (1929: 126). Snyder did not doubt that "races" exist independently of any such choices; "racial" classifications ought, then, to coalesce.

Haldane was explicit about the failure of classifications based on different traits to coincide: "The plain fact is that the distributions of pigmentation and skull-shape are pretty well independent. And it is at once clear that that of blood-groups is independent of either" (1940: 475). This cross-classification of "racial" types provides a potential argument for their nonexistence. Lancelot Hogben's 1931 *Genetic Principles in Medicine and Social Science*, for example, expressed doubt that "racial" classification along genetic lines is achievable even in principle given differences in classifications produced when different combinations of characters are selected—for instance, skin color and head form versus hair texture and nasal index. Hogben treated the blood groups as just one anthropological character among many, arguing that there was no justification for overcoming such discrepancies by taking serological differences as authoritative (Barkan 1992). Haldane's belief that traditional anthropological traits like skin color are often adaptive provided an explanation for the observed discordance of traits in "racial" classification: "if we map the world [using blood groups]," he wrote, "we shall expect to get information of racial origins quite different to that given by such a character as skin colour" (1931[1933]: 67). The distribution of skin color would depend on climate as well as origins, and because pigmentation differences may have evolved fairly rapidly in response to selection pressure, their distribution would provide information only about the recent evolutionary past. The blood groups, in contrast, since they are "not adaptive, or very slightly so," would shed light on "remoter origins" with the result that "[t]he contradiction between the two sources of information is thus only apparent" (1940: 477). Given his view that the blood groups provide "information of a more fundamental character on racial structure" (1940: 477), unlike Hogben, Haldane had no qualms about treating serological differences as authoritative.

The argument that the nonexistence of "racial" types is demonstrated by their cross-classification rests on a typological concept of race. This concept treats "races" as classes whose members share certain traits. This means that individuals belonging to the same "race" would be similar in blood type, facial structure, skin color, hair texture, and so on. With respect to blood types, it suggests "pure races" of *AA*, *BB*, and *OO* individuals, at least in the past. However, beliefs in such "races" were short-lived among serologists who understood the *proportions* of blood group alleles to be characteristic of "racial" types, and groups not individuals to be the units of "racial" classification. The discordance of traits in classification challenges the existence of "racial" types conceived in this way as well. Indigenous peoples of Australia and sub-Saharan Africa would not be combined in the same "racial" type if blood groups were used as a criterion for classification, but they may, if skin color was used. Haldane's preference for a genealogical concept of race legitimized his approach, which viewed the choice of different criteria as picking out "racial" groups at distinct time levels. Criteria with similar temporal significance would be expected to yield "racial" classifications that coalesce. Haldane's approach assumes a typology of well-delineated populations across space and time. When Barkan describes Haldane as a "major critic of racial typology" prior to the Second World War (1992: 162), it bears clarification that "racial typology" in this sense can refer only to the categorization of individual people by similarities in traits believed to reflect shared ancestry. Haldane was *not* a critic of a "racial" typology of groups.

Marks' characterization of serology, particularly Boyd's work, as marginal to physical anthropology by 1945 deviates from the dominant historical interpretation of the mid-twentieth century influence of the evolutionary synthesis on physical anthropology. According to Barkan, pre-war physical anthropology was "a once important branch in human biology that had lost touch with scientific progress. Only after the War was the discipline invigorated and brought up to date with biology" (1992: 160–1). Similarly, Nancy Stepan views the mid-century transition in physical anthropology in terms of an old science, that of "racial biology," giving way to a new science, that of "genetical anthropology":

> [T]he new genetical anthropology represented not merely a correction of old ideas, but the substitution of one way of looking at the biological world by another. The units of analysis, the methods and procedures, and the goals of the new science were quite different from those of the old, and entailed a fundamental alteration in the perception of the biological significance of human races.
>
> (Stepan 1982: 176)

Nevertheless, Stepans' portrayal of the "old racial biology" is remarkably similar to the picture Marks paints of "racial serology":

> In the old racial biology, racial classification was linked directly to the reconstruction of racial history. Since races were thought of as relatively independent biological units, groups of individuals separated by time and space could, nevertheless, be joined together by racial descent if their skulls and other traits were similar.
>
> (Stepan 1982: 180–1)

Marks and Stepans are in agreement that, by the 1960s, physical–biological anthropologists had come to focus their attention on micro-evolutionary processes, studying genetic changes in populations due to mechanisms like mutation, selection, and drift. As Stepans points out, "racial affinity" was no longer the only acceptable explanation for genetic similarities in populations; convergent evolution, once just adaptive noise, became an object of study in its own right.

On this account, Haldane's theoretical interests in origins, migrations, and genealogical relations, at least in *H. sapiens*, place him squarely among the "old racial biologists." However, he is also a transitional figure, given his contributions to theoretical population genetics, his population-based "racial" typology, and his focus on genetic rather than phenotypic properties of populations. Although Marks characterizes Boyd as relegated to the margins of physical anthropology by the end of the war and remaining "intellectually tangential to the main lines of thought in physical anthropology" through the 1960s, in many ways he too is an important transitional figure, more so even than Haldane. In fact, tensions in Boyd's work reflect some of the differences that shape disputes among population geneticists and biological anthropologists today.

The tensions involved in Boyd's work are those of a scientist embedded in, not left behind by, the evolutionary synthesis. In *Genetics and the Origin of Species*, widely regarded as the fundamental text of the evolutionary synthesis, Dobzhansky urged evolutionary geneticists to focus on "the causal rather than the historical problem" (1937: 8). He characterized genetics, like physiology, as a "nomothetic" (law-creating) science and recommended the investigation of "the common properties of living things" rather than the study of "the peculiarities of separate species" through phylogenetic reconstruction (1937: 6). Dobzhansky's favorable review of Boyd's *Genetics and the Races of Man* expressed agreement with Boyd's definition of "races" as genetically distinct "Mendelian populations" kept apart by geography or social forces as well as hope that the cooperation of anthropologists and population geneticists would lead to "important developments in our understanding of human evolution, and particularly of the mechanisms of race formation" (1951: 266). This attention to the "mechanisms of race formation" focuses scientific attention on potential barriers to gene flow and constructs a concept of "race" that is distinct from the genealogical concept of "race" preferred by blood group researchers like the Hirszfelds, Snyder, and Haldane. Applying "the genetic race concept" to *H. sapiens*, Dobzhansky wrote:

> The human species is compounded of numerous subordinate Mendelian populations, which form an intricate hierarchy, beginning with clans, tribes, and various economic and cultural isolates, and culminating in "major" races, and finally the species. Now, not only the major but also the minor populations often differ in gene frequencies. They are "races" by definition.
>
> (Dobzhansky 1951: 265)

In a departure from Marks' skepticism about the reality of higher-order classifications, Dobzhansky held that barriers to gene flow occur at all levels (between continents as well as neighboring villages) which meant a hierarchy of Mendelian populations that combines the smallest groups, panmictic populations, into more comprehensive units.

Dobzhansky's "genetic race concept" lends legitimacy to the attention Boyd's "racial" classification paid to continental differences, and for which he is criticized by Marks and Silverman. Boyd's approach to "racial" classification was largely consistent with the "new systematics" that architects of the evolutionary synthesis like Dobzhansky and Mayr urged biologists to adopt. The aim was to produce "natural" classification systems, whose taxonomic boundaries coincide with actual discontinuities in nature, as a preliminary step in the investigation of dynamic evolutionary processes. Boyd would not have been surprised to find that his "races" corresponded to "the facts of geography"; his a priori assumption was that oceans once constituted geographical barriers to gene flow between populations indigenous to the five continents. Because these barriers have been incomplete and overcome by migration throughout the course of human evolution, isolation has not been "absolute," and there are only quantitative genetic differences between the "races." Hence, although Marks is correct to claim that Boyd imposed "racial" discontinuities on a continuous pattern of blood group frequencies across populations, Marks is mistaken in saying that Boyd did so without awareness. Boyd stated explicitly that "our decision as to what boundary between frequencies is to separate two races remains always a man-made and arbitrary decision" (1950: 273). Marks and Silverman are also correct to claim that Boyd's "racial" classification is circular. Boyd's report that "[t]he method of gene frequencies is completely objective" (1950: 273) ignores the subjectivities associated with judgments of a priori classification already discussed. And yet, the inability to discharge these subjectivities if the circulation of reference is to be maintained casts doubt on whether the circularity involved in the use of a priori categories of classification can be avoided or may be, perhaps, even desirable.

Evidence suggests that Boyd quite consciously sought to adopt the methods and concepts of the evolutionary synthesis despite Marks' claim that he was yesterday's man. Boyd was well acquainted with Dobzhansky's research on the genetics of natural populations and cited him frequently. Boyd's attention to geographical barriers to gene flow and their role in the "racial" differentiation of *H. sapiens* corresponded with Dobzhansky's mapping efforts in *D. pseudoobscura*. His definition of "race" was taken from a 1944 article on the genetics of Drosophila populations by Dobzhansky and Carl Epling: "A race is not an individual, and it is not a single genotype, but it is a group of individuals more or less from the same geographical area (a population), usually with a number of identical genes, but in which many types may occur" (Boyd 1953: 497). This definition foregrounds geographical proximity and relegates genealogy to the background, a background that is nevertheless necessary given that genealogy is part of the fundamental process that structures genetic similarity in virtue of geographical (and reproductive) proximity. Boyd recognized that privileging geographical proximity and genetic similarity over genealogy could result in contradictory "racial" classifications. Unlike Dobzhansky, he was not willing to forego genealogy entirely: "We do not mean to assert that the geneticist can classify mankind with no regard to his recent geographical distribution, and cultural factors such as language, since it is obvious that race, as we understand the term, involves common descent" (1953: 496). "Common descent" served as a constraint for Boyd on "generalizations" based on "abstractions" about "race": "The value of the abstractions will be shown when we apply them to new examples. Thus any combination of gene frequencies which we abstract as characteristic of Africans must not reveal little islands of 'Negroes' in northern Europe or pre-Columbian America" (1953: 496). Boyd was open to Dobzhansky's invitation to address "causal problems" but not led, as a result, to renounce his interest in "historical problems." As we saw, still, in 1950, origins, migrations, and genealogical relations remained of interest to Boyd (Figure 6.9).

Marks' characterization of Cavalli-Sforza as heir apparent to the blood group researchers legitimately draws attention to shared theoretical interests in historical questions concerning origins, migrations, and genealogical relations. But just as Marks' charge that "racial serologists" like Boyd believed in the existence of "qualitatively different major groupings of people, or races" lacks nuance, so does his similar portrayal of Cavalli-Sforza:

> Whether we refer to races as low-tech impressionistic color-coded subspecies as did Linnaeus, or as hi-tech computerized color-coded "ethnic regions" (Cavalli-Sforza *et al.* 1994), the act of imposing qualitative differences on them does not help us understand the biological patterns structuring human variation. What the act represents is the Linnaean, essentialist, pre-evolutionary approach to human diversity.
>
> There is no scientific basis—genetic, phenotypic, or eco-geographic—for asserting that a Persian and a Belgian are qualitatively the same, and a

> Ghanaian and an Ethiopian are qualitatively the same, but a Persian and an Ethiopian are qualitatively different. That is what the natural concept of race would say, and it is false.
>
> (Marks 2000: 9)

Marks finds Cavalli-Sforza, like the "racial serologists," guilty of superimposing qualitative boundaries on patterns of genome diversity that are continuously distributed across space with the unjustified resulting assumption that people belonging to different "racial" groups are absolutely dissimilar. Cavalli-Sforza is no "Linnean essentialist," however; in fact, he appeals to the quantitative pattern of variability in ABO allele frequencies in order to dispel the notion of "pure races":

> Racism has many origins and definitions, but we know that racists often worry about racial "purity." Let us dispense with this aspect first: There are no pure races. . . . It doesn't take much to prove this. In any genetic system, we register a high degree of what is known as *polymorphism*, or genetic variation. . . . For example, the proportions of A, B, and O genes fluctuate from village to village, town to town, and nation to nation. In every microcosm, we find a genetic composition comparable to that of the larger group, albeit a little different.
>
> (Cavalli-Sforza and Cavalli-Sforza 1995: 237–8)

Once again in these disciplinary maneuverings, issues of importance have been overlooked. Marks and Cavalli-Sforza share a taxonomic concept of "race" where the basic units of classification are panmictic breeding populations that are combined in higher-order groups based on patterns of genetic similarity and dissimilarity. *If* "races" were to exist, they would be taxonomic types. For Cavalli-Sforza, given his interest in historical questions, taxonomic divisions could be constructed to represent genealogical relations by choosing appropriate characters for classification and assuming that "genetic distance" accurately reflects time of separation. Despite similarities in the preceding quotes from Dobzhansky and Cavalli-Sforza that might be taken to suggest a shared "race" concept, for Dobzhansky, *all* races were Mendelian populations, or breeding groups, and all genetically distinct Mendelian populations, including panmictic ones, were "races," not units of taxonomic "racial" classification.

In any case, both Marks and Cavalli-Sforza (at least recently) have argued that races do *not* exist. Marks believes that populations are genuine, presumably more-or-less discrete, units of human diversity but that "higher-order classifications of human populations are largely ephemeral" (1995: 115). Marks is especially critical of attempts to classify *H. sapiens* into continental groups given that mitochondrial evidence suggests that all humans are a "subset" of Africans (1996: 358). Cavalli-Sforza treats panmictic populations as real but characterizes attempts to classify "clusters" of populations into races as a "futile exercise" (Cavalli-Sforza *et al.* 1994: 19). This is because any such classification would involve an arbitrary privileging of a given time slice with its particular geographic distribution of populations over another, a concern that coincides with Marks' objection.[13] Additional ironies unite these two parties to debates over the HGDP and the legacy of the human blood group research. One is that there are no scientific referents *without* the subjectivities associated with judgment, for it is these that permit the material extraction that occurs along the chain of reference. Another is that Marks' and Cavalli-Sforza's shared choice of discreteness as the criterion for reality places human populations in just as much trouble as "races."

Conclusion: mapping people, mapping flies

The debate over the historical legacy of the ABO blood group research that has emerged amidst controversies surrounding the Human Genome Diversity Project has a realist tenor. Jonathan Marks emphasizes the failure of abstract categories of serological classification to identify genuine biological objects. This failure, he argues, was a reflection of the social and political biases of blood group researchers who wished to find "races" where there were only populations. L. Luca Cavalli-Sforza believes that the ABO blood group researchers were successful in discovering genuine biological group differences. Today, with improved technologies and the ability to secure data at the level of DNA, he is hopeful that scientists continuing in the tradition of the blood group researchers will be able to reconstruct human evolutionary history by sampling indigenous populations across the globe. Marks and Cavalli-Sforza are in agreement that "objective" data on human genome diversity provide the only basis for a posteriori classification. They disagree about whether the blood group researchers successfully bridged the representationalist gap between abstract words and concrete world.

Bruno Latour's concept of circulating reference promotes a different understanding of scientific objectivity and the problem of representation. Researchers are responsible for constructing chains of reference that connect abstract words to the concrete world via series of numerous small and painstaking steps. Judgments that both Marks and Cavalli-Sforza would regard as a priori and subjective are indispensable to the processes of abstraction and extraction that make each link in the chain possible. These subjectivities of judgment cannot be discharged in the production of a posteriori classifications and tabular and mapping representations of data without the loss of reference. It is, however, possible to ask why certain judgments are made rather than others. At each link of the chain of reference, a range of choices is available to researchers (Figure 6.2). This coheres with the pragmatic approach to explanation we defend in our chapter on mapping Drosophila.

How genes or chromosomes are ordered in space and time, whether or not they become bounded in populations, and the extent to which genetic continuities or discontinuities are privileged depend on pragmatic features arising within specific contexts of investigation. Some philosophers would argue that explanatory content is shaped by context-dependent aims, interests, and values only when humans are objects of knowledge but not otherwise. The suggestion is that the methodological care scientists generally take to ensure the objectivity of their findings becomes overlooked when issues strike close to home. Hence, we have emphasized that explanations in population genetics are pragmatic in flies no less than in humans (Gannett and Griesemer, Chapter 4). It is nevertheless possible that certain aims, interests, and values are more likely to arise in human than in nonhuman research contexts. A pragmatic approach to explanation allows us to make theoretical generalizations about such aims, interests, and values while rejecting traditional assumptions that view them as "contaminants" of "objective" science. Rather than detecting contaminants, recognition that objectivity emerges in scientific work to build circulating reference reveals that subjectivity, in the form of scientific expert judgment, is integral to objective science.

We have seen that Ludwik and Hanna Hirszfeld, Laurence Snyder, J.B.S. Haldane, and William C. Boyd shared theoretical interests in human evolutionary origins, "racial" ties, and migration histories. Thus, the ABO blood group researchers, like A.H. Sturtevant, as we point out in "Classical Genetics and the Geography of Genes," were interested more in "historical problems" than in the causal mechanisms of evolution. Their approach, consequently, is not unlike that taken in Dobzhansky and Sturtevant (1938). In this paper, Theodosius Dobzhansky and Sturtevant present phylogenetic and geographical distribution maps of gene arrangements in chromosomes of two races of *D. pseudoobscura* and combine information provided by these maps to propose a "working hypothesis" concerning the likely evolutionary history of the species. However, comparisons of the use of maps to address "historical problems" in the 1938 Dobzhansky–Sturtevant paper and in the ABO research of the same period reveal some interesting differences in fly and human research contexts. Questions concerning origins and migration histories are addressed at the level of groups in *H. sapiens* and at the level of chromosomes in *D. pseudoobscura*. While there may be underlying assumptions about the continuity of *D. pseudoobscura* populations over time, and evidence of willingness to compare patterns of variability in different chromosomes in order to begin to delineate populations, there is little serious attempt to fix group boundaries based on the evidence available.

Dobzhansky's theoretical interests in the study of *D. pseudoobscura* began to shift around 1936, moving away from his collaborative work with Sturtevant on "historical problems" and toward the investigation of causal mechanisms of evolution in natural populations (Gannett and Griesemer, Chapter 4). It is this approach that was the basis for the Genetics of Natural Populations (GNP) series (Lewontin *et al.* 1981). Dobzhansky evidently believed that geographical variation in the frequencies of chromosomal types in *D. pseudoobscura* and blood group alleles in *H. sapiens* represent analogous processes in both species. Dobzhansky's 1937 *Genetics and the Origin of Species* included charts of blood group frequencies from Snyder; subsequent texts such as the fourth and fifth editions of *Principles of Genetics* (1950, 1958: co-authored with Sinnott and Dunn) included geographical distribution maps of ABO blood group genes originally published by Bertil Lundman and A.E. Mourant. When he discussed "race formation," Dobzhansky presented chromosomal inversion maps for Drosophila in one section and ABO maps for humans in the section immediately following. We have seen that Boyd's 1950 *Genetics and the Races of Man* was, in turn, greatly influenced by Dobzhansky. Again, despite similarities in the approaches of Boyd and Dobzhansky, the investigation of causal mechanisms of evolution differed in people and flies. As in the case of historical questions and the construction of phylogenetic maps, geographical patterns of genetic variability were mapped at the level of chromosomes for *D. pseudoobscura* and at the level of groups in *H. sapiens*. Whereas the geographical inversion maps and geographical frequency maps of Dobzhansky's GNP series emphasize variability within populations, co-temporaneous ABO maps ignore this variability by representing either frequencies of single alleles or homogeneous "racial types." The ABO maps also represent human groups as more-or-less discrete. Only when the focus was on studying genetic drift in *D. pseudoobscura* were efforts made to delineate population boundaries. Generally, in the GNP papers, flies sampled at a given geographical location are taken to be representative of the population in the area without the need to introduce divisions between neighboring populations.

While Boyd shared Dobzhansky's interest in evolutionary mechanisms and favored a geographical–genetic concept of race, unlike Dobzhansky, he was not led to relinquish his interest in historical questions concerning origins, past migrations, and genealogical relations. Historical questions remain at the center of human population genetics research. Cavalli-Sforza, for example, has published a number of phylogenies (e.g. Cavalli-Sforza *et al.* 1994: 78). These phylogenies represent attempts to reconstruct human evolutionary history in terms of branching events that separate human groups. Plans for the HGDP include sampling DNA from individuals belonging to up to 500 indigenous populations in an effort to recover this history (Cavalli-Sforza *et al.* 1991). This demonstrates another important difference between mapping people and mapping flies. *D. pseudoobscura* populations are composed of whatever flies reside in an area at the time they are sampled, for example, those flies that congregate at a particular feeding station. The ABO blood group maps, in contrast, are based on the agglutination reactions of only those individuals whom investigators consider to be indigenous, that is, whose ancestors were "in situ" prior to European colonization. We saw in Boyd's work that this a priori group boundary was justified by researchers' theoretical interest in origins and not recent migrations. But once any such a priori group boundaries are drawn, only some stories become possible and others are ruled out. Inevitably, those who author narratives of evolutionary history will believe that certain moments in our human past are more significant than others. These choices, and the values that inform them, direct the writing of the history of human evolution, a history that, unlike for flies, is written by, for, and about those for whom there exists an interest in such a history.

The deflected continuities uncovered in our companion chapter on flies can now be linked to the historiographic analysis here. Rather than a demonstration that the deflections mark underlying continuities of mapping practice, in this chapter we have argued for a new form of objectivity with judgment rather than against it, building on the insights of Peter Galison, Lorraine Daston and Bruno Latour. Judgment in the twentieth-century science we discuss is the exercise of scientific expertise in the pursuit of scientific work to form chains of "small abstractions" that are integral to the production and maintenance of objectivity. In virtue of the meticulously built and maintained chains through which reference can circulate, objectivity is secured. That is, representations of nature can be retraced to their source objects and objectivity can result because the world can be unpacked from the words provided the judgments that guided chain formation in the first place have not been discharged to the metaphysical ether. Thus, the new objectivity, in virtue of the circulation of reference, is the image of subjectivity, not the break of it.

In our investigation of human blood group mapping, we traced the abstractions and judgments necessary to produce a posteriori classifications and cartographic representations. The circularity of these taxonomic productions is displayed, but unlike the critics of genetic anthropology, we argue that the story of circularity should not be made to tell only a tale of disciplinary rhetoric: the problem of "race" is too important, as is the problem of epistemic virtue in twentieth-century science. Subjectivity cannot be discharged from scientific work, nor would that be a desirable result. To attempt it is to seek a return to nineteenth-century (or earlier) standards of epistemic virtue, to mechanical objectivity or even to artistic genius, rather than to work out a conception of science appropriate to our time and circumstances. To embrace circulation is not to submit to the old charges of subjectivity (or relativism), but to recognize a social transformation of virtue.

Notes

1 This was based on evidence that *AB* individuals do not arise from *R*(*O*) mothers and that *R*(*O*) individuals do not arise from *AB* mothers (Mazumdar 1996).

2 Reardon explains "coproduction" as follows: "detailed empirical work by scholars interested in coproduction has demonstrated that science and society exist in a mutually constitutive and stabilizing relation to one another. . . . In addition to calling into question analyses that reduce science to a knowledge-producing activity separate from society, a coproductionist framework also calls into question analyses that reduce science to social relations" (2002: 15–6).

3 We do not propose to argue that each of the periods described by Daston and Galison can be understood as the transformation of an objectivity/judgment pair rather than of a sequential replacements of epistemic virtues. Here, we argue for a refinement of the complex interplay of objectivity and judgment in the twentieth century.

4 See Griesemer (1990) for another case study of abstraction by extraction.

5 Note that the chain branches—one line goes to Paris and one goes to Manaus. Latour gives the impression that reference circulates along chains, but since these typically branch (and intersect) in scientific practice, reference circulates in complex networks.

6 One might argue that this notion of subjective judgment leading to objectivity is also implicit in nineteenth-century mechanical objectivity, but hidden away in the theory of the instruments (Hacking 1983) which take the human interpreter out of the path from phenomenon to data representation. Rather than artistic judgment in the overt representation of nature, the engineering judgment of the instrument maker is implicit in mechanical objectivity. If one were to trace the circulation of reference in the nineteenth century, it would pass, significantly, through the instruments. Thus, the same argument applied here to the small judgments of the twentieth-century scientific expert to produce circulating reference and objectivity may apply to the nineteenth-century instrument maker as well.

7 It would be inaccurate to assume that this departure of Snyder's from the Hirszfelds can be explained by the greater tendency for Americans to racialize continental differences and for Europeans to racialize national differences. Snyder makes several references to "race" that are quite localized, for example, his indication that, in Syria, "the races divide along religious lines" (1929: 123).

8 Sampling location is in addition to the national identity of the group, for example, "Germans (in Hungary)," "Germans (Berlin)," and "Middle Koreans (Seoul)."

9 As we will see, geographical representations of distributions of group properties similarly must make use of a priori classifications. The "base maps" upon which "thematic" data are plotted must "be a record of the location and identity of geographical features" (Robinson 1982: 16). But locations and identities of such features can only be made on the basis of a priori decisions to represent features in particular ways and according to a chosen system of boundaries, whether political (e.g. national, country), geographic (continents), ethnic, economic, linguistic, religious or otherwise. Such representational choices reflect a priori classifications, for example, that national and racial boundaries coincide or are closely related except for perturbing migration "events." Since it appears likely that the representational practices of genetic anthropology follow those of European ethnographic practices emerging in the nineteenth century (see Robinson 1982: ch. 5), the geographic components of its a priori classifications are likely to be ethno-national-political as we describe in the Hirszfelds' work.

10 According to N. Dwight Harris, the name "Macedonia" was used "in its most restricted—and probably its most correct—meaning to designate that region of the Balkans embraced within the three Turkish vilayets of Salonika, Monastir, and Kosovo, and lying between the districts of Adrianople and Albania" (1913: 205).

11 An outsider's impression of this collection of diverse identities in Salonika is available from war correspondent, G. Ward Price:

> For the spy, Salonica is Paradise. He thrives and multiplies there like a microbe in jelly. If a spy had the chance of creating an ideal environment to work in he could not improve upon Salonica. Imagine a town where the languages commonly and regularly spoken are old Spanish, much adulterated, Greek, Turkish, Italian, Bulgarian. Serb, Roumanian, and French; where every one has changed his subjection at least once during the last five years—from Turkish to Greek—and where before that several thousands of people had all sorts of claims to European nationalities, based on the complicated Turkish system of the Capitulations (under which one brother in the same family would be "French," another "English," another "Italian," perhaps without one of them being able to speak a single sentence in the tongue of the nationality he claimed.
>
> (Price 1918, in Chapter VI, Ourselves and the Greeks: Relations at Salonica)

12 This notion of a deliberate falsehood is also clearly part of cartographic tradition and reflects a form of expert judgment weighing against accurate presentation of mapped data. As Kombst said, writing about thematic maps in 1848, distinct outlines are to be "preferred to an overstudied accuracy in the colouring, which gives only a confused representation" (quoted in Robinson 1982: 139).

13 By conceiving races as monophyletic lineages, Robin Andreasen (1998) successfully responds to these objections to defining races genealogically. On Andreasen's account, the number of races that exist depends on the specifics of the branching process that has occurred during evolutionary history and is not constant but varies between time levels. At any given time level, since these clades represent a nested hierarchy, there is a variable but determinate number of monophyletic lineages that biologists, depending on their research interests, might single out as races. However, there are other problems with Andreasen's approach to defining races as clades (see Gannett 2004).

Bibliography

Andreasen, R.O. (1998) "A New Perspective on the Race Debate," *British Journal of the Philosophy of Science*, 49: 199–225.

Barkan, E. (1992) *The Retreat of Scientific Racism: Changing Concepts of Race in Britain and the United States between the World Wars*, Cambridge: Cambridge University Press.

Bowcock, A. and Cavalli-Sforza, L. (1991) "The Study of Variation in the Human Genome," *Genomics*, 11: 491–8.

Boyd, W.C. (1950) *Genetics and the Races of Man: An Introduction to Modern Physical Anthropology*, Boston: D.C. Heath.

Boyd, W.C. (1953) "The Contributions of Genetics to Anthropology," in A.L. Kroeber (ed.) *Anthropology Today: An Encyclopedic Inventory*, Chicago: University of Chicago Press, 488–506.

Cavalli-Sforza, L.L. (2000) *Genes, Peoples, and Languages*, trans. M. Seielstad, New York: North Point Press.

Cavalli-Sforza, L.L. and Cavalli-Sforza, F. (1995) *The Great Human Diasporas: The History of Diversity and Evolution*, trans. S. Thorne, Reading, MA: Addison-Wesley.

Cavalli-Sforza, L.L., Menozzi, P. and Piazza, A. (1994) *The History and Geography of Human Genes*, Princeton, NJ: Princeton University Press.

Cavalli-Sforza, L.L., Wilson, A.C., Cantor, C.R., Cook-Deegan, R.M. and King, M.-C. (1991) "Call for a Worldwide Survey of Human Genetic Diversity: A Vanishing Opportunity for the Human Genome Project," *Genomics*, 11: 490–1.

Daston, L. (1992) "Objectivity and the Escape from Perspective," *Social Studies of Science*, 22: 597–618.

Daston, L. and Galison, P. (1992) "The Image of Objectivity," *Representations*, 40: 81–128.

Davis, A. (1935) "The Distribution of the Blood-Groups and Its Bearing on the Concept of Race," *The Sociological Review*, 27: 19–34, 183–200.

Dobzhansky, T. (1937) *Genetics and the Origin of Species*, New York: Columbia University Press.

Dobzhansky, T. (1951) "Race and Humanity," *Science*, 113: 264–6.

Dobzhansky, T. and Sturtevant, A.H. (1938) "Inversions in the Chromosomes of Drosophila Pseudoobscura," *Genetics*, 23: 28–64.

Dobzhansky, T. and Epling, C. (1944) *Contributions to the Genetics, Taxonomy, and Ecology of Drosophila pseudoobscura and Its Relatives*, Washington: Carnegie Institution of Washington Publication 554.

Galison, P. (1998) "Judgment against Objectivity," in C.A. Jones and P. Galison (eds) *Picturing Science, Producing Art*, New York: Routledge, 327–359.

Gannett, L. (2004) "The Reification of Biological Race," *British Journal of the Philosophy of Science*, 55: 323–45.

Gerson, E. (1998) "The American System of Research: Evolutionary Biology, 1890–1950," unpublished thesis, University of Chicago.

Gould, S.J. (1983) "The Hardening of the Modern Synthesis," in M. Grene (ed.) *Dimensions of Darwinism: Themes and Counterthemes in Twentieth-Century Evolutionary Theory*, Cambridge: Cambridge University Press, 71–93.

Griesemer, J.R. (1990) "Modeling in the Museum: On the Role of Remnant Models in the Work of Joseph Grinnell," *Biology and Philosophy*, 5: 3–36.

Griesemer, J.R. and Wimsatt, W.C. (1989) "Picturing Weismannism: A Case Study of Conceptual Evolution," in M. Ruse (ed.) *What the Philosophy of Biology Is, Essays for David Hull*, Dordrecht: Kluwer Academic Publishers, 75–137.

Haldane, J.B.S. (1931) "Prehistory in the Light of Genetics," *Proceedings, Royal Institution of Great Britain*, 26: 355; reprinted in *Science and Human Life* (1933), New York: Harper & Bros.

Haldane, J.B.S. (1940) "The Blood-Group Frequencies of European Peoples, and Racial Origins," *Human Biology*, 12 (4): 457–80.

Harris, N.D. (1913) "The Macedonian Question and the Balkan War," *American Political Science Review*, 7 (2): 197–216.

Hirszfeld, L. and Hirszfeld, H. (1919a) "Essai d'application des méthodes sérologiques au problème des races," *L'Anthropologie*, 29: 505–37.

Hirszfeld, L. and Hirszfeld, H. (1919b) "Serological Differences between the Blood of Different Races: The Results of Researches on the Macedonian Front," *Lancet*, 2: 675–9; reprinted in S.H. Boyer, IV (ed.) (1963) *Papers on Human Genetics*, Englewood Cliffs, NJ: Prentice-Hall, 32–43.

Hogben, L. (1931) *Genetic Principles in Medicine and Social Science*, London: Williams and Norgate.

Jubien, M. (1997) *Contemporary Metaphysics*, Oxford: Blackwell Publishers.

Kirsh, N. (2003) "Population Genetics in Israel in the 1950s: The Unconscious Internalization of Ideology," *Isis*, 94: 631–55.

Landsteiner, K. and Levine, P. (1928) "On the Racial Distribution of Some Agglutinable Structures of Human Blood," *Journal of Immunology*, 16 (2): 123–31.

Latour, B. (1999) *Pandora's Hope: Essays on the Reality of Science Studies*, Cambridge, MA: Harvard University Press.

Lawler, S.D. and Lawler, L.J. (1957) *Human Blood Groups and Inheritance*, 2nd edn, Cambridge, MA: Harvard University Press.

Lewontin, R.C., Moore, J.A., Provine, W.B. and Wallace, B. (eds) (1981) *Dobzhansky's Genetics of Natural Populations, I–XLIII*, New York: Columbia University Press.

Marks, J. (1995) *Human Biodiversity: Genes, Race, and History*, New York: Aldine de Gruyter.

Marks, J. (1996) "The Legacy of Serological Studies in American Physical Anthropology," *History and Philosophy of the Life Sciences*, 18: 345–62.

Marks, J. (2000) "Human Biodiversity as a Central Theme of Biological Anthropology: Then and Now," *Kroeber Anthropological Society Papers*, 84: 1–10.

Mazumdar, P.M.H. (1996) "Two Models for Human Genetics: Blood Grouping and Psychiatry in Germany between the World Wars," *Bulletin of the History of Medicine*, 70: 609–57.

Mourant, A.E. (1961) "Blood Groups," in G.A. Harrison (ed.) *Genetical Variation in Human Populations*, New York: Pergamon Press, 1–15.

Paul, D.P. (1994a) "Eugenic Anxieties, Social Realities, and Political Choices," in C.F. Cranor (ed.) *Are Genes Us? The Social Consequences of the New Genetics*, New Brunswick, NJ: Rutgers University Press, 142–54.

Paul, D.P. (1994b) "Is Human Genetics Disguised Eugenics?" in R.F. Weir, S.C. Lawrence and E. Fales (eds) *Genes and Human Self-Knowledge: Historical and Philosophical Reflections on Modern Genetics*, Iowa City: University of Iowa Press, 67–83.

Paul, D.P. (1995) *Controlling Human Heredity: 1865 to the Present*, Atlantic Highlands, NJ: Humanities Press.

Price, G.W. (1918) *The Story of the Salonica Army*, New York: Edward J. Clode. Available at http://www.ku..edu/~libsite/www/Salonica/salonTC.htm (accessed March 3, 2003).

Reardon, J.E. (2002) "Race to the Finish: Identity and Governance in an Age of Genetics," unpublished thesis, Cornell University.

Roberts, Leslie (1991) "Scientific Split Over Sampling Strategy," *Science*, 252: 1615.

Robinson, A.H. (1982) *Early Thematic Mapping in the History of Cartography*, Chicago: University of Chicago Press.

Silverman, R. (2000) "The Blood Group 'Fad' in Post-War Racial Anthropology," *Kroeber Anthropological Society Papers*, 84: 11–27.

Sinnott, E.W., Dunn, L.C. and Dobzhansky, T. (1950) *Principles of Genetics*, 4th edn, New York: McGraw-Hill.

Sinnott, E.W., Dunn, L.C. and Dobzhansky, T. (1958) *Principles of Genetics*, 5th edn, New York: McGraw-Hill.

Snyder, L.H. (1925) "Human Blood Groups and Their Bearing on Racial Relationships," *Proceedings of the National Academy of Sciences*, 11: 406–7.

Snyder, L.H. (1926) "Human Blood Groups: Their Inheritance and Racial Significance," *American Journal of Physical Anthropology*, 9 (2): 233–63.

Snyder, L.H. (1929) *Blood Grouping in Relation to Clinical and Legal Medicine*, Baltimore: Williams and Wilkins.

Stoneking, M. (2001) "Single Nucleotide Polymorphisms: From the Evolutionary Past," *Nature*, 409: 821–2.

Wilkinson, H.R. (1951) *Maps and Politics: A Review of the Ethnographic Cartography of Macedonia*, Liverpool: University Press.

Wyman, L.C. and Boyd, W.C. (1935) "Human Blood Groups and Anthropology," *American Anthropologist*, 37(2): 181–200.

7 Mapping as technology

Genes, mutant mice, and biomedical research (1910–65)

Jean-Paul Gaudillière

Introduction

In March 1951, William Loomis, who was working as an expert for the Natural Sciences Division of the Rockefeller Foundation, visited the Jackson Memorial Laboratory in Bar Harbor, Maine. The "Jackson" as it was then known was the largest American center for maintaining, studying, and selling genetically controlled, that is, inbred strains of mice. Since the early 1930s it had combined the functions of laboratory, resource center, and production plant. These operations had been supported by numerous grants from the Rockefeller Foundation, the total amount of which came to more than half a million dollars. Loomis had been sent to Maine because Clarence Cook Little, the Managing Director of the Jackson, had mailed the Rockefeller Foundation an application for $175,000 to support diverse research projects linking cancer genetics, cytology, biochemistry, and reproductive physiology.

When he returned to the Rockefeller offices, Loomis gave a devastating account of his visit.

> Their specialty has always been mammalian genetics, which, in fact, has seemed not so much to come down to chromosomal mapping, which is close to impossible, with 40 chromosomes in the diploid phase, but rather to the inbreeding in the brother–sister mating of various strains of mice. (…) To WL's mind the truly unique field they have at hand is that of determining the influence of the mother's ovary, uterus and milk on the character of the progeny. (…) The best of the Jackson is selling useful strains of mice for cancer research. The worst is the research on maternal inheritance. The JML has produced very little first class research.[1]

Consequently, Loomis said, nothing approaching such a big grant should be considered by the Foundation. As had happened several times in the history of the laboratory, the Rockefeller Natural Science Division approved funding on a smaller basis with the argument that the center was providing—with its controlled model organisms—a very valuable service to the biological and medical communities.

Although, in the present time of automated sequencing and large-scale genome analysis, Loomis' comments about the complexity of mouse chromosomes and the difficulty of mapping look badly informed, they were for their time well grounded. Loomis' identification of chromosomal mapping as a key element of modern genetic research was then a common assumption. Mice were however not part of the standard pattern illustrated by the publication of numerous chromosomal maps for flies, maize, and other plants. It was only 20 years after the Second World War that the Jackson scientists proved Loomis' statement wrong by circulating a chromosomal map of the mouse locating 140 different genes (Staff of the Jackson Laboratory 1965).

When it came to chromosomal mapping, therefore, mice were not flies. Geneticists as well as historians of science have often commented on the contrasting fate of model organisms in genetics (Sinnott and Dunn 1939; Morse 1978; Burian 1993; Geison and Laubichler 2001). In order to account for these trajectories, biological specificity is often commented upon. Mice are mammals and not insects. They breed slowly, and have small progenies. Consequently, large breeding ventures are time, labor, and money consuming. Given this, it is hardly surprising that mutants surfaced rarely, and that mousers worked on different problems to those pursued by observers of a "breeding reactor" like the fruitfly. This biological interpretation should however be qualified. Mapping the mouse was never impossible, it just required other means and practices than those developed for Drosophila, the reference case.

This chapter focuses on the history of inbred mice as a means of making both the origins and centrality of mapping practices in twentieth-century genetics, less straightforward. Two assumptions are, in this context, important. First, the mouse as a biological and material entity was nothing if not unique and stable. It was the product of a complex process of selection and tinkering. It was a technological object living in a multilayered and highly artificial environment—a system of laboratory work—which was largely responsible for defining the animal model, and what it was good for. Second, the effects of the material infrastructure on the development of mouse genetics cannot be isolated from issues of representation, scientific sociability, institutional patterns, and commercialization. R. Kohler's book on the fly group is certainly the most convincing attempt so far at combining several of these levels of analysis (Kohler 1994). The case of mice, however, reveals a segment of American genetics, which did not resemble the world of the Drosophilists. This was a world of scientists trading with specialists of human diseases. Mouse geneticists were certainly doing research on genes. But they were not only doing that. They also modeled pathologies, an activity for which they organized the production and sometimes the sales of genetically controlled mice. The existence of this world, thus, puts into question many elements of our Drosophila-centered history of genetic mapping.

Inbreeding, and physiological studies within the Bussey school

During most of the twentieth century, mice were not primarily genetic tools, but rather seen as models of human pathologies. This is aptly illustrated by their status within the first institution devoted to the genetics of small mammals, the laboratory headed by William Castle at Harvard University School of Applied Biology located at the Bussey Institution. The Bussey campus was an outpost of Harvard University located in Jamaica Plains, where Castle, then Professor of Zoology, emigrated in 1908 to develop genetics.

W. Provine has discussed Castle's shift from Zoology to Mendelian studies of inheritance (Provine 1986). In the context of this chapter, we just need to remember that Castle was ambivalent to Mendel's laws and some basic assumptions of the new genetics. On the one hand, he accepted the idea of segregating factors. On the other hand, Castle viewed segregation patterns as nothing but universal. Castle and his students worked on rats, guinea pigs, rabbits, as well as mice. Many experiments revolved around the problem of the transmission of quantitative and continuous characters, showing blending rather than segregation. Mendelizing work concentrated on studies of coat color. Castle himself developed a broad and comprehensive scheme in which eight Mendelian factors participated in the genetic determination of coat color in guinea pigs (Provine 1986).

At the Bussey Institution, the first PhD on mice was a study of this sort, focusing on the color of the fur. Completed by C.C. Little, this work was, to a large extent, an adaptation of Castle's scheme to whatever variants of mice Little could collect, when visiting the local merchants of fancy animals. Little's coat color system included six out of the eight Mendelian factors introduced by Castle. In addition to this successful but unsurprising analysis, Little discussed two problems (Little 1913). The first was the physiological relation between genes and the production of pigments. Building on an interpretation already advanced by Cuenot in relation to the yellow color of mice, Little proposed a link between genes, pigment, and enzymes. He, however, thought that this particular problem should be left to the biochemist: the biologist's role was to document the physiological effects of hereditary factors.

The second innovative dimension of Little's work as an undergraduate was of a more lasting importance and dealt with breeding technologies. Like most Castle's students, Little was trained by maintaining stocks. This was viewed as a means of giving students a pragmatic insight into what research project's were doable (Dunn 1962). Building on Johanssen's recent work, Little embarked on an attempt at producing pure lines of mice by means of inbreeding, that is, systematic mating within the same litter. Inbreeding was not a prerequisite for him to undertake a Mendelian study of inheritance in mice. Little's thesis in fact relied on strains supposedly inbred by fanciers for commercial purposes and did not mention his own inbred lines. The technology of inbreeding, however, proved critical in creating a junction between the genetics of mice and cancer research, or more precisely between genetics and the study of transplanted tumors.

Observation had been made in the early twentieth century, that the transplantation of tumors was more successful between mice or rats of the same race, that is, if one used mice from the same colony, usually designated by the colony's geographic origin. This race effect was not immediately understood in genetic terms. Interest in hereditary factors emerged when the pathologist Leo Loeb found that a spontaneous tumor of Japanese waltzing mice, a strain bred for a "waltzing" trait (a defect of the inner ear) by professional animal breeders, could be transplanted with a high degree of success in these mice (Loeb 1908). Loeb himself was not immediately attracted to genetic investigation, but Harvard pathologist E.E. Tyzzer took over Loeb's experimental system (Gaudillière and Löwy 1998). By the time he embarked on the study of hereditary factors in the genesis of spontaneous tumors, Tyzzer was director of the laboratory of the Harvard Cancer Commission. His official goal was

> to determine if the susceptibility to an inoculable tumor is transmitted in accordance with the principles of heredity such as are embodied in Mendel's laws (...) The waltzing tumor was especially adapted for the study of the problem at hand on account of the uniformity of the results obtained from its inoculation into different varieties of mice.
>
> (Tyzzer 1909)

Tyzzer crossbred Japanese waltzing mice with common albino mice and studied the susceptibility of the offspring to the Japanese tumor. He was unable, however, to develop an interpretation of his results that would fit a distribution of Mendelian factors. His conclusion in 1909 was that, successful transplantation of tumors in mice depended upon three factors: the method of inoculation, the character of the individual tumor employed, and the "nature of the soil upon which the tumor is implanted" (Tyzzer 1909). Racial differences were important but their role was unclear.

The study of the inheritance of susceptibility to transplanted tumors took a new turn when Tyzzer started to work with Little, capitalizing on the latter's experience in inbreeding. In 1913, Little had obtained an homogenous stock of common mice, the dilute brown race (dba), that he took into Tyzzer's laboratory in order to study transplantation in hybrids that come from mating with the Japanese waltzing mice. The use of dilute brown mice was a way to narrow down the variability of experiments. It was highly successful: tumors from the waltzing strain were rejected in dba stocks; they took in waltzing mice; and were partly accepted in first generation hybrids. Little commented:

> the stocks used are genetically favorable for obtaining uniform and reliable experimental results. It seems important to emphasize this phase of the work, for if mixed or relatively impure races are used, variable and inconclusive results are almost certain to be obtained. We feel that the material used is of sufficient constancy and definiteness to lend strength to any experimental results obtained in the study of its hereditary behavior.
>
> (Little and Tyzzer 1916)

Tyzzer and Little concluded that tumor susceptibility was controlled by multiple hereditary factors, in this case probably as many as 12–14.

This collaboration resulted in a significant displacement of the inheritance problem. The local but successful routinization of transplantation experiments, achieved by using a single tumor type and "inbred" hosts, actually turned the homogeneity problem upside down. In the 1920s a majority of specialists agreed that hereditary factors influenced the success of tumor transplantation. It became less clear, however, whether scientists who observed the fate of grafted tumors were studying the transplantation of foreign tissues or cancer. It was generally agreed that since "resistance" against transplanted tumors was not specific to cancer tissues, the phenomenon was of little interest to clinicians. Consequently, in the 1920s and 1930s, leading scientists in the domain of experimental cancer research seldom viewed transplanted tumors as an adequate model for studying the genesis and development of malignant growths. They employed transplanted tumors (e.g., Ehrlich's carcinoma in albino mice) as biochemical, physiological or cytological models. Simultaneously, transplantation became a means of assessing the purity of the genetic background. Inbred mice thus became highly valuable tools for controlling the role of genes, and enhancing the replicability of biomedical experiments. Little concentrated his mouse research on the genetics of cancer (Rader 1998; Gaudillière 1999). He explained that

> studies with inoculated tumors give information as to the genetic nature of normal tissue and normal growth; studies with spontaneous tumors give information as to the genetic nature of the process involving the failure of growth control. Each supplements and amplifies the other.
>
> (Little 1923)

The linkage of inbred mice and cancer studies, however, was not the complete story. Karen Rader has analyzed how the Bussey Institution provided a home for early mousers (Rader 1995, 1998). She shows both, the importance of mouse genetics before Second World War and the absence of a significant mapping enterprise. As mentioned in the introduction to this chapter, it is tempting to explain this pattern by invoking the difficulty of obtaining mutants. During the 1920s and 1930s, the number of mutants described in the literature remained very small, and nobody assembled an infrastructure large enough to overcome the scarcity of mapping material. The history of the laboratory mouse, Rader recounts, was plagued with problems of stocks. Little tried to help by turning the Cold Spring Harbor Station for Experimental Evolution into a small reserve where mousers could locate some of their stocks. This arrangement did not last long as Little, in the 1920s, embarked for an administrative career of university president. All along the 1920s, the mousers repeatedly complained against their poor working conditions, particularly the difficulty to find space and means for breeding and maintaining the animals. In 1925, Leslie Dunn accordingly wrote a long letter to his mentor, Castle urging him to do something for a former student of Morgan, Leonell Strong, who was looking for a new job since the administration of his college would no longer let him carry out his work on mice.

> Just before I went I had a letter from Strong (L.C. of St Stephens) saying that he was out of a job for next year. The college has decided that it can't carry his mouse experiments any longer, which in view of the smallness of the place and the fact that it is primarily a teaching institution for classical studies is not

> surprising. (. . .) I suggested that the Mayo, the Rockefeller or the Crocker were the most likely place to turn to, and that he write you for advice. I thought also that if he could get a temporary grant to take care of his family and his work, you might be able to take him in until he found a place.[2]

The mutant problem, however, is more than a question of biological traits. Mice were bad breeders. They did not easily produce many mutants, but they do. Feasibility should be seen as a historical problem: mapping was doable but required different resources to those mobilized in the genetic history of Drosophila. In the 1920s, mice were not flies because one did not really want them to become flies.

Within this perspective, K. Rader has discussed the patterns of sociability prevailing in the Bussey school (Rader 1998). She contrasts the ethos of diversity, autonomy, and flexibility, which reigned within Castle's laboratory, with the division of labor and resources which typified the Morgan mapping enterprise. The latter favored collective and integrated forms of research, the former resulted in more dispersed projects on various models. Evidence for this interpretation may be found in the repartition of mammalian organisms between Castle's students. The same person could alternatively work on different animals, while different workers usually investigated unrelated rodents. Castle himself favored rabbits and rats, Sewall Wright worked on guinea-pigs only, Leslie Dunn and Georges Snell concentrated on mice.

The line of interpretation proposed here is complementary to Reader's, and consists of suggesting that mice were employed for purposes other than studying the structure of genes. As exemplified by the case of Little's inbred stocks, laboratory mice were animal models rather than model organisms. The experimental work done with them was closely related to medical research, and did not lend in itself to chromosomal mapping. One approach to investigating this question is to check the ways in which inbred mice were, or were not, linked with the mapping technologies originating in the Morgan group. It then appears that the first phase of mouse genetics was dominated by what may be called a physio-pathological perspective. Such a configuration did not only prevail in the career of researchers like Little, who operated at the boundary between biology and pathology. It also pervaded the work of scientists like Leslie Dunn, who did not work on problems directly related to medicine. Two examples may help discuss the issue.

Leslie Dunn was the first of Castle's students to find an academic niche where he could do proper research. In 1928 he replaced Morgan at Columbia University. In Dunn's laboratory, problems in the inheritance of color variations remained high on the agenda. Coat color studies were often placed in the context of developmental biology. As Dunn wrote in a famous paper on spotting patterns of the house mouse:

> The processes which lead to the formation of patterns during ontogeny in animals are at present very imperfectly understood (. . .) patterns at the marking of the skin and hair in mammals we have almost no knowledge of; yet

> they provide a rich and varied material from which it would be possible to discover some steps of the steps (*sic*) by which one part or area of the body comes to differ from another. Many of these patterns are hereditary (...) Thus to our interest in them for the light they may throw on some of the problems of individual development is added at once a new problem, how the genes influence a specific pattern.
>
> (Dunn 1937a: 15)

Biological action was at the center. Moreover, in a very interesting inversion of Morgan's hierarchy of functional and structural analysis, Dunn stated that the latter could only be cleared when the former had been worked out: "Questions concerning the allelism and location of the genes wait upon such knowledge of their individual effects" (Dunn 1937a: 17).

Coat color studies were thus viewed as a very elegant and sophisticated system for investigating the interactions between genes.

> A thorough study of the variations in a group of related characters in any organism will usually reveal an intricate series of interactions between the component factors. As an example we shall choose the house mouse, for in this animal a large number of spontaneous variations have provided the opportunity for a genetic analysis of the factors affecting coat color. (...) In fact the wild coat color itself is found to depend on the presence and interactions of all of the factors named. Thus, in order to produce the agouti pattern there must be present the factors for color (C), agouti (A), black (B), dark eye (P), dense color (D), and solid color (S). (...) Were knowledge complete, it is probable that the list of factors necessary for the production of the agouti pattern would be much longer and that the letters of the alphabet would be exhausted.
>
> (Sinnott and Dunn 1939)

One original aspect of this research was the role attributed to modifier genes. The notion was taken from Castle. In 1924, while Dunn was expanding his mouse research, gradually leaving the genetics of chicken, Castle wrote him: "I think your plan for studying pattern modifiers in mice is a good one and I think the matter a fundamental genetic problem. That is why I am harnessing away at the same question in rabbits."[3] Modifier genes supposedly affected the expression of other genes. But how could they be identified? How could one differentiate their effects from mere phenotypic variations? Dunn's response was no less procedural than Morgan's approach to localization. Dunn designed special stocks and special crossings, and these were aimed at affecting the variable expression of genes.

One of the most interesting example was the study of *S*, the spotting gene of the mouse (Dunn 1937a). *S* was associated with strains of mice selected by fanciers and sold on the market under the name of "pied" mice. These were animals with patches of black and white hair, the white-spotting being located in particular areas—the feet, the tail, the belly, the nose and middle of the back—thus forming a white belt. Spotting could be more or less intense. Geneticists tried to reduce this variability by inbreeding and selection, thus producing strains "breeding true to greater or lesser of white spotting" (Dunn 1937a). Within these lines, the remaining variability was classified, environmental or developmental, while differences between the lines were described as hereditary. As several of these lines originated in the apparently homogeneous piebald strains, *S* (spotting) was not viewed as the one single gene controlling de-pigmentation.

Practically speaking, the search for modifier genes was based on the "recognized technique of experimental breeding" (Dunn 1937a). Since the phenotypic trait to be analyzed was color variation, quantitative procedures for measuring spotting were developed in the laboratory. One of them was the preparation of dried skins, followed by planimeter measurements. Precise quantification on living animals was not deemed feasible or necessary, and so numbers were obtained by dividing the body into twenty parts and counting how many of them, respectively, were white and colored (Figure 7.1).

The work concentrated on the production of genetically pure strains showing stable spotting patterns. Inbred all-white animals were then crossed with various types of spotted lines and back-crossed in order to show that a few genes were involved as shown by the frequent recovery of the all-white parent type in the F2 generation. The "modifiers" were then "extracted and accumulated" in pure stocks with a new series of crossings concentrating on the analysis of dark *SS* animals obtained after crossing *Ss* × *Ss* animals in which "modifiers" had been introduced by repeated

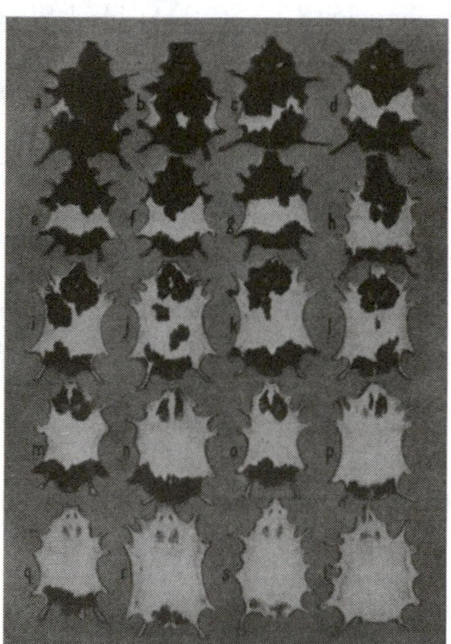

Figure 7.1 In Dunn's group at Columbia, pied mice were investigated for their variable coat color patterns, which manifested gene interactions in the production of physiological events and morphological traits. This figure illustrated several publications on spotting. (From Dunn 1937b.)

back-crossing with all whites. Dunn argued that these animals exemplified two particular forms of relation between phenotype and genotype. The first type was *gene interaction*. In contrast to Bridges' understanding of modifiers, this was a physiological, rather than a genetic phenomenon.

The spotting modifiers could affect both the *S* and *s* alleles, and did not display the sort of specificity emphasized by the Drosophila workers. The second sort of relation was the modification of dominance, which was illustrated by the ability of the *modifier complex* to increase the spotting range of *Ss* animals, which were practically identical to the *SS* mice in the absence of modifiers.

A second group of investigations concentrated on the *W* gene originating in a strain, showing white spotting, that Little had isolated in 1915. *W* produced spots in black mice. *WW* animals were anemic and barely viable, *ww* animals were all-black, while only *Ww* displayed the so-called variegated pattern. The level of spotting was again extremely variable. Using mice of the *WwSS* type, Dunn selected the most variable offspring, thus increasing the extent of spotting from 1% of the fur to 90% after 14 generations. These hyper-variegated animals were then inbred (Dunn 1937b). For all practical purposes, the second group of modifiers included all the variability factors extracted and stabilized during these crossings. Since these modifiers had no visible effect in the black animals carrying no *W* mutation, Dunn argued for specific interaction in the sense of Bridges.

> The modifying genes accumulated by selection in the light variegated WwSS race are multiple and probably recombine at random with each over and with W. By themselves they produce little or no spotting even when several are homozygous. (...) The m(W) genes interact with W in a very striking way to produce when several are homozygous a maximal variegated spotting effect which renders nearly the whole pelt white. They do not interact thus with any other gene and the relation is a specific one.
>
> (Dunn 1937b: 59)

Within this physiological culture, linkage studies played a limited role. Back-crossing and other Morganian techniques were employed as tools to check the specificity of effects and the autonomy of new genetic factors. Thus, there was no attempt to localize the modifier, or other genes. This does not mean that linkage tests and crossing over rates had no place at all in the Bussey community. It rather means that they were not associated with the mapping perspective, and perceived as tools for individualizing the various hereditary factors participating in the making of a peculiar phenotype. Within the context of the piebald study, Castle thus wrote Dunn:

> I have been thinking about your all-white mice obtained as a selection product of piebald. The case reminds me much of the reputed origin of Vienna White in rabbits as a selection from Dutch toward the whitest condition attainable. (...) Is it not possible that in your race, which originated in the selection toward all-white, you had a gene like the VW of rabbits? As only the linkage test with English and angora served to establish the distinctiveness

> of VW in rabbits, so you might establish the relation of your all-white gene to ordinary piebald by the linkage test involving hairless. If it is distinct this test should prove it.[4]

One should make clear that the practice of mouse genetics, however, echoed some aspects of the Drosophila research. Practically speaking, coat color studies relied on "the recognized techniques of experimental breeding" as Dunn explained, and also on the collection of variants (Dunn 1937a). Castle's correspondence, thus, testifies of a not so rare circulation of mutants. After his former student Leslie Dunn succeeded Morgan, exchanges between Columbia University and the Bussey Institution were quite important. Castle regularly requested particular strains, especially coat color mutants. Requests traveled back and forth: "I wonder if you or Dr Keeler have on hand any self-brown mice of which you could spare a male and a female or more if possible"[5] wrote Dunn as he was investigating the white spotting pattern. Within this community of shared resources, it was understood that shipments should be reciprocated without reservation. As Castle once explained: "We are grateful for your generosity in sharing this and other stocks of mice with us, and we shall be more than glad to be able to return the favor."[6] Moreover, the existence of an informal network of users resulted in the fact that, the mice boarding the train from New York to Boston and vice versa could originate from or end up in other laboratories. "As to the short-tailed mice, we just supplied Green, last week with a small stock, which he needed for some experimental work, and which he said you could not supply at the time" wrote Castle in the same letter. In contrast to the Drosophila exchange system, this circulation was, however, only minimally organized. Up to the 1940s there was no newsletter informing the mouse people about who kept which mutant, while no one attempted to organize a reference collection or resource center. The circulation of mutant mice may, therefore, best be described as a gift economy rooted in a culture of curiosity. Written exchanges were dominated by the description of rare and interesting specimens. As Castle wrote after the discovery of new color variant:

> There seems to be little doubt that we have this time the true *black-and-tan* of the house mouse, and that it is an exact homologue (or analogue?) of the *black-and-tan* in rabbits. I am certain that Pincus has among his stocks some light-bellied agouti (Feldman's stock) and I will ask him to send you some. They, rather than the ordinary agouti of mice, would seem to correspond to the gray of rabbits.[7]

Curiosity was also leading to offers of service:

> We received yesterday seven or eight short eared male mice from Miss Lynch. These came through in good condition and are certainly quite distinct from anything you have seen. Would you like to have a couple of these at once? If so I will have them sent to you.[8]

By the mid 1930s, greater use of linkage tests affected these circulation patterns. More frequent supply was needed to conduct the crossings.

> We had a nice shipment of flexed tail mice from Hunt yesterday—very interesting—you should have seen them. He is working on some possible linkages and we shall work on others. Could you spare us for the purpose a pair or so of black-eyed-whites (with the lethal gene)? Also have you a gray race? Snell wants a few gray females to use in crossing with hairless from non-agouti (which you gave us). If you can spare us some, we should be pleased to get them. Just send or collect anything available. If you have anything that you haven't in the mouse line, we shall be pleased to supply you.[9]

Linkage groups thus surfaced within the Bussey School, but they were comparatively late products. Their appearance may be taken as a reaction to the mounting status of the fly group. By the late 1920s, another student of Castle, George D. Snell, completed a thesis on linkage in mice. This work included the first table of linkage groups in the mouse ever published (Figure 7.2).

Back crosses, cross-over analyses, distance calculations had been imported from the Drosophila mapping system, the scale, however, remained much smaller. Most of Snell's table was a compilation of scattered crossings, which had been completed during the first two decades of mouse genetics. No more than five linkages could be mentioned and only three chromosomal distances had been computed. Snell himself had only established three linkages. This was nonetheless the result of the not so quick task of monitoring more than 5,000 crossings. In his correspondence, Castle was quite explicit about the material difficulties of the enterprise. When Snell had just completed his thesis, Castle wrote Dunn:

> A letter just received from Gates states that he would be willing to undertake a linkage test between waltzing and the two types of hairless, which Snell has been testing out during the past two years for linkage with factors others than waltzing. We have had such poor success in raising waltzers, probably because our temperature control is not accurate enough, that these particular linkages have not been worked out. Gates has some of the Riga stock, but not your hairless variety. I wonder if you could supply him with some. Our own stock is extremely low.[10]

Mapping the mouse was thus certainly feasible, but it required a different form of work than that of mapping the Drosophila chromosomes. The threshold to be crossed was both cultural and technological, as shown by the developments within what was in the 1930s, the single center organizing the maintenance of mouse mutants—the Jackson Laboratory.

CHROMOSOME	GENE	SYMBOL	NAME	CROSSOVER PERCENT
1	1	P	Dark-eye	
		p	Pink-eye	
				19.06 in female
	2	C	Full color	13.89 in male
		c^{ch}	Chinchilla	
		c^{d}	Extreme dilution	
		c	Albinism	
				2.5
	3	S^{h}	Non-shaker	
		s^{h}	Shaker	
2	4	A^{y}	Yellow	
		A^{w}	White-bellied agouti	
		A	Agouti	
		a^{t}	Black-and-tan	
		a	Non-agouti	
3	5	B	Black	
		b	Brown	
4	6	D	Density	
		d	Dilution	
				0.06
	7	S^{e}	Normal-ear	
		s^{e}	Short-ear	
5	8	S	Self	
		s	Piebald	
				9.8 in female
	9	H^{r}	Haired	2.6 in male
		h^{r}	Hairless	
6	10	W	Black-eyed white	
		w	Self	
7	11	V	Normal walking	
		v	Waltzing	
8	12	R	Rodded retinae	
		r	Rodless	
				12 ?
	13	S^{l}	Non-silver	
		s^{l}	Silver	
9	14	N	Naked	
		n	Normal coat	
?	15	H	Normal head	
		h	Haemoragic head	
?	16	T	Tailless	
		t	Normal tail	
?	17	D^{w}	Non-dwarf	
		d^{w}	Dwarf	

Figure 7.2 Snell's first assessment of linkage studies in the mouse published as part of his thesis work. The synthesis took the form of a table and no more than five linkages could then be documented. (From Snell 1931.)

Mouse genetics as tool: the Jackson Biomedical Culture

The Jackson Memorial Laboratory was created in 1929 as a research site, where scientists would explore "man's knowledge of himself, of his development, growth and reproduction . . . and of his in-born ailments through research with genetically controlled experimental animals" (Holstein 1979). In Little's eyes, as well as in the eyes of his wealthy industrial patrons, research on the etiology of cancer was critical to the development of the laboratory. The center focused largely on biology-based experimental medicine. Gathering new tools was viewed as a means of furthering this target. One typical event was to recruit Leonell Strong, the earlier cited student of T.H. Morgan, who had developed an inbred strain of mice, in which 90% of the females were affected by mammary tumors. These animals embodied a genetic cause for cancer. They were employed in large numbers in the laboratory to mimic human breast cancer and render the putative relationship between cancer genes, hormones, and environmental factors (Gaudillière 1999).

Production tasks escalated in the 1930s as the Jackson scientists started to distribute their mice to outside workers (Rader 1995). A few figures highlight this development. In 1932, three years after the construction of the first building at Bar Harbor, a dozen scientists and technicians were breeding 20,000 mice a year for local usage only. In 1933, the US Public Health Service Cancer Laboratory at Harvard Medical School was the premier outside destination of the so-called Jax mice, yet this institution barely imported a few thousand animals employed as models of carcinogenesis. Other major consumers were experimental pathologists using homogeneous "normal" white mice. In contrast to the Jackson workers, they did not work on cancer or genetic disorders, but on infectious diseases like yellow fever, typhoid, tuberculosis, and so on. For instance, the scientists at the International Health Division of the Rockefeller Foundation were by that time buying 20,000 Jackson mice a year.[11] Up to the late 1930s, sales roughly covered 10–20% of the Jackson budget. This means that the growth of the Jackson Memorial Laboratory was mainly paid for, by individual philanthropy and by the Rockefeller Foundation.[12]

Although selling the mice did not meet the local financial need, commercial production changed the face of the laboratory. Initial work had been organized around a handful of research-maintenance units, that is, one scientist and one or two technicians, using and breeding a few strains that they would eventually pass to other researchers. By the late 1930s, after the first big supply contract with the Rockefeller Foundation had been signed, two types of settings emerged.[13] On the one hand, there were laboratories linked to research stocks. On the other hand, there was a production site where the most requested generic mice were multiplied by caretakers. Genetically controlled breeding pairs moved from the former to the latter.

Although C.C. Little viewed the production activities as having "a good effect on morale and keeps everyone in close contact with the animal stock," he did not think of himself and of his colleagues as instrument-makers.[14] The research agenda was biomedical, even though the dual nature of the site triggered particular innovations. For instance, specific interests in breeding and husbandry, produced objects such as the agent causing mammary tumors in the C_3H strain (Gaudillière 1999). What would become a famous cancer virus originated in vertical transmission patterns: it was passed to suckling newborns in the milk of contaminated nursing mothers. The Jackson workers collaborated with half a dozen medical institutions. These exchanges neither focused on the supply of animals nor addressed issues in formal genetics. The local scientists kept working on a wide range of topics including growth, development, and the etiology of several human diseases. Until the Second World War, in spite of a large production infrastructure, the Jackson was primarily a modeling center. Mapping seemed to be off their horizon.

In 1945, however, the staff of the Jackson Laboratory edited a special issue of *The Journal of Heredity* devoted to mouse genetics. The issue included a two-page insert entitled "A Chromosome Map of the House Mouse." The so-called map actually described ten linkage groups, of which five presented only the minimal requirement of two genes. The total number of mutants (32) was small enough to have each locus associated with a drawing or a photograph of its corresponding mutant phenotype (Figure 7.3).

The map had one more noteworthy feature. Most of the data originated in laboratories other than the Jackson. The Jackson scientists had isolated none of the mapped mutants, and they had contributed only two linkages. The 1945 map nonetheless testified to a changing status of mouse genetics.

Within the Jackson, George Snell promoted the mapping culture. After his thesis on linkage and a short-term college experience, Castle's former student moved to Little's laboratory. There, he did not try to scale-up linkage studies into a mapping project. Following his arrival, Snell was given technical and administrative tasks. He reorganized the production section of the laboratory. The task was made urgent by expanding sales, and Snell systematized the separation of research and production stocks.[15] His second job was to coordinate the preparation of the Jackson manual on the laboratory mouse, as well as the 1945 issue of *The Journal of Heredity*. Snell's research work was at that time described as a combination of formal genetics and maintenance: "For his and other genetic studies, Dr Snell has been carrying and improving 14 stocks with 30 mutant genes as well as 3 translocation stocks" (Jackson Report 1943). Keeping an eye on production, he nonetheless contributed to the search for new mutants. In the late 1940s and early 1950s, the Jackson workers more regularly reported the discovery of mutated strains. This, as well as the experimentation on linkages, however, remained a technical component of the modeling strategy.

Interesting new mutants were those, which could be used either for investigating physiological problems or for modeling pathologies. A typical example was, in 1950, the discovery of *obese* by Snell's collaborator Margaret Dickie, an assistant then involved in the supervision of research stocks. The isolation of the mutant was followed by a decade-long study of obesity, which was conducted in collaboration

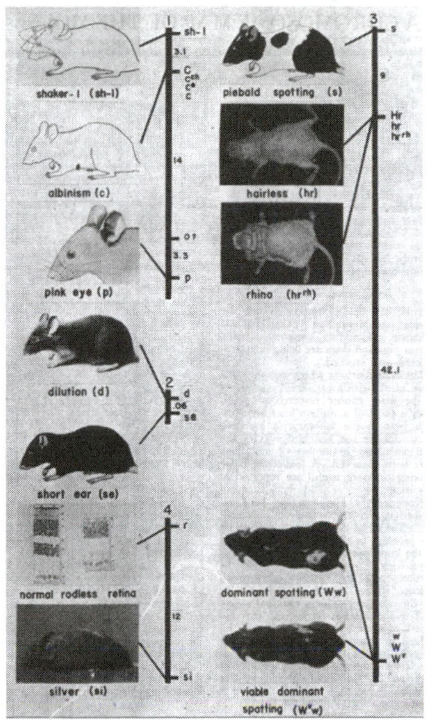

Figure 7.3 In 1945, the staff of the Jackson Memorial Laboratory coordinated a special issue of *The Journal of Heredity* on mouse genetics. This review included a vivid representation of the mouse chromosomes. (From Staff of the Jackson Laboratory 1945.)

with the Harvard Department of Nutrition (Gaudillière 2000). Research into the localization of *ob* played no part in this venture.

The isolation of *luxoid* by Margaret Green (1955) is worth mentioning in the context of this discussion, since it is one of the rare instances when—because of the biomedical agenda—the mapping of genes and the mapping of embryological territories came in contact. *Luxoid* was found in 1950, in a strain of mice employed for investigating mammary tumors. The mutant showed strong anomalies of feet, limbs, vertebrae, and ribs. These manifestations were similar to those found in another mutation—*luxate*—described by the British mouser T.C. Carter working at the Edinburgh Institute of Animal Genetics. The first report on *luxoid*, therefore, needed to substantiate the claim for novelty. Anatomical differences existed, but given the wide range of effects of both mutants, these differences were not strong enough to convince other geneticists that the genes involved were actually different. In continuity with the instrumental use of linkage tests, genetic localization was for this purpose deemed critical. As crossing results suggested that *lu* and *lx* did not segregate with the same markers, both mutants were attributed specific genes. The possibility that both genes belonged to the same linkage group was open. For the Jackson geneticists, the most important aspect of *luxoid* remained its morphological closeness to *luxate*. Based on extensive dissections, *lu* and *lx* were presented as having opposite effects on the development of the skeleton. The former increased the number of vertebrae and (partly fused) ribs, while the latter reduced both. These patterns were interpreted in terms of the relationship between an embryological inductor and potent tissues. An increased (or decreased) number of the vertebral structures were modeled in terms of a posterior (or anterior) displacement of the limb potent tissue (or limb inductor) (Green 1955). Spatially distinct *lu* and *lx* genes thus determined spatially distinct arrangements of presumptive territories.

One may mention two additional symptoms of the instrumental status of the mapping technologies at Bar Harbor. First, in contrast to the Edinburgh school of mouse genetics (which included T.C. Carter, D.S. Falconer, and M.F. Lyon), which started to systematize localization research after Second World War by means of radiation treated mice, the Maine mousers did not develop mapping strains until the late 1950s. The mutants employed by Snell were simple testing strains bearing two markers, which were sufficient for achieving classical three-point-tests. Consequently, the Jackson geneticists rarely reported distance data. One exception was the linkage study of *pirouette* (Dickie 1946). However, generally the scientific reports did not mention the construction of the sort of complex mapping devices designed in Edinburgh, that is, stocks juxtaposing four to six mutations in a single linkage group to be employed for screening large sections of the genetic map at once (Carter 1952).

More importantly, the Jackson mousers made no use of radiation and radioactive isotopes to produce new and more numerous mutants. The procedure could have made mapping ventures more tempting. It was explicitely ruled out by Little. The issue came under discussion in 1948, as the Atomic Energy Commission expanded its production of isotopes, and advertised their uses in biological research. Little wrote,

> In considering the prompt and generous offer of space at the Brookhaven Laboratory, the Trustees realized that if the Jackson Laboratory colony of mice was brought into any possible contact with radioactive isotopes (…) the one adequate material would be jeopardized. (…) The Trustees have therefore decided to exclude from the Jackson Laboratory all the radioactive isotopes, and all animals or material exposed to them. (…) Since production of mutations, and other cytogenic or histogenic changes may be increased above their normal rate of incidence by exposure to irradiation, a large control population is the only way in which valid and measurable 'normal' incidence can be established.[16]

Isotopes were banned in the name of the most valuable products of the Jackson: genetic control and genetic purity. The effects of radiation on the genetic material were therefore to be researched by others, in the first place by the Atomic Energy Commission geneticists.

From this discussion, one may conclude that, the biomedical culture of the Jackson and the modeling *habitus* led to forms of work, experimental techniques, and thinking habits which proved incompatible with the structural approaches of gene mappers. While true, this statement is at the same time incomplete. A few developments in the immediate postwar period testify to an emerging mapping spirit within the arena of mouse genetics. One development, which remains to be properly investigated, was the appearance of projects linking mutant production and genetic localization within the context of radiation studies sponsored by the US and British atomic authorities. A second change was the establishment of a newsletter, which helped to organize the dispersed community of mousers.

The issue of linkage information surfaced in the late 1930s. Thinking of rationalizing the exchange of mutants, L. Dunn—who was probably the most Morganian among the mousers—sought to delegate the editing of a Mouse Newsletter. In 1937, he wrote the young William Gates, then at Louisiana State University:

> I am reminded by the receipt of codified linkage data for the fowl from Warren that the people working with mice began the same type of circular report, which has apparently been given up. (...) You probably have your hands full, but if the opportunity arose and you were able to correspond with some other people who are working in similar problems, I am sure all would welcome a resumption of the type of thing that you used to do. (...) The people at Little's laboratory keep records of data but aren't primarily interested in mutations other than those useful for cancer work, but Couldman seems sufficiently interested to represent that laboratory if you need someone there.[17]

Gates proved amenable to the proposal. During the following spring, he wrote all the laboratories involved in mouse genetics. A first circular was sent out in July 1938, offering to gather information on current projects and available stocks. As a testimony to the social prerequisite for any mapping venture, Gates added: "An interesting item, which I think a group of this kind can accomplish is to tabulate the present linkage information in mice."[18] Gates' project did not expand beyond the stage of collecting data for a putative survey of mouse genetics. When the war broke out, nothing had been published. Snell decided to resume the task. In 1941, he circulated the first mimeographed *Mouse Genetics News*. During the war and its aftermath, this issue was reprinted several times with unevenly updated information. The real start of the Mouse Newsletter took place in 1949, when the information service was taken over by Dunn, and relocated at Columbia.

In contrast to the *Drosophila Information Service*, the mouse journal focused on the accurate description of existing stocks, and on bibliographical information. The main effect of this newsletter was to facilitate both the development of homogenous nomenclature, and the circulation of inbred strains. Descriptions of research results and projects occupied little space. Linkage data surfaced here and there, when Dunn's correspondents considered that they were worth mentioning. Until the mid-1950s, a few centers including Columbia, Edinburgh, and the various laboratories involved in radiation studies actually engaged in building a loose mapping collective.

A third, and more critical, sign of growing interest in mapping was the postwar invention of a powerful hybrid, a form of biomedical mapping, originating in the renewal of transplantation studies. In 1938, the immunologist P.A. Gorer, then at the Lister Institute in London, published a paper linking transplantation studies, blood group research, and hereditary transmission (Gorer 1938). The article reported a series of experiments suggesting that in albino mice, the genetic ability to resist a tumor specific to that strain, segregated with a particular antigen, called type II. This antigen was characteristic of mouse red cells, and detectable by means of agglutination reactions. Gorer thus translated Little's old assumption about the genetic basis of tumor transplantation, into a modern hypothesis on the genetic control of antigenic molecules. As he expanded this correlation, Gorer was regularly invited to visit the Jackson Laboratory.

He first came for a sabbatical in 1946–47, during which he worked on genes, transplantation, and inbred strains. The product of his association with Snell was a *dispositif* for mapping the newly labeled mouse histocompatibility genes (Snell 1948). Building on Snell's experience of linkage and inbreeding technologies, the collaborating biologists invented a visualization system for the postulated transplantation genes. Gorer had introduced the basic procedure by combining the inoculation of reference tumors with blood typing. In Bar Harbor, this was complemented with genetic tools. In particular, the transmission of Gorer's type II factor was linked to the transmission of the *fused* mutation. The latter was a genetic marker of easy use since *fused* provoked (dominant) malformation of the tail. Once the linkage was recognized, Snell generalized the procedure to develop a genetic screen for other alleles. Further, he also mobilized the Jackson know-how into a second direction. Linkage tests were completed with a protocol for selecting *isogenic* strains, that is, strains differing by one histocompatibility factor (Figure 7.4).

The procedure aimed at importing one foreign histocompatibility gene at a time in a given strain A. The test for such successful importation was the production of hybrids between A animals and an inbred strain acting as a putative source of transplantation genes. F1 animals, which proved able to resist a tumor specific to strain A, were preserved. An homogenous genetic background of the A type would then be restored by continuous breeding with A mice. Benefiting from the Jackson stocks, Snell could start isogenic strains from 100 inbred lines. Five years later, by the mid-1950s, the procedure had proved highly successful since half of these strains had reached or passed the twelfth generation, then taken as the threshold for genetic homogeneity.

One may call this package of animal resources, breeding, variation, and testing procedures, an immunogenetic system. Its productivity was not only manifested in the number of isogenic lines that the Jackson initiated, but also in Snell's literary production. It is worth noting that the deciphering of the mouse histocompatibility

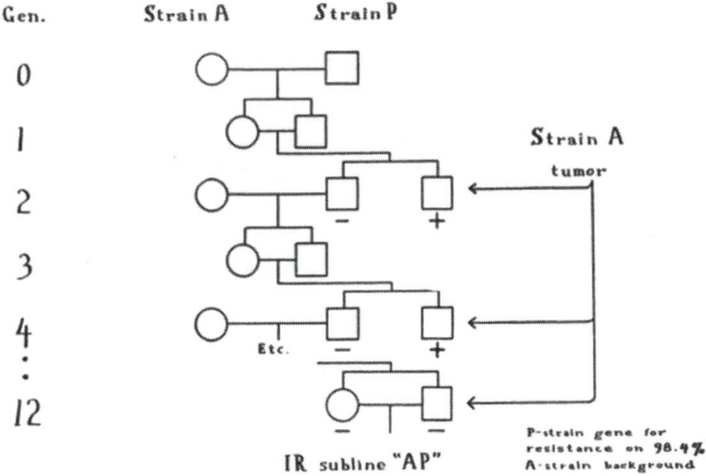

Figure 7.4 Producing isogenic strains, that is, mouse strains differing by just one histocompatibility factor was one of the key aspect of Snell's mapping practice at the Jackson Laboratory. (From Snell 1953.)

complex—in contrast to the collective nature of Drosophila mapping—remained Snell's affair. It is not that isogenic lines did not circulate. The correspondence between Snell, Gorer and Little, which has been left at Bar Harbor, document regular exchanges and friendly relationships.[19] A relatively stable division of labor, nonetheless, emerged. During the decade 1950–60, Snell published twice as many articles as Gorer's group. Both performed crossings and immune reactions, but the latter focused on the characterization of antigens and immunology testing. The former was most systematic in his exploitation of the isogenic lines and F1 tests, producing several H locus and two dozen alleles (Snell 1958).

To what extent was Snell's enterprise, a mapping project rather than the mobilization of linkage technologies, analogous to what had previously been done at Columbia or at the Jackson? Two features are important in this respect. First, Snell's research on histocompatibility shared an emphasis on gene localization with early chromosomal mapping. Snell perceived that sort of structural analysis as a prerequisite and a clue to functional studies. Second, the search for the *H* genes implied a process of reduction akin to the translation of phenotypes into a one-dimensional alignment of hereditary factors. It is true that the histocompatibility project initially did not translate into inscriptions that one would at first sight call maps. Rather, the outcome consisted of tables listing strains, alleles, and typing results, more precisely tables of antigenic components and alleles (Figure 7.5).

The individualization of the latter, however, relied on linkage data, and rough localization. In that sense, these lists were—like maps—aligning the genetic factors. But Snell's tables aligned the *H* factors in a second more innovative way.

Allele	Antigenic components												Typed strains
H-2^{a}	C	D	E	F	–	H	–	K	M	–	–	–	A AKR.K
H-2^{b}	–	D^{b}	E	F	–	–	–	–	–	–	–	–	A.BY C57BL/6 C57BL/10 B10.BY B10.LP
													C57L C3H.SW D1.LP LP 129
H-2^{c}		D											D1.C
H-2^{d}	C	D	E^{d}	F		H	–	–	M	–	–	–	BALB/c C57BL/6Ks B10.D2 B10.SW DBA/2 ST.T6
H-$2^{d'}$	C	D'	E^{d}	F				–	M				YBL/Rr YBR/Wi
H-2^{e}	C		E	F		–							STOLI
H-2^{f}			E?		G	H	I						A.CA B6.M
H-2^{k} and	C	–	E	–		H		K	–	–	–	–	AKR AKR.ALB CBA CHI C3H C3H.K C57BR/a
H-$2^{k'}$													C57BR/cd C58 D1.ST ST
H-2^{m}		–	E					K	M				AKR.M
H-2^{p}	C	–	E					–		P	–	–	P
H-2^{q}	C	–	E			–		–	M	–	Q	–	B6.Y C/St DBA/1
H-2^{r}	C?	–			–		–	K					LP.RIII RIII/Wy
H-2^{s}	C	–	E		G	–	–	–	–	–	–	S	A.SW
Crossover	C	D^{b}	E	F				K					From $(H\text{-}2^{a}/H\text{-}2^{b})F_1$
Crossover	C	D	E	F				–					From $(H\text{-}2^{a}/H\text{-}2^{b})F_1$
Crossover	–	D^{b}	E^{d}	F				–					From $(H\text{-}2^{d}/H\text{-}2^{b})F_1$

Figure 7.5 Mapping the histocompatibility genes resulted in a new form of tables, which linked strains, genetic alleles, and serological typing results. (From Snell 1953.)

The correspondence between alleles and antigens was presented as a representation of the linear relationship between genes, gene products, and surface macromolecules. This suggestion was a direct echo of the practice of biochemical mapping, the widely discussed alignment of genes, enzymes, and metabolic pathways, introduced by Beadle and Tatum in the course of their Neurospora work.[20]

One last feature highlighting the biomedical nature of Snell's mapping project is that histocompatibility research was perceived as leading to an increased ability to control the fate of grafts and cellular immunity. The basic reasoning consisted in saying that knowing and manipulating the *H* genes would help work aimed at fighting indigenous cancers. As Snell wrote:

> A great body of evidence has been built up, which demonstrates that the tendency of a given strain to accept or reject a transplanted mass of tumor is largely determined by the nature of the two histocompatibility genes. (...) A change in the histocompatibility gene may occur by mutation and suddenly shift the entire characteristics of a mouse stock. (...) Related to the study of genetic control of tumor growth are the attempts to immunize against tumors.[21]

This was no simple rhetoric. The Jackson geneticists made numerous attempts to increase the resistance to transplanted tumors, initially by inoculating tumor extracts and antiserums, later by working on adoptive cellular immunity.

Although transplantation research paved the way to a form of genetic mapping, the irony of the Jackson history however is that systematic chromosomal study of the mouse was not undertaken as a follow-up. Instead, it emerged out of the use of inbred mice for modeling human cancer. As discussed later, the changing scale of biomedical research was at the roots of this unexpected development.

Scaling-up: mapping in the era of big biomedecine

In the 1930s, the search for anticancer drugs was seen as a marginal, slightly disreputable subject doomed to failure (Bud 1978). Surgery and radiation were the treatments of choice. By contrast, after the Second World War, professionals as well as lay people shared the feeling—partly based on the recent success of antibiotics—that the control of malignant diseases by means of drugs was imminent. Moreover, this control would be achieved by the establishment of large-scale cooperative programs modeled on the collaboration between state research agencies, hospitals, and industry which characterized the development of penicillin during the War (Löwy 1996; Gaudillière 2002).

In the early 1950s, this feeling was transformed into a political issue. The continuous pressure of Congress, together with growing demands of non-National Cancer Institute specialists, and of the chemical industry, led in 1955 to the development of the Cancer Chemotherapy National Service Center (CCNSC). The explicit aim of the new body was, in the words of one of its main organizers: "to set up all the functions of a pharmaceutical house," namely the synthesis of candidate molecules, the pre-clinical testing of these chemicals, and the clinical trials of the most promising drugs.

Pre-clinical screening of drugs, unlike clinical research, can be relatively easily adapted to standardized, industry-like patterns of production (Gaudillière and Löwy 1998). The achievement of uniformity among experimental mice was one of the important elements in such adaptation. The CCNSC decided that three transplantable tumors would be employed in all the laboratory tests of drugs. The basic scheme was that, molecules inhibiting the growth of these tumors in mice would be good candidates for clinical trials. The decision to use tumors transplanted in inbred strains of mice immediately created a need to enlarge the production of such animals. From 1956 onward, the CCNSC collaborated with the Jackson Memorial Laboratory to elaborate minimal standards for laboratory animals and develop a mouse production infrastructure.

Mass production was first conducted in Bar Harbor, and was later extended to commercial laboratories (Zubord 1966). All the animals used in screening tests had to be supplied by producers accredited by the CCNSC, and all the demands for the supply of mice were processed through the CCNSC's Mammalian Genetics and Animal Production Section. The Jackson workers were responsible for organizing the control of genetic purity. The most important task was to supply the other commercial breeders with certified, breeding pairs of mice to be put at reproductive work. The CCNSC thus opened a specialized market, which made possible the large-scale production of "more uniformly healthy, well fed mice, with known genetic background and variability."[22]

A few years later, US specialists in drug therapy of cancer, strongly criticized CCNSC methods of screening for anti-tumor drugs. Aware of poor correlation between the anti-cancer activity observed in the three screens system and the results of the first clinical trials, scientists associated with the CCNSC program, proposed enlarging the assay system in order to include other tumors and animals.

These changes in the organization of CCNSC services did not, however, end the controversy between the scientists and doctors, who on the one hand advocated an industrial-type selection of cancer-inhibiting compounds, and on the other hand supported a more traditional style of investigation, based on clinical expertise. Tinkering with the screening procedure however induced the CCNSC directors to argue that—besides concrete (and debatable) achievements in the organization of efficient testing for anti-cancer drugs—their program brought important benefits to the scientific community as a whole. One of the most important results of the chemotherapy screening program, they explained, was

> the development of enough high-quality animal resources to meet the needs of the program and the entire scientific community. The program was a key factor in anticipating and providing such resources for the major expansion of biomedical research in the past decade.
>
> (Zubrod 1966)

The impact of this industrial research operation on the community of mousers was very important. The CCNSC-based mass-production did make some inbred strains widely available to biomedical scientists, but it also altered the nature of the Jackson operations. In 1955, the Jackson Laboratory sold 200,000 mice. Five years later, the production of inbred animals or first generation hybrids for cancer research reached one million.

Scaling up required more production rooms, more technicians and caretakers, cheaper and simpler means for bedding, feeding, and housing the mice. But, expansion was not only a matter of increasing quantity; it also implied the challenge of maintaining quality. In lieu of guaranteeing the uniformity of dozens of thousands of animals, the laboratory was to operate on a plant size and standardize many hundreds of thousands of mice. Scaling up the production of mice by two orders of magnitude meant increased risks of contamination, diseases, and unnoticed variations in the living material. Scaling up required increased control of living conditions, increased control of the personnel, and a well-organized control of quality. In other words, mass-production changed the definition of tasks, the organization of the laboratory, and the division of labor. The production of standard testing mice for cancer research thus established the animal, technical and human infrastructure which was indispensable for a large mapping venture.

At Bar Harbor, a reformed production scheme operated from 1956–57 onward, after the signature of a major contract with the CCNSC.[23] This scheme relied on the coordination of three departments: (a) the foundation stocks where scientists and technicians maintained pedigreed and systematically controlled animals from every inbred strain; (b) the research expansion stocks and production expansion stocks where technicians produced hundreds of breeding pairs a year; and (c) the production stocks, where caretakers and fore(wo)men put these pairs to reproductive work.

In the newly built mouse production rooms, not only new mice, but novel forms of work emerged. Caretaking was not "taylorized" in the sense of time-motion studies, but task distribution became much more specific. Local recommendations added to the general rules set up by the CCNSC. Critical to the success of the operation was keeping records of mouse circulation, as when moving pairs from the production expansion stocks to the production rooms. As a booklet for new Jax workers explained:

> Each complete litter not used to make new breeding pairs within the production expansion stocks should be put into a pen marked with a small card noting strain, pedigree number of parents (female number is always written first), birth date of offspring, number of males and females. (...) Arrange these animals in trios and in brother–sister pairs for the production stocks supply assigning to each mating an identifying number. (...) These identifying numbers follow these animals throughout their existence in the production colony.[24]

Breeding cards showing the complete records of an animal's life were kept on permanent file, coded and transferred onto IBM cards for statistical analysis. This increased control of the mice, both generated and required new data and new knowledge of husbandry, statistical normality, and variation.

Accordingly, a few engineers were employed to conduct studies of breeding behavior, longevity, nutrition, causes of death, and growth rates. They soon joined colleagues in the other production centers to develop a laboratory animal care society. Further, in contrast to what might have been expected from the prevailing concern with homogenous, large-scale production, the development of the research expansion stocks actually opened a new space for innovation, at the boundary between the laboratory and the plant. In this space, a few researchers were responsible both for systematic quality control based on grafting assays and for the selection of scientifically interesting stocks. Following the mid-1950s reorganization, the Jackson workers paid special attention to variants and they entered a world inhabited by dozens of mutant strains of mice. With the changing scale of production and increased attention to abnormalities in large stocks, a threshold was passed: the zone between the laboratory and the plant started to produce numerous good mutants for both chromosome mapping and for biomedical research (see Figure 7.6(a) and (b)).

This pattern may be illustrated by the origins of the mouse mutants described after 1945 (Table 7.1).

Rather than initiating a radical departure from previous research habits or accepted paradigms in genetics, this mutational explosion of the late 1950s/early 1960s resulted in the generalization of an integrated program of research with the mutants. This program combined modeling and mapping. The quantitative change (more mutants) had qualitative consequences since it made possible the transition from linkage studies to an organized mapping enterprise. Although the biomedical status of most mouse mutants did not vanish (Gaudillière 2001), a new

(a)

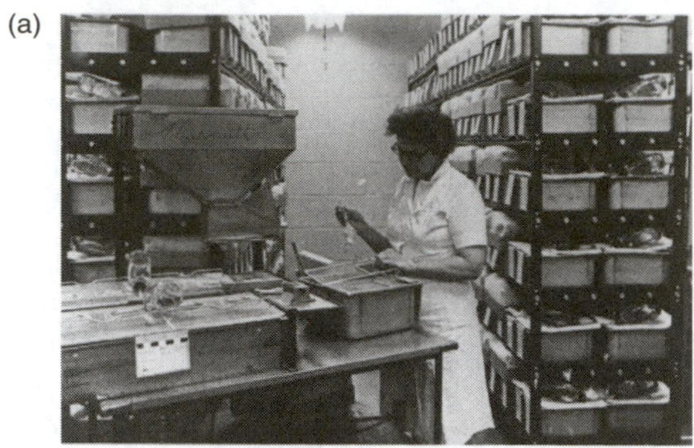

(b)

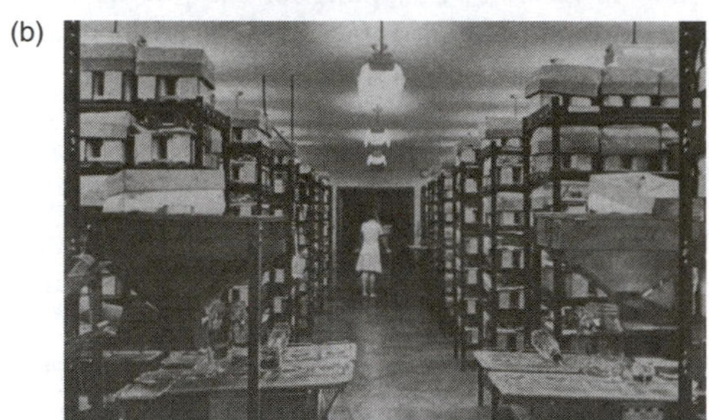

Figure 7.6 (a) and (b) The changing scale of mouse production at the Jackson Laboratory did not only mean scaling-up technologies (for instance through the building of new breeding rooms), but implied a new gaze at variants. (Reproduced with permission of the Jackson Laboratory Library Archives.)

Table 7.1 Mouse mutants described after 1945

	Jackson	*Other centers*	*Pathological mutants*	*Neurological mutants*	*Skeleton mutants*	*Total*
1946–50	0	12	6	0	2	12
1951–55	11	37	24	9	9	48
1956–60	15	49	34	12	10	64
1961–65	48	68	52	19	11	116

Source: Green, E. (ed.) (1966) *Biology of the Laboratory Mouse*, Jackson Memorial Laboratory.

research layer was nonetheless added with the establishment of a Jackson mouse mutant stocks center. The center was funded by the National Science Foundation, and played a key role as a mapping resource center.

The idea of establishing such a facility echoed previous attempts to expand the Jackson laboratory. During the 1940s, Little had approached the Rockefeller

Foundation to discuss the creation of Jackson units for inbred guinea pig, inbred rabbit, and inbred dog genetics. Although seriously considered, the scheme failed. Little's proposal ended up in a limited program for breeding dogs, which the Rockefeller Medical Sciences Division supported as an attempt at developing research into the genetics of behavior.

As described in the first funding application to the NSF, the mouse mutant center too was to combine production and research. Its most important function was to maintain all "good mutants, i.e. mutants for easily recognizable single genes," including "stocks with multiple mutations" which were intentionally "constructed or under construction for efficiently testing a new mutation for linkage with markers of the known linkage groups of the mouse."[25] Margaret Green, the head of the new center, thus organized the collection of strains not available at the Jackson, and their maintenance. Becoming a resource center, however, meant that the Jackson was to make all these stocks available on request. Tensions with the commercial side of the enterprise were somehow inevitable. They took the form of having some mutants like *obese, hairless* or *dwarf* being part of the NSF funded collection while being produced on a larger scale within the mutant production stocks established by Green in conjunction with the production department of the laboratory. One must, however, notice that conflicts of interest were rare. Few mutants were both, in great demand and difficult to breed. Orders from most outside customers were usually limited to a small number of breeding pairs. Among all the mutants discovered at Bar Harbor during the first five years of operation of the mutant center, one single strain—i.e. *diabetes*—actually crossed the threshold of the mutant center to join obese, hairless, dwarf, and muscular dystrophy mice massively sold on the research market.

The contribution of the mutant center to mapping was not only to provide animal material. It publicized the existence of mutants by producing a complement to the *Mouse Newsletter*. Since the late 1940s, news about who was maintaining what mutants, as well as about the isolation of new variants, had vastly expanded. The collection of information about dozens of centers had become more difficult. The task of establishing regularly consolidated lists of stocks was apparently so tedious that nobody complained when the Jackson workers proposed replacing the newsletter. As part of its operations, the mutant center circulated a simpler list of inbred strains indicating who could supply them, in case the Jackson could not. The staff of the center also became responsible for compiling the Standardized Nomenclature of Inbred Strains.

In a vein quite similar to that of the Jackson's practice in cancer research, claims about the ability of the mutant research center to supply up-to-date research resources were substantiated by local scientific results. Local linkage studies provided the background for selecting good mutants and developing complex mapping stocks. This led to a rapid and simultaneous growth of animal capital, linkage reports, and mouse genetic maps. In 1960, when the mutant center was established, the core stocks were composed of 73 mutants out of the 190 existing variants. In 1970, the center maintained 125 mutants out of 400 classified variations. Testing tools were of two sorts: (a) stocks "for efficiently testing new mutations for linkage with markers of the 19 known linkage groups. These stocks contain nearly all the 'good' markers in useful locations"; (b) "with several markers in the same linkage group to facilitate determination of the linear order of a new mutant, once its linkage group has been established." Moreover, the mouse mutant center had by then developed new strains characterized by one or several chromosomal translocations, which were viewed as landmarks for a cytological map. In 1950–54, 32 papers on linkages between

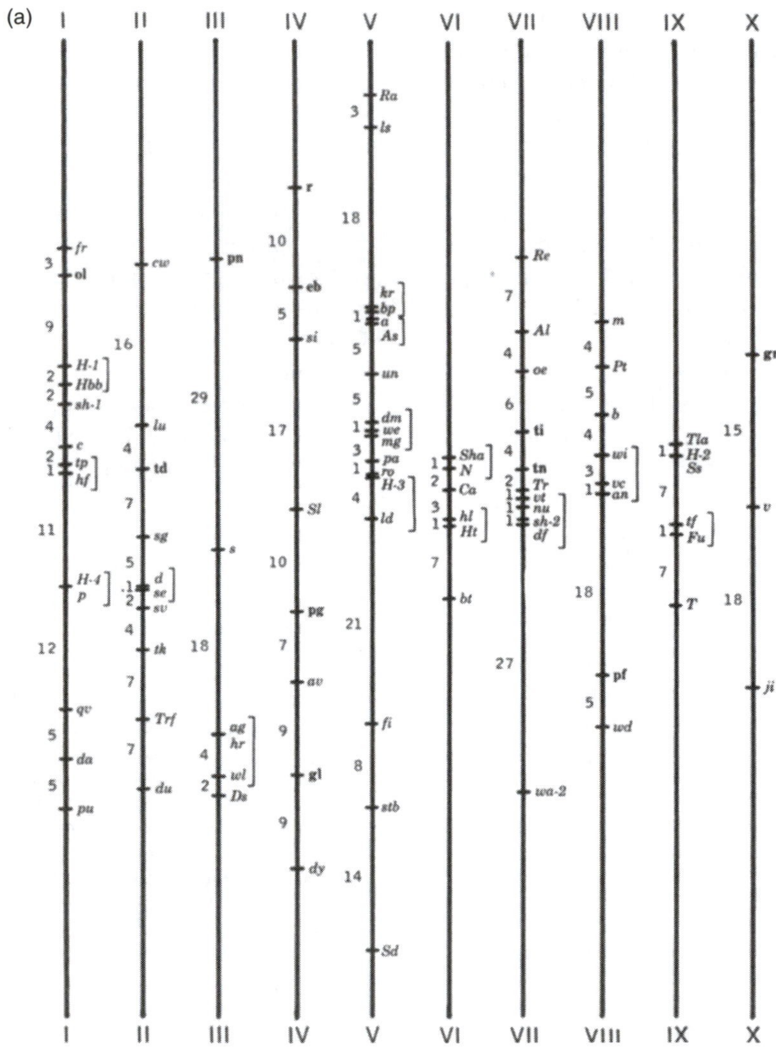

Figure 7.7 (a and b) In 1965, the map of the mouse chromosomes drawn by the Jackson workers included one hundred loci. It was in all respects analogous to the Drosophila chromosomal maps. (From Staff of the Jackson Laboratory 1965.)

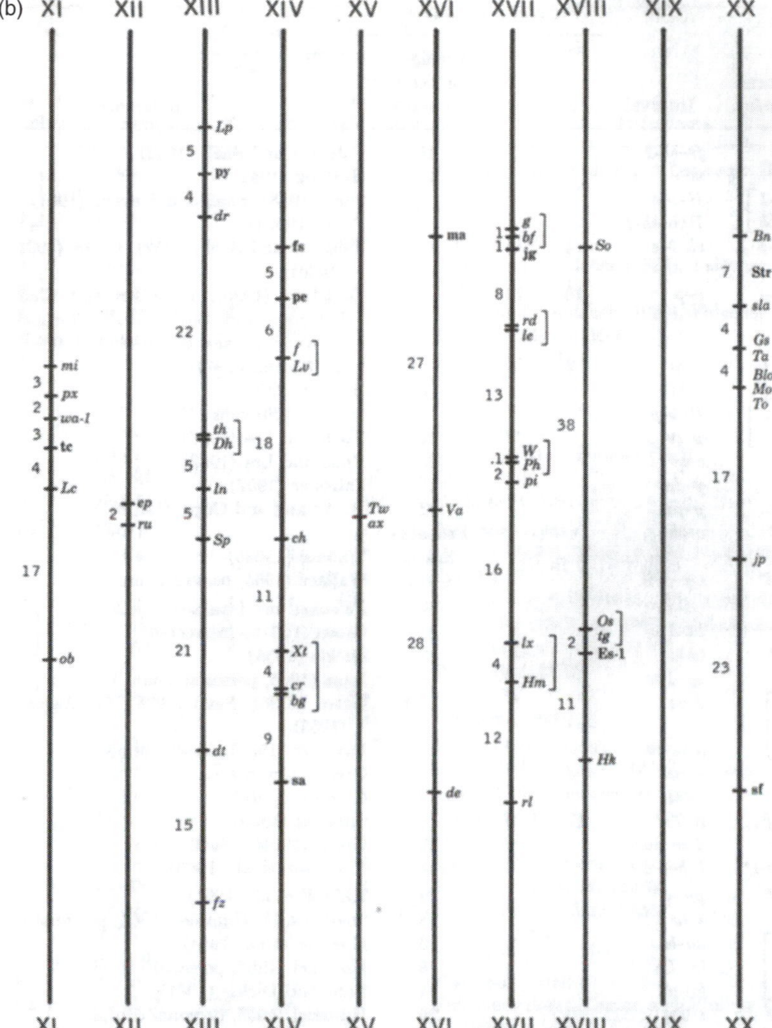

Figure 7.7 Continued

genes and chromosomal localization were published, four of which were authored by Jackson scientists. In the years 1955–59, the respective figures were 34 and 6. By contrast, in the years 1960–64, the number of linkage reports (most of them in the *Mouse Newsletter*, since such information was no longer viewed as worth an entire article) doubled (61) with one-third (22 publications) coming from the Jackson mutant center. Meanwhile, the map of mouse genes had become a pure localization device reporting chromosomal location and linear distances between genes (Figure 7.7 (a) and (b)).

Conclusion

The first conclusion to be taken from this *flanerie* across the worlds of mammalian genetics is that Morgan's style of research did not translate well into mouse language. For decades, observers of heredity in mice did not view linkage studies and chromosomal localization as worthwhile projects in their own right. They borrowed linkage techniques and notions of chromosomal genetics, but they did not consider that a systematic organization of the knowledge on mouse genes in the form of linear maps was worth the investment of resources, which was required to render mice similar to flies. The history of the mouse thus reminds us that the genetic cultures and genetic practices of the twentieth century are more diverse than anticipated from a Drosophila-centered view of the field.

Mice were not viewed as analogous to flies. As mentioned in the introduction to this chapter, the basic properties of the organisms are often evoked when explaining this contrast, particularly when one comes to the mutant problem. Certainly, the history of genetics would have been different if mice had been good breeders. However, biological constraints should not be taken out of context. Genetic mapping was neither the straightforward use of material resources, nor the simple outcome of observation. It is a form of work, a historically located system of practice, which combines epistemic, literary, social, and technological layers.

Mice were not produced like flies, at least until the post-war boom in biomedical research changed the status of mice. Within the Jackson Laboratory, a systematic mapping project based on the selection, breeding, and crossing of a significant number of mutants did surface in the 1960s. The uses of inbred strains in cancer research then led to the development of a large production infrastructure, which in turn created new spaces for the isolation and maintenance of mutants. The fate of laboratory mice was not equivalent to that of laboratory flies, because the former were tools rather than problems, because they were technological objects. Within this context, the production of the organism was not a metaphore. It was a matter of scaling-up, building plants, and organizing sales. Technology should however not be reduced merely to engineering and marketing. The technological side of mapping includes production rooms, but also norms of standardization, quality control protocols, and new ways of looking at variations. The mapping of mice did not follow the mapping of flies, because mice were constructed as human beings. Mice were initially not mapped, because the genetics to be done with them was not chromosomal genetics. Inbred mice emerged in the research landscape as models of pathological processes. They were mammals akin to the human body. This biomedical construction of the laboratory mouse did not only imply that the most interesting—and most searched-for—strains were those of medical and pathological interest. It also means that, as illustrated by the culture of the Bussey school, mouse genetics was dominated, by a form of physiological genetics. Questions about phenotype determination, then provided a broader and more straightforward zone for trading with medicine.

Before the era of the big biomedecine, the use of mice as models actually created niches for particular forms of mapping. These were impure practices exemplified by Snell's research in immunogenetics. These *mélanges* articulated structural genes and medical aims, linkage techniques and biochemistry, moral and commercial economies. In that sense, they anticipated the biotechnological and medical dynamics of contemporary genomics. Somehow, in the end, history repeats itself.

Notes

1 W.F. Loomis diary, R.G. 1.1, 200, Box 144, folder 1779, Rockefeller Archives Center (RAC).
2 L.C. Dunn to W.E. Castle, May 15, 1925; American Philosophical Society (APS), Dunn papers, DB 917.
3 W.E. Castle to L.C. Dunn, October 28, 1924, APS, Dunn papers, DB 917.
4 W.E. Castle to L.C. Dunn, October 17, 1930, APS, Dunn papers, DB 917.
5 L.C. Dunn to W.E. Castle, November 4, 1930, APS, Dunn papers, DB 917.
6 W.E. Castle to L.C. Dunn, December 20, 1933, APS, Dunn papers, DB 917.
7 W.E. Castle to L.C. Dunn, June 29, 1928 APS, Dunn papers, DB 917.
8 W.E. Castle to L.C. Dunn, February 13, 1923, APS, Dunn papers, DB 917.
9 W.E. Castle to L.C. Dunn, February 13, 1929, APS, Dunn papers, DB 917.
10 W.E. Castle to L.C. Dunn, October 7, 1929, APS, Dunn papers, DB 917.
11 J. Bauer to W.W. Weaver, March 24, 1937, RAC, RG 1.2, 100 IHD Laboratory.
12 On this see W.W. Weaver's correspondence, RAC, RG 1.1, 200, Box 143, folder 1774.
13 *Genes, Mice and Men: A Quarter-Century of Progress at the R.B. Jackson Memorial Laboratory*, Bar Harbor, 1954, Archives of the Jackson Laboratory (AJL).
14 C.C. Little to W.W. Weaver, December 4, 1937, RAC, RG 1.1 series 200, Box 143, folder 1774.
15 Jackson Laboratory Annual Reports for 1938–39, 1940–41, 1943, AJL.
16 Annual report of the Jackson Memorial Laboratory, 1948–49, AJL.
17 L.C. Dunn to W. Gates, January 14, 1937, APS, Dunn papers, DB 917.
18 W. Gates to "Mousers," July 2, 1937, APS, Dunn papers, DB 917.
19 C.C. Little to P.A. Gorer, December 9, 1953; P.A. Gorer to C.C. Little, April 5, 1954, AJL.
20 Snell did not try to push his system into a simple one to one relationship. Histocompatibility genes were viewed as genetically simple but molecularly complex since they seemed to control several antigens. Snell did not try to disentangle this pattern by looking for smaller levels of genetic analysis. Since the combination of genetic and serologic techniques sufficed in circumventing the practical difficulties created by such an overlap, loose alignment remained the rule.
21 Annual Report of the Jackson Memorial Laboratory, 1951–52, AJL.
22 The National Program of Cancer Chemotherapy: Information Statement, *Cancer Chemotherapy Reports*, 1959, pp. 43–64.
23 Minutes of the CCNSC Chemotherapy Review Board, 1959. List of mouse supply contracts. NCI Archives, AR 002397.
24 Guide to New Personnel in Jackson Laboratory Research Expansion Stocks and Production Expansion Stocks, 1959, AJL.
25 Jackson Memorial Laboratory, "Research Proposal to the National Science Foundation," November 1960, AJL.

Bibliography

Bud, R. (1978) "Strategies in American Cancer Research After World War II," *Social Studies of Science*, 8: 425–59.

Burian, R.M. (1993) "How the Choice of Experimental Organism Matters: Epistemological Reflections on an Aspect of Biological Practice," *Journal of the History of Biology*, 26: 351–67.

Carter, T.C. and Falconer, D.S. (1952) "Stocks for Detecting Linkage in the Mouse, and the Theory of Their Design," *Journal of Genetics*, 50: 307–23.

Clause, B.T. (1993) "The Wistar Rat as a Right Choice: Establishing Mammalian Standards and the Ideal of the Standardized Mammal," *Journal of the History of Biology*, 26: 329–49.

Dickie, M. (1946) "Linkage Studies with the Pirouette Gene in the Mouse," *Journal of Heredity*, 37: 335–7.

Dunn, L.C. and Charles, D.R. (1937a) "Studies on Spotting Patterns: I. Analysis of Quantitative Variations in the Pied Spotting of the House Mouse," *Genetics*, 22: 14–43.

Dunn, L.C. (1937b) "Studies on Spotting Patterns: II. Genetic Analysis of Variegated Spotting in the House Mouse," *Genetics*, 22: 43–64.

—— (1962, reprinted 1991) *A Short History of Genetics*, Ames: Iowa State University Press.

Gaudillière, J.-P. (1999) "Circulating Mice and Viruses: The Jackson Memorial Laboratory, the National Cancer Institute, and the Genetics of Breast Cancer," in M. Fortun and E. Mendelsohn (eds), *The Practices of Human Genetics*, Dordrecht: Kluwer Academic Publishers, 89–124.

Gaudillière, J.-P. and Löwy, I. (1998) "Disciplining Cancer: Mice and the Practice of Genetic Purity," in J.-P. Gaudillière and I. Löwy (eds), *The Invisible Industrialist: Manufactures and the Production of Scientific Knowledge*, London: Macmillan, 209–49.

—— (2000) "Making Mice and Other Devices: The Dynamics of Instrumentation in American Biomedical Research, 1930–1960," in B. Joerges and T. Shinn (eds), *Instrumentation Between Science, State and Industry*, Dordrecht: Kluwer Academic Publishers, 175–96.

—— (2001) "Making Heredity in Mice and Men: The Production and Uses of Animal Models in Postwar Human Genetics," in I. Löwy and J.-P. Gaudillière (eds), *Heredity and Infection: A History of Disease Transmission*, London: Routledge, 181–202.

—— (2002) *L'invention de la biomédecine: La France, l'Amérique et la production des savoirs du vivant, 1945–1965*, Paris: La Découverte.

Geison, G. and Laubichler, M.D. (2001) "The Varied Lives of Organisms: Variation in the Historiography of the Biological Sciences," *Studies in History and Philosophy of the Biological and the Biomedical Sciences*, 3: 1–29.

Gorer, P.A. (1938) "The Genetic and Antigenic Basis of Tumor Transplantation," *Journal of Pathology*, 54: 691–7.

Gorer, P.A., Lyman, S. and Snell, G.D. (1948) "Studies on the Genetic and Antigenic Basis of Tumor Transplantation: Linkage between a Histocompatibility Gene and 'fused' in Mice," *Proceedings of the Royal Society*, Ser. B., 135: 499–505.

Green, M.C. (1955) "Luxoid—A New Hereditary Leg and Foot Abnormality," *Journal of Heredity*, 46: 91–9.

Holstein, J. (1979) *The First Fifty Years at the Jackson Laboratory*, Bar Harbor: The Jackson Laboratory.

Kohler, R. (1994) *Lords of the Fly: Drosophila and the Experimental Life*, Chicago: The University of Chicago Press.

Little, C.C. (1913) *Experimental Studies of the Inheritance of Coat Color in Mice*, Washington: Carnegie Institution Publications.

Little, C.C. (1923) "The Relations of Genetics to the Problem of Cancer," *Harvey Lectures 1921–1922*, Philadelphia: Lippincott, 65–88.

Little, C.C. and Tyzzer, E.E. (1916) "Further Experimental Studies of the Inheritance of Susceptibility to a Transplantable Tumor," *Journal of Medical Research*, 33: 393–427.

Loeb, L. (1908) "Über Entstehung eines Sarcom nach Transplantation eines Adenocarcinoms einer japanischen Maus," *Zeitschrift für Krebsforschung*, 7: 80.

Löwy, I. (1996) *Between Bench and Bedside: Science, Healing and Interleukine 2 in a Cancer Ward*, Cambridge: Harvard University Press.

Morse III, H.C. (ed.) (1978) *Origins of Inbred Mice*, New York: Academic Press.

Provine, W.B. (1986) *Sewall Wright and Evolutionary Biology*, Chicago: The University of Chicago Press.

Rader, K. (1995) *Making Mice: C.C. Little, the Jackson Laboratory, and the Standardization of* Mus musculus *for Research*, PhD dissertation, University of Indiana.

—— (1998) "The Mouse People: Murine Genetics Work at the Bussey Institution, 1909–1936," *Journal of the History of Biology*, 31: 327–54.

Sinnott, E.W. and Dunn, L.C. (1939) *Principles of Genetics*, New York: MacGraw Hill.

Snell, G.D. (1931) "Inheritance in the House Mouse: The Linkage Relations of Short-Ear, Hairless, and Naked," *Genetics*, 16: 42–74.

—— (1948) "Methods for the Study of Histocompatibility Genes," *Journal of Genetics*, 49: 87–108.

—— (1953) "The Genetics of Transplantation," *Journal of the National Cancer Institute*, 14: 691–700.

—— (1958) "Histocompatibility Genes of the Mouse: II. Production and Analysis of Isogenic Resistant Lines," *Journal of the National Cancer Institute*, 21: 843–77.

Staff of the Jackson Memorial Laboratory (1945) "A Chromosomal Map of Genes of the Mouse," *Journal of Heredity*, 36: 271–2.

Staff of the Jackson Memorial Laboratory (1965) *The Biology of the Laboratory Mouse*, Bar Harbor.

Tyzzer, E.E. (1909) "A Series of Spontaneous Tumors in Mice with Observation on the Influence of Heredity on the Frequency of Their Occurrence," *Journal of Medical Research*, 20: 479–519.

Zubrod, C.G. (1966) "The Cancer Chemotherapy Program 1965," *Cancer Chemotherapy Reports*, 50: 397–401.

Commentaries

Genetic mapping

Approaches to the spatial topography of genetics

David Turnbull

On July 7, 2000 the journal *Science* celebrated the publication of the map of the human genome. A quick visual survey shows that this issue had nine advertisements with some kind of allusion to maps in them; almost all of them utilizing an image of the earth from space, the ultimate panoptic icon, the entire world from one spot. But, there were also sixteen articles devoted to some form of mapping in the sense of detailing spatial topography, from plate subduction to protein folding. In addition, *Science* has a regular column "Science's Compass." The article celebrating the publication of the genome map was titled "Finally: The Book of Life and Instructions for Navigating it," invoking a trite, but seductive metaphor that is basically cartographic. Mapping and its attendant cartographic metaphors, are clearly some of the most profoundly important ways in which we conceive and understand the gene and also how we represent nature. The ubiquity and power of the map in our thinking calls for a close examination of how our representations of nature are affected by our mapping practices. Are invocations of mapping and map terminology simply handy tropes, or do they reveal a more profoundly cognitive spatiality? Or again, do our signifying practices and our mental processes interact and coproduce one another in some complex way? The workshop on Mapping Cultures of the Twentieth Century Genetics at the Max Planck Institute for the History of Science in Berlin raised a number of pointed questions about the role and nature of mapping, both in genetics and science generally. What is a map? What do maps do? Is there really any mapping going on? Is mapping specific to particular styles of doing genetic work? Are maps really necessary or are they just scaffolding? How do we move between and/or combine maps? Are genetic maps another capitalistic form of imperialism opening up territory for exploitation? Is mapping somehow linked to centralization in science? Is mapping fundamental to turning biology into informatics? What sorts of spatial and temporal narratives are invoked in mapping? What are we doing as historians, sociologists, philosophers or cultural analysts, in mapping cultures? Are we, like geneticists, doing some form of ontic politics, bringing into existence epistemic objects and reifying them? Is there an attached reflexive problem? Can we somehow put our understanding of mapping to use, can we on the one hand understand the processes of science better, can we, on the other hand, find different ways of imaging and ordering the world?

This chapter approaches the broad question of "what is the role of mapping in the human genome project?" by suggesting a number of ways we can conceive the nature of mapping and the mapping of nature and how such conceptions have been transformed in the development of genomics and proteomics. Much of the discussion about mapping is skewed by its cartographic origins. The emphasis has been on understanding topographical maps as forms of representation; for example, Harley and Woodward provide the broadest of classic definitions in their foundational series in the history of cartography: "Maps are graphic representations that facilitate a spatial understanding of things, concepts, conditions, processes, or events in the human world" (Harley and Woodward 1987: xvi). We could of course readily substitute natural for human in that definition. Extremely important critiques have been developed from this approach especially those building on the trenchant deconstructive work of Brian Harley which have largely concentrated on exploring how maps embody forms of power and what the possibilities are for resistance (Wood 1992; Harley 2001).

Inclusive as Harley and Woodward's definition is, it is important to develop a much broader, less representationalist approach. Mapping is an activity, it is performative, embodying skills and practices, and is central to all our ways of being, knowing, experiencing, and creating meaning, especially in the ways we naturalize the social and socialize the natural. Mapping like language is fundamental to a variety of processes: mathematical, linguistic, cognitive, semiotic, behavioral, political, communicative, aesthetic, and narratological. The reason for the centrality of mapping in such a variety of human intellectual, and technical practices is, I would argue, because it is basic to two key activities and processes for entities like ourselves that are embodied minds in an environment—that is movement and spatiality. But, just as language is fundamental to all the basic human activities and is also profoundly variable across cultures, so is mapping both fundamental and variable.

A recent, major transition within socio-cultural analysis generally has been the "spatial turn" (Shapin 1998) but there has as yet been little recognition of the deep underlying spatial commonalities, in a large number of disparate areas of research, that have come to see mapping as central. Such areas include: cognitive linguistics, mental mapping in geography, cognitive psychology, spatial cognition, AI, sociology of knowledge, anthropology of space, philosophy of science, genetic mapping, geography: cultural and physical, cartography, geographic information systems (GIS), cyberspace, science, and cultural studies, metamapping of mapping and the massive proliferation of mapping in all areas of science that Hall points out in his *Mapping the Next Millennium* (Hall 1992).

The following sections propose a formulation of a range of general claims about how maps provide for ways of reading, performing, representing and possessing, "nature" and where possible, illustrate them from a fairly general reading of the genetic mapping literature.

Maps as representations

It has long been recognized that maps cannot be simply "accurate representations." The questions of selection, generalization, scale, projection, frame, and code, all contribute to the recognition that maps are conventional and can be only evaluated against specific human purposes and criteria (Keates 1996). Nonetheless, a history of cartography as one of increasing map accuracy has become metonymic for scientific progress generally and has contributed to the resilience of positivism (Edney 1993). The problems of this representationalist position are classically undermined by such questions as Mandelbrot's "how long is the coastline of Britain?" (Mandelbrot 1983) and re-emphasized by the recent survey of Norway's coastline revealing it to be a staggering 45 percent longer than previously calculated. On Mandelbrot's analysis, of course, as we increase the accuracy or the resolution, by shortening our measuring sticks or increasing magnification, the coastline does not become a more precisely determined length but becomes instead infinitely long. Our devices for measuring the world frame our understanding of nature but cannot by themselves lead to greater correspondence with reality, rather they require the proliferation of evermore sophisticated technical devices and social strategies to keep our conceptions and nature in line, which simultaneously allows for the possible emergence of alternative spaces and representations (Turnbull 1998).

Maps as discursive devices for making connections and assemblages

A primary cognitive function of maps is the arrangement of apparently unrelated, disparate and distant items, events, ideas or processes in a spatial array so that otherwise unperceived connections can be made between them (Turnbull 1993). As David Harvey argues, "the discursive activity of mapping space is a fundamental prerequisite to the structuring of any kind of knowledge... Social relations are always spatial and exist within a certain produced framework of spatialities... [they are mappings] of some sort, symbolic material or figurative" (Harvey 1996: 111–12, cited in Wald 2000).

This suggests that mapping is fundamental to cognition, narration, discourse, and language use.

Knowledge production is not simply an idealistic linking of ideas; it is also a social process of linking people, practices and places—of creating a knowledge space. All knowledge is produced by particular groups of people at particular sites with particular skills, techniques, and technologies. These local knowledges have to be assembled, and maps are a classic example of the kinds of devices that enable knowledge to move. The resulting assemblages form a knowledge space in which particular ways of knowing, performing and interacting are normalized (Turnbull 1996a, 2000a).

For Latour maps are a key device for turning the world into a laboratory where the fragmented bits of nature become assemblable, amenable to measurement and alignment, in a network of inscriptions in the agonistic struggle. "Scientists master the world, but only if the world comes to them in the form of two-dimensional, superposable, combinable inscriptions." "That is immutable mobiles which when cleverly aligned produce the circulating reference" (Latour 1999: 29, 307).

However, the conditions for establishing maps as immutable mobiles and assemblage devices require considerable amounts of social labor. For topographical maps to become combinable the landscape has to be literally bound together with a network of surveyed triangles, national surveys have to be linked, and time has to be standardized (Turnbull 1996a). Spatiality itself is transformed; land, boundaries and ownership are coproduced with the mapping process (Thongchai 1994). Knowledge then, in all cultures, in all eras and at all levels is bound up in forms of space and movement.

Maps as devices to materialize questions

Robert Kohler in *Lords of the Fly* extends the Bachelardian thesis (Bachelard 1985) that techniques and instruments are frozen theory, and shows how genetic maps were coproduced in the process of transforming the fruit fly into a piece of standardized apparatus.

> Standard drosophilas were constructed from stocks that produced recombination data conforming most closely to Mendelian theory. Their chromosomes were a bricolage, artfuly put together from useful pieces of chromosomes of various mutant stock and cleaned by selective inbreeding of the genetic noise that messed up genetic mapping. The purposes and key concepts of mapping were thus built into domesticated drosophilas.
>
> (Kohler 1994: 23)

This exemplifies Hans-Jörg Rheinberger's general claim that "an experimental system is a device to materialize questions. It cogenerates the phenomena or material entities and the concepts they come to embody" (Rheinberger 1998: 288). Maps are thus a key component of experimental science which depends on the transformation of nature into a "manipulable system" (Stokes and Turnbull 1990).

Maps as tools for control, appropriation, and ideological expression

For Donna Haraway, the control that maps provide is not so much technical as political and instrumental, "cartography is perhaps the chief tool-metaphor of technoscience" (Haraway 1997: 163). She sees the narrative of genome mapping as a "process of bodily specialization akin to enclosing the commons in land, through institutions of alienable property, and in authorship, through institutions of copyright" (Haraway 1997: 163). A position akin to Harley's and to Nelkin and Lindee who argue that "the genome—when mapped and sequenced—will be a powerful guide to moral order... The apparent precision of a map may make invisible the priorities and interests that shaped it" (Nelkin and Lindee 1995: 8).

For Abby Lippman, genetic "mapping stories" "objectify the body and make the genome, rather than the person the focus of medical attention. They extend to its limit Foucault's conception of the medical/objectifying gaze" (Lippman 1992: 1470). While Rosner and Johnson manage to combine all of the preceding factors in an account following Harley, and Law and Whittaker (Law and Whittaker 1988).

> Like imperialist maps these genome maps are claims to ownership not only of the specific sites of genes that scientists have identified (with the fortunes that can come from patents) but also of the power and status associated with making sense of what has been unknown, with imposing order on chaos, with telling a plausible story, with—as Harley says—'structuring the world.'
>
> (Rosner and Johnson 1995)

Mapping as a fundamental cognitive process

All of the aforementioned, rely heavily on the notion of stories or narratives, but leave untheorized the actual activity of mapping itself. The work of two cognitive linguists, Gilles Fauconnier and Mark Turner, throw very interesting light on what the mental activity of mapping consists in, and how deeply imbricated it is in the fundamental process of making meaning. Fauconnier argues that mapping is not just a metaphor or an analogy, but is at the heart of meaning construction and is central to all forms of reasoning. A mapping in the most general mathematical sense is finding a correspondence between two sets and then assigning to each element in the first a counterpart in the second. Mappings operate to build and link mental spaces. Mental spaces are partial structures that proliferate when we think and talk, allowing a fine grain partitioning of our discourse and knowledge structures. Mapping, creating, and linking domains are prelinguistic processes that provide a cognitive substrate for language; reasoning and interfacing with the world and help account for the poorly understood human ability to resolve massively underspecified conditions (Fauconnier 1997).

Mark Turner describes the same prelinguistic cognitive processes in more literary terms. He claims that, small spatial stories and parables—the projection of one story on another, or what Fauconnier calls linking domains or mapping—are the root of the human capacities for thinking, knowing, acting and possibly even speaking. Most of our experience, our knowledge, and our thinking are organized as stories. The mental scope of story is magnified by projection—one story helps make sense of another (Turner 1996: v, 15).

The strength of Fauconnier and Turner's rather abstracted approach is that it succinctly links the narratological and the spatial into a performative understanding of mapping. As de Certeau notes, a metaphor in modern Greek is a conveyance, a device for moving through space, for establishing connections between spatially disparate places (de Certeau 1984). So, metaphors and their deployment in narratives have the function of maps—making connections and creating knowledge spaces. Topographic maps are themselves narratives, bringing the landscape into knowledge in the process of traveling through it (Carter 1990; Turnbull 2002).

Or as Hans-Jörg Rheinberger and Charles Galperin put it at the MPI workshop, they are narratives of position, pathways and order that provide location in space and time.

Mapping and knowledge spaces

As Adam Bostanci points out, the concept of mapping the human genome was not primarily concerned with representation, but was used to coordinate the disparate research groups and approaches in the human genome project (Bostanci, volume 2). Brian Balmer has mapped or, more properly, "metamapped" the way researchers, disciplines, and techniques were assembled to create the Human Genome Project and the ways in which that, in turn, shaped the nature of the project. In effect, the process of assemblage and the project coproduced each other creating an intellectual or knowledge space—a space which sociological analysts have brought into existence through their mappings. But, such spaces are always sites of contestation. Balmer, for example, holds that one of the stakes at issue was whether mapping *per se* was in itself a worthwhile pursuit. In his view, the Human Genome Project is a "boundary object" linking "communities of practice" (Balmer 1996).

Mapping as boundary objects—devices for handling multiplicity, heterogeneity, and messiness

James Griesemer and Leigh Star's invocation of "boundary objects" as entities in science on which there is no fixed agreement, but which have sufficient stability to enable communal research, is extremely important in the genetic context (Star 1989). Raphael Falk, Evelyn Fox Keller, Richard Burian, and Hans-Jörg Rheinberger have all pointed out that there is no agreement on what a gene is (Burian 1985; Falk 1996; Fox Keller 2000; Rheinberger 2000), a high stakes and highly controversial claim. Coyne, in contrast, holds that "the gene is a perfectly good working term for biologists, especially when defined as a piece of DNA that is translated into messenger RNA" (Coyne 2000).

Fox Keller claims that there are radically distinct uses of the term; one a

> . . . structural entity maintained by the molecular machinery of the cell so that it can be faithfully transmitted from generation to generation; and the other a functional entity that emerges only out of the dynamic interaction between and among a great many players.
>
> (Fox Keller 2000: 71)

Falk, Fox Keller, and Rheinberger also point out that we have achieved a vast amount without any agreement or even large-scale effort to work out what a gene is.

It seems to me that in addition to the spatiality of knowledge, the ubiquity of this deep heterogeneity in scientific knowledge is the most profound insight to come out of science studies. It has been acknowledged and given a variety of labels across the board by historians, philosophers and sociologists, yet it is as yet merely recognized rather than profoundly understood (Falk 1996; Rouse 1996; Turnbull 2000b). It does after all confound many highly cherished beliefs about the rationality and unity of science, but especially that "doing nature" consists in creating a one-to-one mimetic correspondence between nature and our representations. This raises the possibility then, that it may be the process of mapping itself in genome research that allows for this non-problematic lack of agreement and specificity of the gene as a biological function. This would indicate that, as Rheinberger suggests, a gene is a classic boundary object, like a photon, an electron, or a Newtonian gravitational force about which you "feign no hypotheses" but measure its effects whilst knowing that there are unresolved contradictions and paradoxes. But, it may be that the answers to the question Rheinberger asks about the "epistemology of the vague and the exuberant" (Rheinberger 2000: 222), are to be found in the practices, and spatial stories that are inherent in genetic mapping. So, an attendant key question emerges, how does mapping affect the ontology of the gene, does it contribute to the creation of the concept of the gene as being a structure at a specific place whilst bracketing its dynamic character in the cell processes and in the interactions of the environment? In a wider focus, does the spatio/narratological character of knowledge practice provide a way to understand its heterogeneity?

Maps as spatial and temporal narratives

Curiously, when Francis Collins and Craig Venter gave their public address at AAAS 2001, announcing the decoding of the human genome, neither mentioned the word map. Frank Collins described it as "the book of life composed of three books; a history book of human evolution, a manual of gene structures, a medical text book with 62 pages of minutiae." Craig Venter denied that it is the book of life

> ...we won't find the instructions for building the heart or the brain here. Genes are part of our everyday language so we expected lots of genes for everything, in fact we are not hard wired. The complexity comes from gene regulation. Its a recorded history soon we will have an exact time line of human development.
>
> (ABC 2001)

It would seem that for Collins and Venter, genetic spatiality is displaced by, or perhaps allows for, the emergence of an evolutionary narrative of temporality. Indeed, this is now apparent in the subordination of archeology and prehistory to the narrative of archeogenetics with stories of mitochondrial Eves and Y chromosome Adams and the transformation of human history into a map (Olson 2002).

According to Jay Clayton, genetic research deploys a particular narrative of temporality that he calls "genome time"—a "perpetual present" in which what is inscribed in the genes is, was, and always will be (Wald 2000: 698). This serves to displace an evolutionary sense of time and is another example of the complex interactions and displacements of spatial and temporal narratives, which may also be reflected in the differing structural and functional conceptions of the gene found by Fox Keller. Patricia Wald contrasts Clayton's genome time with the predictive "time of the geneticists"—the perspective of the "future perfect," which she sees as being in oscillation with the perpetual present of genome time.

> Implicit in the mapping of the human genome is the possibility (often disclaimed) that geneticists will be able to alter their perspective of human fate ... not only being able to predict the expression of certain genes (simple future), but of being able to specify those predictions temporally and understand the conditions of gene expression in order to look forward as though looking back (future perfect).
>
> (Wald 2000: 698–9)

Genetic mapping thus has deeply embedded narratives of both spatiality and temporality.

Unmapping and remapping

This leads to Rosner and Johnson's profound question, is there only one story to tell? What happens when dissidents attempt to create a counter-narrative, to assert a different set of borders, and draw a map of their own, one that has nothing to do with the current "central bastions" of standards and measures (Rosner and Johnson 1995: 121)? Barton and Barton propose a change of design standards and reshaping the metaphor to "map as collage" in order to address the suppression of the spatial or synchronic perspective (Barton and Barton 1993).

Chaudhuri aptly uses the term "unmapping" to name the process where "the stereotype is *simultaneously* [my italics] evoked and undermined, recalled and revised" (Chaudhuri 1991: 204). As Harvey claims:

> The imaginary of spatiality is of crucial significance in the search for alternative mappings of the social process and its outcomes. The structures of many social and literary theories are in this regard, often secret mappings of otherwise intractable processes and events.
>
> (Harvey 1996: 112)

So if the key question is not "what is a map?" but "what is mapping?" and if, as Turner and Fauconnier argue, mapping is telling one story in terms of another, then unmapping becomes a way of showing that the apparent fixity of the mapping of the story–story relationship can be changed, other stories can be related, other domains can be mapped on to each other.

Corner suggests that mapping is an

> ... extremely shrewd and tactical enterprise, a practice of relational reasoning that intelligently unfolds new realities out of existing constraints, quantities,

> facts and conditions. The artistry lies in the use of the technique in the ways in which things are framed and set up.
>
> (Corner 1999: 251)

So, just as we seem to get more epistemic fecundity out of holding conflicting definitions of genes in tension with one another, so too should we gain heuristic power from holding differing mappings in tension with one another. One possible resolution of the modern/postmodern dilemma which could open a path towards "transmodernity" may lie in embracing the "agonistic pluralism" of heterogeneity and establishing a "third space" in which it would be possible to keep open opposing spatialities rather than in attempting a uniform rationality or unity (Dussel 1993). The spatial and narratological practices of mapping are currently among the best prospects to allow an exploration of such complex interstitial spaces (Turnbull 2002).

Evolution, mapping, narrativity, and reflexive difficulties

In conclusion, returning to some of the questions raised at the start, it seems that in a peculiar way there is little mapping going on in genetics, at least if we restrict mapping to the spatial representation of causal processes. Strictly speaking, genetic mapping is about the location and ordering of genetic markers and is a practical requirement for making the experimental work of sequencing genes, feasible. The more profound forms of spatiality that will require mapping of a very different order is yet to come in the burgeoning field of proteomics, where the folding and topology of the protein has causal effects. However, on a more liberal interpretation of mapping in genetics, I think the foregoing discussion shows that maps do indeed play an absolutely central role in coordinating the work, bringing genes into existence, and in making them manipulable, mobile, and assemblable.

However, maps perform nature in varied and particular ways. They serve to create a narrative of potential completeness, they define a landscape, designate the kinds of features it may have. They provide blanks and the capacity for filling them in. On David Gugerli's account maps do this by creating an "optically consistent space," with a "fiction of homogeneity" and a "politics of truth" (Gugerli, volume 2). But, as has been argued, genetic maps are not the only spatial and temporal narratives available, there are alternatives, there are narratives of dialectical and interactive processes, which raise the possibility of differing spatialities, temporalities and narratives being performed at the same time.

This conclusion does, however, raise deeper questions concerning the origins of language, narrative, and mapping. In particular, it points to reflexive difficulties inherent in evolutionary explanations of the human condition, that is time-factored, spatial narratives of our capacity to create historical explanations, make maps, tell stories.

Simon Winchester's book *The Man who Changed the World* tells the story of William Smith and the first geological map, the first map to spatialize time and provide for the possibility of historical explanation in the natural sciences. This map poses a reflexive conundrum in that the bringing into being of evolutionary and geological time through a form of spatial narrative reflects a human mental capacity which is itself the product of evolutionary processes (Gould 2001: 56).

The seeming paradox can only partly be resolved in evolutionary terms, necessitating some of the creative tension mentioned earlier to be handled adequately. A potential story can now be told about the development of narrativity and hence of our history telling and mapping capacities in terms of the coevolution of time-factoring and space-making with language and technology. Our capacities for making connections literally and cognitively, between materials and between ideas originated in string and stories, a co-production dating back 40,000 years.

We are "story telling animals," as Alisdair McIntyre pointed out (McIntyre 1981), a central narrative capacity that we developed with art and speech and story telling is a mode of time factoring. According to Alexander Marshack, we were recording the cycles of the sun and the moon on pieces of bone as far back as 25,000 years ago (Marshack 1972). We did this because we order our lives; give our lives meaning, purpose, significance, and shape by ordering or factoring them in time. Hence, time is central to all story telling (Ricoeur 1984), but, equally central is mapping. As mentioned earlier small spatial stories—the linking of domains or mapping—are the root of the human capacities for thinking, knowing, acting, and possibly even speaking (Turner 1996; Fauconnier 1997).

Patricia McNeil has very persuasively and thoroughly explored what she describes as the "gradual elaboration of narrative scripts from everyday routines and gestural word/signs over time into conventionally-sanctioned, archetypal narrative plots" (McNeil 1996: 332). McNeil argues that around 40,000 BC, a cultural explosion occurred with the co-construction of tools, technology, language, and narrative expression (McNeil 1996: 347). But, the key technological innovation which our "lithic" preoccupations have led us to overlook is string, a development so important that we should follow Elizabeth Barber in calling it the "string revolution" (Barber 1994: 44). String was arguably one of the most significant and least recognized of all technologies. It, like stories, was essential to the making of connections, joining things together and allowing us to move and carry things. Stories and string brought about the coproduction of, mapping and weaving, and with them, narratives of spatiality and temporality.

It is in this interaction between story telling and weaving that I think there is something important to be learnt. Weaving and story telling have a common origin reflected in the Latin *texere* from which text and textile are both derived. The anthropologist Tim Ingold, discussing weaving in another context, offers the insight that making is a form of weaving rather than the other way round.

> To emphasise making is to regard the object as the expression of an idea; to emphasise weaving is to regard it as the embodiment of a rhythmic movement. Therefore to invert making and weaving is also to invert idea and movement, to see the movement as truly generative of the object rather than merely revelatory of an object that is already present, in an ideal, conceptual or virtual form, in advance of the process that discloses it.
>
> (Ingold 2000: 346–7)

Ingold claims that there are three points about skill which are exemplified in basket weaving, but which are nevertheless common to the practice of any craft, any process of making:

> First the practitioner operates within a field of forces set up through his or her engagement with the material; secondly the work does not merely involve the mechanical application of external force but calls for care, judgement and dexterity; and thirdly the action has quality, in the sense that every movement, like every line in a story, grows rhythmically out of the one before and lays the groundwork for the next.
>
> (Ingold 2000: 346–7)

Weaving, making and narrative, from this perspective, are thus essentially based in bodily movements and hence in the coproduction of spatiality and temporality, since as Ingold puts it, "places do not have locations but histories. Bound together by the itineraries of their inhabitants, they exist not in space but as nodes in a matrix of movement" (Ingold 2000: 219). As de Certeau remarks "every story is a travel story—a spatial practice" (de Certeau 1984: 115–6).

So, spatiality and temporality are inherent in both our ways of making and of making sense and have evolved with our capacities for speech and movement, hence some of Gould's paradox dissolves. But, we are left with the reflexive difficulty that our ways of telling stories and of mapping—of invoking historical explanations and spatial relationships—are deeply intermeshed. But they are not universal in form, they vary with differing ways of knowing and being in the world. The strategy most suitable for handling these problems and the one most likely to reveal the concealed spatio-temporal narratives, is the "bothness" of Dussel's "agonistic pluralism," of holding the differing narratives of genetics and other explanations of human behavior in tension and telling more than one story at a time.

Bibliography

ABC *Science Show*, February 24, 2001.

Bachelard, G. (1985) *The New Scientific Spirit*, Boston: Beacon Press.

Balmer, B. (1996) "Managing Mapping in the Human Genome Project," *Social Studies of Science*, 26: 531–74.

Barber, E. (1994) *Women's Work: The First 20,000 Years*, New York: W.W. Norton & Co.

Barton, B. and Barton, M. (1993) "Ideology and the Map: Toward a Postmodern Visual Design Practice," in N. Blyler and C. Thralls (eds) *Professional Communication: The Social Perspective*, Newbury Park: Sage.

Burian, R. (1985) "On Conceptual Change in Biology," in D. Depew and B. Weber (eds) *Evolution at a Crossroads: The New Biology and the New Philosophy of Science*, Cambridge: MIT Press.

Carter, P. (1990) "Plotting: Australia's Explorer Narratives as 'Spatial History'," *Yale Journal of History*, 3: 91–107.

Certeau, M. de (1984) *The Practice of Everyday Life*, Berkeley: University of California Press.

Chaudhuri, U. (1991) "The Future of the Hyphen: Interculturalism, Textuality and the Difference within," in B. Marranca and G. Dasgupta (eds) *Interculturalism and Performance: Writings from PAJ*, New York: PAJ Publications.

Corner, J. (1999) "The Agency of Mapping: Speculation, Critique and Invention," in D. Cosgrove (ed.) *Mappings*, London: Reaktion Books.

Coyne, J. (2000) "The Gene is Dead: Long Live the Gene," *Nature*, 408: 26–7.

Dussel, E. (1993) "Eurocentrism and Modernity," *Boundary*, 2: 65–76.

Edney, M.H. (1993) "Cartography without 'Progress': Reinterpreting the Nature and Historical Development of Mapmaking," *Cartographica*, 30: 54–68.

Falk, R. (1996) "What is a Gene?" *Studies in History and Philosophy of Science*, 17: 133–73.

Fauconnier, G. (1997) *Mappings in Thought and Language*, Cambridge: Cambridge University Press.

Fox Keller, E. (2000) *The Century of the Gene*, Cambridge: Harvard University Press.

Gould, S.J. (2001) "The Man Who Set the Clock Back," *New York Review of Books*, XLVIII: 51–6.

Hall, S.S. (1992) *Mapping the Next Millennium: The Discovery of New Geographies*, New York: Random House.

Haraway, D. (1997) *Modest_Witness@Second_Millenium. FemaleMan©_Meets_OncoMouse™*, New York: Routledge.

Harley, J.B. (2001) *The New Nature of Maps: Essays in the History of Cartography*, Baltimore: Johns Hopkins University.

Harley, J.B. and Woodward, D. (eds) (1987) *The History of Cartography, Vol. 1: Cartography in Prehistoric, Ancient and Medieval Europe and the Mediterranean*, Chicago: University of Chicago Press.

Harvey, D. (1996) *Justice, Nature and the Geography of Difference*, Cambridge, Mass: Blackwell.

Ingold, T. (2000) *The Perception of the Environment: Essays on Livelihood, Dwelling and Skill*, London: Routledge.

Kohler, R. (1994) *Lords of the Fly: Drosophila Genetics and the Experimental Life*, Chicago: University of Chicago Press.

Latour, B. (1999) *Pandora's Hope: Essays on the Reality of Science Studies*, Cambridge: Harvard University Press.

Law, J. and Whittaker, J. (1988) "On the Art of Representation: Notes on the Politics of Visualisation," in G. Fyfe and J. Law (eds) *Picturing Power: Visual Depictions and Social Relations*, London: Routledge.

Lippman, A. (1992) "Led (Astray) by Genetic Maps: The Cartography of the Human Genome and Cartography," *Social Science and Medicine*, 35: 1469–76.

McIntyre, A. (1981) *After Virtue: A Study in Moral Theory*, Notre Dame: University of Notre Dame.

McNeil, L. (1996) "Homo Inventans: The Evolution of Narrativity," *Language and Communication*, 16 (4): 331–60.

Marshack, A. (1972) *The Roots of Civilization: The Cognitive Beginnings of Man's First Art, Symbol and Notation*, New York: McGraw Hill.

Mandelbrot, B. (1983) *The Fractal Geometry of Nature*, New York: W.H. Freeman and Co.

Nelkin, D. and Lindee, S. (1995) *The DNA Mystique: The Gene as a Cultural Icon*, New York: W.H. Freeman and Co.

Olson, S. (2002) *Mapping Human History: Discovering the Past through Our Genes*, Boston: Houghton Mifflin.

Rheinberger, H.-J. (1998) "Experimental Systems, Graphematic Spaces," in T. Lenoir (ed.) *Inscribing Science: Scientific Texts and the Materiality of Communication*, Stanford: Stanford University Press.

—— (2000) "Gene Concepts: Fragments from the Perspective of Molecular Biology," in P. Beurton, R. Falk and H-J. Rheinberger (eds) *The Concept of the Gene in Development and Evolution*, Cambridge: Cambridge University Press.

Ricoeur, P. (1984) *Time and Narrative*, Vol. 1, Chicago: University of Chicago Press.

Rosner, M. and Johnson, T.R. (1995) "Telling Stories: Metaphors of the Human Genome Project," *Hypatia*, 10: 104–29.

Rouse, J. (1996) *Engaging Science: How to Understand its Practices Philosophically*, Ithaca: Cornell University Presss.

Shapin, S. (1998) "Placing the View from Nowhere: Historical and Sociological Problems in the Location of Science," *Transactions of the Institute of British Geographers*, 23: 5–12.

Star, S.L. (1989) "The Structure of Ill-Structured Solutions: Boundary Objects and Heterogeneous Distributed Problem Solving," in L. Gasser and N. Huhns (eds) *Distributed Artificial Intelligence*, New York: Morgan Kauffman Publications.

Stokes, T. and Turnbull, D. (1990) "Manipulable Systems and Laboratory Strategies in a Biomedical Research Institute," in H.L. Grand (ed.) *Experimental Inquiries: Historical, Philosophical and Social Studies in Science*, Dordrecht: Kluwer Academic Publishers.

Thongchai, W. (1994) *Siam Mapped: A History of the Geo-Body of a Nation*, Honolulu: University of Hawaii Press.

Turnbull, D. (1993) *Maps are Territories: Science is an Atlas*, Chicago: Chicago University Press.

—— (1996) "Cartography and Science in Early Modern Europe: Mapping the Construction of Knowledge Spaces," *Imago Mundi*, 48: 5–24.

—— (1998) "Mapping Encounters and (En)countering Maps: A Critical Examination of Cartographic Resistance," in S. Gorenstein (ed.) *Research in Science and Technology Studies: Knowledge Systems*, Stanford Connecticut: JAI Press.

—— (2000a) *Masons, Tricksters and Cartographers: Comparative Studies in the Sociology of Scientific and Indigenous Knowledge*, Reading: Harwood Academic Publishers.

—— (2000b) "Rationality and the Disunity of the Sciences," in H. Selin (ed.) *Mathematics Across Cultures: The History of Non-Western Mathematics*, Dordrecht: Kluwer Academic Publishers.

—— (2002) "Travelling Knowledge: Narratives, Assemblage and Encounters," in M.-N. Bourget, C. Licoppe, and H.O. Sibum (eds) *Instruments, Travel and Science: Itineraries of Precision from the Seventeenth to the Twentieth Century*, London: Routledge, 273–94.

Turner, M. (1996) *The Literary Mind*, New York: Oxford University Press.

Wald, P. (2000) "Future Perfect: Grammar, Genes and Geography," *New Literary History*, 31: 681–708.

Wood, D. (1992) *The Power of Maps*, New York: The Guilford Press.

Mapping as a cultural practice

Jens Lachmund

As a sociologist of knowledge I am currently engaged in a study of the mapping culture of a field of biological expertise which is very different from the strands of research which form the focus of this volume. My study examines the role of maps and mapping practices in ecology, more specifically, ecological studies of the flora and vegetation of German cities. In the interdisciplinary field of urban ecology, such maps have become a major form in which knowledge about urban ecosystems is produced, as well as one of the means by which such knowledge is translated into urban planning and conservation procedures. In this reflection, I will use the example of the mapping culture of urban ecology to discuss the way in which cartography has been involved in the constitution of scientific knowledge and to invite some comparison between ecological mapping and genetic mapping.

Traditionally, maps have been seen as neutral forms of representation of natural space and the location of phenomena within. Accordingly, the history of mapping was seen as a continuous process of developing ever more precise and more complete depictions of the world. Differences in the ways of constructing maps, such as alternative systems of projection or the choice of topographical signatures, have been considered as purely technical matters which did not interfere with the representational function of the map. In contrast, a more critical view of maps and mapping has been developed by cultural theorists such as Henry Lefèbvre (1991), Michel de Certeau (1998), and, more recently, James Scott (1998). For these authors, maps are not just neutral media of representation of a pre-given reality. Rather, they construct a specific version of that reality which is characterized by standardization and geometrical abstraction and which serves the needs of state power.[1] Although this is an important move beyond the somewhat naïve realism of the traditional view, this critique of mapping is based on a very general argumentation and does not tell us much about the ways in which maps actually work in concrete social and political settings. Moreover, the critique of mapping as an abstraction remains, based on the idea that there is a kind of pre-given reality outside, in the world that serves as a yardstick from which to judge the content of maps.

I intend to illustrate a perspective on mapping which avoids both the idea of precise representation as well as the critique of abstraction. In this respect, important work has been done by recent analyses of the visual and textual rhetoric of maps which have often drawn upon semiotic approaches (Harley 1989; Wood 1992). In contrast, I argue here for an understanding of mapping as a cultural practice, broadly conceived of as a locally enacted nexus of doings, sayings and related material objects. The "practical turn" which has characterized much of recent social and historical studies of science has given considerable attention to the practical nature of knowledge production in the sciences (cf. Lynch 1985; Lynch/Woolgar 1990; Pickering 1995; Rouse 1996; Knorr-Cetina 1999). Rather than focusing on institutions and social groupings of sciences, these studies have traced the day-to-day activities of science as they are performed in laboratories, research hospitals or other "places of knowledge" (Shapin/Ophir 1991). In a similar way, my study on ecological mapping aims at a historical understanding of the actual technical, social, and political processes in which certain representations that pass as maps have been produced, circulated, and imbued with meaning in the scientific culture under consideration. I will now discuss three ways in which a notion of maps as cultural practices might yield insights into the nature of mapping and cartographic knowledge. First, the role of diversity in mapping practices; second, the way in which mapping itself is enacted as a cultural category, and third, the stabilization of cartographic meaning in the context of practical infrastructures.

The diversity of maps

Seeing mapping as a cultural practice implies that there are different possible ways of cartographic organization of reality. How a certain segment of geographical space is depicted on a map, is determined neither by the natural world itself, nor by the intrinsic properties of geometric measurement. Rather, it is an articulation of the choices and mapping conventions of map-makers and their communities of practice. Different ways of mapping therefore, produce different realities, and it is thus from the diversity of mapping practices that we can learn about the diversity of the ways in which sciences make up the world.

The maps which have been produced in the ecological surveys I have studied, are all based on widely shared principles of Western cartography. They have a homogenous scale and projection. They are oriented to the North. They use a number of codified signatures such as lines, colors, and point symbols representing various topographical and ecological features. Since they are drawn on official ordinance survey sheets, they reproduce a certain vision of the topography of the area with streets, houses, rivers, woods, railway-tracks etc. as their primary features. This sets these maps apart from many other forms of cartographic depiction. The choice of another scale or projection scheme would have allowed other relationships between the objects to become visible. The choice of objects depicted on the maps is also highly selective. For example, ordinance survey maps show Christian churches but no mosques. More dramatically, these maps differ from many non-Western ways of mapping as well as from recent attempts to develop alternative forms of mapping which aim at representing the embodied experience and the imaginative qualities of space. Examples of the latter would be the 1960s situationist's psychogeographic maps of cityscapes or the so-called "Parish Maps" which have recently been designed by British artists and citizens groups in British neighborhoods.[2]

Ecologist's maps however differ from ordinary ordinance survey maps in that they include a variety of elements which form the center of concern for the ecologists who work with them. They are "thematic maps," focusing specifically on plants and animals. In this respect, further differences exist in the ways in which these maps are organized. Often, they are distribution maps of certain species of plants or animals. A geometrical grid is used to divide the map into squares. Those squares in which a certain species is present are marked by a point. Hence, these maps provide a synoptic view of the distribution pattern of that species in space that otherwise would not have been observable. Another kind of map shows ecological habitats or "biotopes" of these species as non-geometrical territorial units. They use lines, colors or hachures to delineate the area under consideration into areas which are considered as showing a characteristic composition of plant and animal species, so-called "biotope types." These maps are of a higher degree of generalization, as data on the geographical distribution is no longer shown separately. Another striking contrast to point maps is the way in which territorial units are defined. In contrast to the purely mathematical construction of grid-squares, they are neatly delineated according to topographical patterns of the landscape which are seen as being correlated to changes in plant composition, for example, water, forests, agricultural areas, urban green areas and between different types of settlement areas within the city.

Mapping as a cultural category

This diversity of mapping practices not only shows how different realities are made up in different contexts of scientific activity, but also raises the question of what makes the map different from other forms of representation. What distinguishes a map from, let's say, a photograph, a painting or statistical figure? What do we mean if we talk about genetic research as a form of mapping? To what extent does it make sense to use mapping as an analogy or metaphor to understand research fields other than "real" cartography? And what makes that term metaphoric in contrast to accounts of "real" maps? Besides this, there are also various borderline cases which we might hesitate to call maps at all, although they seem to perform more or less the same function. Would you, for example, call a globe or a GIS-database a map?

Wouldn't it be necessary to come up with a clear-cut definition which would escape this linguistic messiness in order to be able to talk about maps in a scientifically solid way? We might search for some definitional criteria such as flatness, geometricity, or more generally, the attempt to represent the spatial relations between the phenomena mapped. We might also think of mapping as a kind of scientific activity which is primarily descriptive and which aims at a comprehensive inventory of a segment of reality rather than developing explanatory models. However, a notion of mapping as a cultural practice would suggest that another tack could be taken. We might better turn the category of the map itself into the phenomenon to be studied, either historically or ethnographically. What constitutes under which circumstances, a map, and for whom? What are the epistemic, moral and social consequences of such categorizations? This would mean tracing the various "family resemblances"—to take up Wittgenstein's (1963) apt expression—which allow us in everyday life to lump together things as maps and to distinguish them from their various counterparts. Moreover, we might also look at cases when the category of mapping is contested or invoked explicitly by certain actors in order to strengthen claims of knowledge? For example, the French photographer Nadar, who in 1859 took the first aerial photograph from a balloon above Paris, later claimed to have produced a map. Considering aerial photographs as maps, remained a common trope of the propaganda for using these images in military recognition, geographical research, and planning. At the turn of the twentieth century, the development of photogrammetrical analysis and sophisticated practices of photo-interpretation, however, eroded this simple analogy between the aerial photograph and the cartographic map. Although they share many properties of maps, aerial photographs were no longer seen as maps in themselves. Rather, they became considered technological means of map production. We might wonder, if the invocation of the map analogy in contemporary genetics performs a similar rhetorical function for fostering that project and its techno-political claims. Likewise, we might expect that the future development of these technologies will at some point erode the evidence this category actually has for understanding genetics.

The stabilization of cartographic knowledge

The conception of mapping as a cultural practice not only allows us to make sense of the diversity of mapping possibilities; it is also a way of accounting for the way in which certain maps, and not others, are produced and stabilized as an authoritative representation of reality. Some authors have argued that maps should be viewed as rhetorical devices whose content and form are largely determined by the interests of the map-maker and his or her attempt to convince an audience (Harley 1989; Wood 1992).[3] Although I do not wish to deny the role of interests in selecting maps and mapping strategies, an understanding of mapping as a cultural practice allows us a more complex understanding of the processes in which certain maps become stabilized as representations of reality and why other possible ways of mapping do not. In order to understand these processes, we have to look at the way in which they link up with other components of the cultural contexts in which they are embedded. This is not to argue that maps and mapping practices are caused by these contextual conditions; rather it sees them as being articulated within a larger infrastructure of practical activities.[4]

First, what enters a map as a piece of information and how this is displayed on the map depends to a large extent on the practicalities of the processes in which the map has been produced. We might think here of the practical activities of surveying in which landscapes are measured and topographic objects are selected. In the case of thematic maps, such as those produced by the ecologists, maps are the result of extensive inspection tours, fieldwork on selected sample areas, and in many cases, the interpretation of aerial photographs. Contingencies such as time pressure, organizational routines, the skills of the individual observer, and the observability of the phenomena on which the mapping project focuses, make this a highly selective process of knowledge formation. For example, these maps typically include more data about plants than about animals, because the former are easier to observe and to localize on the map. Moreover, visible features of the landscape such as rivers, streets, and hedges which are also easy to display on the map, are often used to draw the boundaries between different landscape types. If ecological maps are produced primarily by the interpretation of aerial photographs, this also has important consequences for the scale down to which phenomena can be recognized, as well as for the selection of the criteria according to which land-use types are delineated and classified.

Second, maps usually form part of larger systems of information gathering and storing which require a certain amount of standardization. The storage of information in archives and databases, the translation of information from one form into the other, and finally, any form of comparative analysis of the mapping contents—are all only possible if information has been formatted in a homogenous way. One of the primary requirements of the production of cartographic knowledge therefore, is the need to align these newly developed maps with the already existing formats of mapping. When, for example, ecologists use official ordinance survey maps as a point of reference for their own maps, it provides them with a standard format of geometrical and cartographic conventions. This makes the ecological maps comparable with each other, with the ordinance survey maps themselves and also with thematic maps on other topics which have been produced on the same base. Likewise, the categories which have been used for classifying phenomena on the maps, such as the biological classification of maps or the use of land-use categories for the classification of territorial units, also act as means of standardization which align the information produced with existing practices of representation. Moreover, in the previous decade, it also became important to reconcile the way in which ecological maps are organized with the standards of data processing in programs of digital cartography and geo-information systems (GIS).

Third, maps are often related to political projects of governing the spaces they focus on. Many authors have shown that maps were constitutively involved in the constitution of nation-states and the appropriation of colonial territories. Likewise, thematic maps produced in various sciences, were not free from political implications. Ecologists became interested in mapping the city in the 1970s and 1980s at just the same time as landscape planning and nature conservation appeared as new issues on the agenda of urban politics in Germany. Maps in this context were an important means of claims-making and they helped ecologists to create political alliances with policy-makers and activists. Moreover, as ecologists were often called upon as expert advisors, ecological maps of the city were also produced for policy institutions which often involved close cooperation between map-makers and government officials.

As with fieldwork and information-systems, governmental practices represented a further infrastructural context, maps had to be aligned to. On the one hand, these maps were constitutive for the new practices of governing space. Thus, the delineation of cities according to biotope-types not only created new objects of ecological knowledge, the latter also became political entities to which certain administrative and legal regulations applied. For example, if the map identified a certain part of the city as an ecologically valuable biotope, building on this site became restricted. It might even have resulted in turning the area into a nature reserve. On the other hand, the need to inform governmental and legal practices of the city administration had far-reaching implications on the ways in which the city was mapped. Thus, political activist groups or the city administration often tended to influence mapping projects in such a way as to focus primarily on species and areas which were politically contested or of direct relevance to urban planning. The way in which map-makers chose between the two main strategies of ecological mapping mentioned earlier also reflected their attempt to meet the requirements of urban governance. Whereas more academic studies of the bio-geography of the city which were only loosely connected to governmental issues, tended to produce point-maps, policy-related mapping projects used to focus on territorial units. In contrast to point-maps, they were seen as more suitable for delineating homogenous territories on which certain political dispositions could be deployed. The land-use categories on which biotope-maps were based, resonated well with the categories used in urban planning schemes. Furthermore, the high degree of generalization of these maps helped attune them to the skills and practices of the administrative personnel.

The field-activities of producing maps, information-systems and governmental procedures are examples of the various practical infrastructures within which maps are constructed and stabilized. Examining the way in which they interact with the form and the content of maps helps us to understand how these maps acquire meaning and how they become stabilized, at least for some time, as meaningful representations of reality. Seeing mapping as a cultural practice thus allows us to account both for the diversity as well as for the stabilization of cartographic meaning.

Concluding remarks

Very similar problems as those which I have addressed with respect to the mapping of geographical space, and more particular the mapping of the flora and fauna of cities, can also be observed in the field of genetic mapping. Not only were there, as Gannett and Griesemer's chapter makes clear, many direct connections between projects of genetic mapping and the mapping of plant and animal distribution in geographical space. The case-studies in this volume also show the rich diversity of the ways in which genes and genomes themselves have been represented at different times and in different places. As some of the chapters make clear, this is not only a matter of different theoretical interpretations. As with the maps discussed in this reflection, this diversity can also be observed with respect to the material and symbolic forms in which genetic knowledge has been encoded (see specifically the contributions by Gannett/Griesemer, this volume and de Chadarevian, volume 2). Our understanding of contemporary genetic knowledge might thus benefit from a similar approach to the way in which these maps are enacted in cultural practice: What are the different forms in which these representation have been constructed? What do they emphasize? What are they silent about? What is the extent to which they are labeled as maps, and what are the consequences of such labeling? What are the practical infrastructures which lead to the construction and stabilization of specific genetic maps at the expense of others? How have they been aligned to the context of knowledge production? How do they fit into larger information-systems? What governmental strategies are they linked to? Many of these issues are addressed throughout the chapters of this volume. Asking these questions in a comparative way not only enables us to see the similarities between many of the practical problems the two research fields are faced with, it also allows us to more systematically explore the many differences which exist between these two mapping cultures. Such differences are not only to be found in the visual content of the maps themselves, but in the whole infrastructure in which they are embedded. What, for example, does it mean for the way in which maps are constructed and stabilized if their context of production is not fieldwork but, as in much of genetic mapping, experimental laboratory practice? This is, of course, not the place to fully explore these issues. What I intended to show in this reflection was simply that a notion of science as a cultural practice might help to generate new questions about maps and mapping that might be helpful for the historical and sociological understanding of ecological maps as well as the representations of modern genetics.

Notes

1 For Lefèbvre maps fall under the category of "representations of spaces" (1991: 233) of planners and technocrats which he contrasts with the lived experience of space (representational spaces) by the people. Certeau contrasts the synoptic view of a city as it was given from the top of the World Trade Center with the symbolic appropriation of space by the people walking in the streets. For Scott, modernist maps and other representations create abstract state spaces and policies which ignore the local knowledge of residents.

2 Parish Maps have been produced since the late 1980s by local artists and residents. This project has been launched by the British environment and arts organization Common Ground. See Crouch, D. and Matless, D. (1996).

3 But see also the critique of a "conspiracy"—model of the politics of mapping see Black, J. (1998) *Maps and Politics*, Cambridge: Cambridge University Press.

4 It is a widely held idea in science and technology studies that knowledge claims and technological artifacts become stabilized as a result of contextually bounded processes of the fixation of meaning. See for example, Pinch, T. and Bijker, W. (1987) "The Social Construction of Facts and Artifacts: Or How the Sociology of Science and the Sociology of Technology Might Benefit from Each Other," in W.E. Bijker, T. Hughes, and T. Pinch (eds) *The Social Construction of Technological Systems*, Cambridge: MIT Press. For a broader discussion of practical infrastructures in the shaping of knowledge see Bowker, G.C. and Star, S.L. (1999) *Sorting Things Out: Classification and Its Consequences*, Cambridge: MIT Press.

Bibliography

Black, J. (1998) *Maps and Politics*, Cambridge: Cambridge University Press.

Bowker, G.C. and Star, S.L. (1999) *Sorting Things Out: Classification and its Consequences*, Cambridge, MA: MIT Press.

Certeau, M. de (1998) *The Practice of Everyday Life*, Minneapolis: University of Minnesota Press.

Crouch, D. and Matless, D. (1996) "Refiguring Geography: Parish Maps of Common Ground," *Transactions of the Institute of British Geography*, NS 21, 236–55.

Harley, B. (1989) Deconstructing the Map, *Cartographica*, 26(2): 1–20.

Knorr-Cetina, K. (1999) *Epistemic Cultures*, Cambridge: Harvard University Press.

Lefèbvre, H. (1991) *The Production of Space*, Oxford: Blackwell.

Lynch, M. (1985) *Art and Artifact in Laboratory Life*, London: Routledge & Paul.

Lynch, M. and Woolgar, S. (1990) *Representation in Scientific Practice*, Cambridge: Harvard University Press.

Pickering, A. (1995) *The Mangle of Practice*, Chicago: Chicago University Press.

Pinch, T. and Bijker, W.E. (1987) "The Social Construction of Facts and Artifacts: Or How the Sociology of Science and the Sociology of Technology Might Benefit from Each Other," in: W.E. Bijker, T. Hughes and T. Pinch (eds) *The Social Construction of Technological Systems*, Cambridge: MIT Press.

Rouse, J. (1996) *Engaging Science*, Ithaka: Cornell University Press.

Scott, J. (1998) *Seeing Like a State: How Certain Schemes to Improve the Human Condition have Failed*, New Haven: Yale University Press.

Shapin, S. and Ophir, A. (1991) "The Place of Knowledge," *Science in Context*, Special Issue 4, 1.

Wittgenstein, L. (1963) *Philosophical Investigations*, Oxford: Basil Blackwell.

Wood, D. (1992) *The Power of Maps*, London: Blackwell.

Index